current procedural terminology

cpt®

2012

Changes

An Insider's View

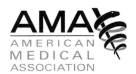

AMA

AMERICAN
MEDICAL
ASSOCIATION

ISBN: 978-1-60359-569-8
AC34: 11-P-004:11/11

Contents

Foreword

The American Medical Association is pleased to offer *CPT® Changes 2012: An Insider's View*. Since this book was first published in 2000, it has served as the definitive text on additions, revisions, and deletions to the CPT code set.

In developing this book, it was our intention to provide CPT users with a glimpse of the logic, rationale, and proposed function of CPT changes that resulted from the decisions of the CPT Editorial Panel and the yearly update process. American Medical Association (AMA) staff members have the unique perspective of being both participants in the CPT editorial process and users of the CPT code set. *CPT Changes* is intended to bridge understanding between clinical decisions made at the CPT Editorial Panel regarding appropriate service or procedure descriptions with functional interpretations of coding guidelines, code intent, and code combinations necessary for users of the CPT code set. A new edition of this book, like the codebook, is published annually.

To assist CPT users in applying new and revised CPT codes, this book includes clinical examples that describe the typical patient who might receive the procedure and detailed descriptions of the procedure. Both of these are required as a part of the CPT code change proposal process and are used by the CPT Editorial Panel in crafting language, guidelines, and parenthetical notes associated with the new or revised codes. In addition, many of the clinical examples and descriptions of the procedures are used in the AMA/Specialty Society RVS Update process for conducting surveys on physician work and in developing work relative value recommendations to the Centers for Medicare and Medicaid Services (CMS) as part of the Medicare Physician Fee Schedule (MPFS).

We are confident that the information contained in *CPT Changes* each year will prove to be a valuable resource to CPT users not only as they apply changes for the year of publication but also as a resource for frequent reference as they continue their education in CPT coding. The AMA makes every effort to be a voice of clarity and consistency in an otherwise confusing system of health care claims and payment, and *CPT Changes 2012: An Insider's View* demonstrates our continued commitment to assist users of the CPT code set.

Using This Book

This book is designed to serve as a reference guide to understanding the changes contained in *Current Procedural Terminology (CPT®) 2012* and is not intended to replace the CPT codebook. Every effort is made to ensure accuracy; however, if differences exist, you should always defer to the information contained in the *CPT 2012* codebook.

The Symbols

This book uses the same coding conventions that appear in the CPT nomenclature.

- ●   Indicates that a new procedure number was added to the CPT nomenclature

- ▲   Indicates that a code revision has resulted in a substantially altered procedure descriptor

- ✚   Indicates a CPT add-on code

- ⊘   Indicates a code that is exempt from the use of modifier 51 but is not designated as a CPT add-on procedure/service

- ►◄   Indicate revised guidelines, cross-references, and/or explanatory text

- ⊙   Indicates a code that typically includes moderate sedation

- ⁄   Indicates a code for a vaccine that is pending FDA approval

- #   Indicates a resequenced code

- ○   Indicates a reinstated or recycled code

Whenever possible, complete segments of text from the CPT codebook are provided, however, in some cases the text has been abbreviated.

The Rationale

After each change or series of changes is a rationale. The rationale is intended to provide a brief explanation as to why changes occurred but may not answer every question that may arise as a result of the changes.

Reading the Clinical Examples

The clinical examples and their procedural descriptions included in this text with many of the codes provide practical situations for which the new and/or revised codes in the *CPT 2012* codebook would be appropriately reported. It is important to note that these examples do not suggest limiting the use of a code but only represent the typical patient and service or procedure. They do not describe the universe of patients for whom the service or procedure would be appropriate. In addition, third-party payer reporting policies may differ.

The Tabular Review of the Changes

The table beginning on page 325 allows you to see all of the code changes at a glance. By reviewing the table you can easily determine the level to which your particular field of interest has been affected by the changes in the *CPT 2012* codebook.

CPT Codebook Text and Guidelines

In *CPT Changes 2012*, guideline and revised CPT codebook text appears in brown indented type. Any revised text, guidelines, and/or headings are indicated with the ►◄ symbols. This convention in *CPT Changes 2011* differs slightly from the CPT codebook. Within the codebook, symbols are placed at the beginning and end of a paragraph that contains a revision or revisions. *CPT Changes 2012* offers readers a more detailed view of the changes to the codes and guidelines. In this book, the revision symbols (►◄) are placed around each specific change.

Introduction

The "Instructions for Use of the CPT Codebook" has been updated to include language defining "physician and other qualified healthcare professionals."

Instructions

Select the name of the procedure . . .

It is important to recognize . . .

▶A "physician or other qualified healthcare professional" is an individual who is qualified by education, training, licensure/regulation (when applicable), and facility privileging (when applicable) who performs a professional service within his/her scope of practice and independently reports that professional service. These professionals are distinct from "clinical staff." A clinical staff member is a person who works under the supervision of a physician or other qualified healthcare professional and who is allowed by law, regulation, and facility policy to perform or assist in the performance of a specified professional service, but who does not individually report that professional service. Other policies may also affect who may report specific services.◀

Instructions, typically included as parenthetical . . .

✍ Rationale

In the "Introduction" of the CPT codebook, language has been added to the "Instructions for Use of the CPT Codebook" defining "qualified healthcare professional."

The new language defines the appropriate reporting of services performed by either qualified health care professionals or supervised clinical staff members, who may provide portions of a service under the supervision of a qualified provider but may not individually report services with CPT codes.

The revision was necessary to clarify the sections of CPT that include "or other qualified health care professional" as questions often arise regarding professionals who are qualified and licensed to perform a service, but not independently report that service and those nonphysician health care professionals who are able to perform a professional service within their scope of practice and independently report a professional service.

Evaluation and Management

A few revisions have been made in the Evaluation and Management section, some of which include: (1) typical times added to the initial observation codes 99218-99220; (2) editorial revisions to the Prolonged Services codes 99354-99359 and introductory guidelines to clarify the definition of direct patient contact and removal of physician-specific references in the title and code descriptors, as well as the addition of the language "other qualified health care professionals" to the introductory guidelines; and (3) revisions made to the Inpatient Neonatal Intensive Care Services and Pediatric and Neonatal Critical Care Services guidelines.

Evaluation and Management (E/M) Services Guidelines

New and Established Patient

►Solely for the purposes of distinguishing between new and established patients, **professional services** are those face-to-face services rendered by a physician and reported by a specific CPT code(s). A new patient is one who has not received any professional services from the physician or another physician of the **exact** same specialty **and subspecialty** who belongs to the same group practice, within the past three years.◄

►An established patient is one who has received professional services from the physician or another physician of the **exact** same specialty **and subspecialty** who belongs to the same group practice, within the past three years. See Decision Tree.◄

In the instance where a physician is on call for or covering for another physician, the patient's encounter will be classified as it would have been by the physician who is not available.

No distinction is made between new and established patients in the emergency department. E/M services in the emergency department category may be reported for any new or established patient who presents for treatment in the emergency department.

►The decision tree on page 5 is provided to aid in determining whether to report the E/M service provided as a new or an established patient encounter.◄

🖎 Rationale

The New and Established Patient definitions in the Evaluation and Management Guidelines have been revised providing further clarification of professional services rendered by physicians in regard to specialties and subspecialties. The revision includes the addition of the terms *exact* and *subspecialty* to specifically indicate that the professional services would be from a physican or another physician of the "exact" same specialty "and subspecialty" who belongs to the same group practice within the past three years. This revision clarifies that, although the physician may be of the same specialty, differences among subspecialties might require a significant new patient workup and should therefore be considered a new patient service rather than an established patient service. The Decision Tree for New vs Established Patients has also been added back to the E/M guidelines.

Hospital Observation Services

Initial Observation Care

NEW OR ESTABLISHED PATIENT

▲99218　**Initial observation care,** per day, for the evaluation and management of a patient which requires these 3 key components:

- **A detailed or comprehensive history;**

- **A detailed or comprehensive examination; and**

- **Medical decision making that is straightforward or of low complexity.**

Counseling and/or coordination of care with other providers or agencies are provided consistent with the nature of the problem(s) and the patient's and/or family's needs.

Usually, the problem(s) requiring admission to "observation status" are of low severity. Physicians typically spend 30 minutes at the bedside and on the patient's hospital floor or unit.

▲99219　**Initial observation care,** per day, for the evaluation and management of a patient, which requires these 3 key components:

- **A comprehensive history;**

- **A comprehensive examination; and**

- **Medical decision making of moderate complexity.**

Counseling and/or coordination of care with other providers or agencies are provided consistent with the nature of the problem(s) and the patient's and/or family's needs.

Usually, the problem(s) requiring admission to "observation status" are of moderate severity. Physicians typically spend 50 minutes at the bedside and on the patient's hospital floor or unit.

▲99220　Initial observation care, per day, for the evaluation and management of a patient, which requires these 3 key components:

- **A comprehensive history;**

- **A comprehensive examination; and**

- **Medical decision making of high complexity.**

Counseling and/or coordination of care with other providers or agencies are provided consistent with the nature of the problem(s) and the patient's and/or family's needs.

Usually, the problem(s) requiring admission to "observation status" are of high severity. Physicians typically spend 70 minutes at the bedside and on the patient's hospital floor or unit.

✎ Rationale

Typical times have been added to the initial observation codes 99218-99220 based on a crosswalk from the Hospital Inpatient Services codes.

Prolonged Services

Prolonged Service With Direct Patient Contact

▶Codes 99354-99357 are used when a physician or other qualified health care professional provides prolonged service involving direct patient contact that is provided beyond the usual service in either the inpatient or outpatient setting. Direct patient contact is face-to-face and includes additional non-face-to-face services on the patient's floor or unit in the hospital or nursing facility during the same session. This service is reported in addition to the designated evaluation and management services at any level and any other services provided at the same session as evaluation and management services. Appropriate codes should be selected for supplies provided or procedures performed in the care of the patient during this period.◀

▶Codes 99354-99355 are used to report the total duration of face-to-face time spent by a physician or other qualified health care professional on a given date providing prolonged service in the office or other outpatient setting, even if the time spent by the physician or other qualified health care professional on that date is not continuous. Codes 99356-99357 are used to report the total duration of time spent by a physician or other qualified health care professional at the bedside and on the patient's floor or unit, in the hospital or nursing facility on a given date providing prolonged service to a patient, even if the time spent by the physician or other qualified health care professional on that date is not continuous.◀

Code 99354 or 99356 is used to report the first hour of prolonged service on a given date, depending on the place of service.

▶Either code should be used only once per date, even if the time spent by the physician or other qualified health care professional is not continuous on that date. Prolonged service of less than 30 minutes total duration on a given date is not separately reported because the work involved is included in the total work of the evaluation and management codes.◀

Code 99355 or 99357 is used to report each additional 30 minutes beyond the first hour, depending on the place of service. Either code may also be used to report the final 15-30 minutes of prolonged service on a given date. Prolonged service of less than 15 minutes beyond the first hour or less than 15 minutes beyond the final 30 minutes is not reported separately.

The use of the time based add-on codes requires that the primary evaluation and management service have a typical or specified time published in the CPT codebook.

▶The following examples illustrate the correct reporting of prolonged physician or other qualified health care professional service with direct patient contact in the office setting:◀

+▲99354   Prolonged service in the office or other outpatient setting requiring direct patient contact beyond the usual service; first hour (List separately in addition to code for office or other outpatient **Evaluation and Management** service)

(Use 99354 in conjunction with 99201-99215, 99241-99245, 99324-99337, 99341-99350, 90809, 90815)

+▲99355   each additional 30 minutes (List separately in addition to code for prolonged service)

(Use 99355 in conjunction with 99354)

+▲99356 Prolonged service in the inpatient or observation setting, requiring unit/floor time beyond the usual service; first hour (List separately in addition to code for inpatient **Evaluation and Management** service)

▶(Use 99356 in conjunction with 99218-99220, 99221-99233, 99251-99255, 99304-99310, 90822, 90829)◀

+▲99357 each additional 30 minutes (List separately in addition to code for prolonged service)

(Use 99357 in conjunction with 99356)

Prolonged Service Without Direct Patient Contact

▶Codes 99358 and 99359 are used when a prolonged service is provided that is neither face-to face time in the office or outpatient setting, nor additional unit/floor time in the hospital or nursing facility setting during the same session of an evaluation and management service and is beyond the usual physician or other qualified health care professional service time.◀

▶This service is to be reported in relation to other physician or other qualified health care professional services, including evaluation and management services at any level. This prolonged service may be reported on a different date than the primary service to which it is related. For example, extensive record review may relate to a previous evaluation and management service performed earlier and commences upon receipt of past records. However, it must relate to a service or patient where (face-to-face) patient care has occurred or will occur and relate to ongoing patient management. A typical time for the primary service need not be established within the CPT code set.◀

▶Codes 99358 and 99359 are used to report the total duration of non-face-to-face time spent by a physician or other qualified health care professional on a given date providing prolonged service, even if the time spent by the physician or other qualified health care professional on that date is not continuous. Code 99358 is used to report the first hour of prolonged service on a given date regardless of the place of service. It should be used only once per date.◀

Prolonged service of less than 30 minutes total duration on a given date is not separately reported.

Code 99359 is used to report each additional 30 minutes beyond the first hour regardless of the place of service. It may also be used to report the final 15 to 30 minutes of prolonged service on a given date.

Prolonged service of less than 15 minutes beyond the first hour or less than 15 minutes beyond the final 30 minutes is not reported separately.

Do not report 99358-99359 for time spent in medical team conferences, on-line medical evaluations, care plan oversight services, anticoagulation management, or other non-face-to-face services that have more specific codes and no upper time limit in the CPT code set. Codes 99358-99359 may be reported when related to other non-face-to-face services codes that have a published maximum time (eg, telephone services).

▲99358 Prolonged evaluation and management service before and/or after direct patient care; first hour

+▲99359 each additional 30 minutes (List separately in addition to code for prolonged service)

(Use 99359 in conjunction with 99358)

⊘=Modifier 51 Exempt   ⊙=Moderate Sedation   ✚=Add-on Code   𝑵=FDA approval pending

✎ Rationale

The Prolonged Services codes 99354-99359 and the accompanying introductory guidelines have been editorially revised to clarify the definition of direct patient contact and remove the reference "face-to-face." Further clarifications include removal of physician-specific references in the title and code descriptors and the addition of the language "other qualified healthcare professionals" to the introductory guidelines. In addition, codes 99356 and 99357 have been revised to include observation as a setting for prolonged services. The parenthetical note following code 99356 has been revised to include the observation codes as appropriate for use in conjunction with 99356. This parenthetical note includes the initial observation codes 99218-99220 and lists the subsequent observation codes (99224-99226) as part of the 99221-99233 range.

Inpatient Neonatal Intensive Care Services and Pediatric and Neonatal Critical Care Services

Pediatric Critical Care Patient Transport

The following codes (99466, 99467) are used to report the physical attendance and direct face-to-face care by a physician during the interfacility transport of a critically ill or critically injured pediatric patient 24 months of age or younger. For the purpose of reporting codes 99466 and 99467, face-to-face care begins when the physician assumes primary responsibility of the pediatric patient at the referring hospital/facility, and ends when the receiving hospital/facility accepts responsibility for the pediatric patient's care. Only the time the physician spends in direct face-to-face contact with the patient during the transport should be reported. Pediatric patient transport services involving less than 30 minutes of face-to-face physician care should not be reported using codes 99466, 99467. Procedure(s) or service(s) performed by other members of the transporting team may not be reported by the supervising physician.

For the definition of the critically injured pediatric patient, see the **Neonatal and Pediatric Critical Care Services** section.

The direction of emergency care to transporting staff by a physician located in a hospital or other facility by two-way communication is not considered direct face-to-face care and should not be reported with 99466, 99467. Physician-directed emergency care through outside voice communication to transporting staff personnel is reported with 99288.

Emergency department services (99281-99285), initial hospital care (99221-99223), critical care (99291, 99292), initial date neonatal intensive (99477) or critical care (99468) are only reported after the patient has been admitted to the emergency department, the inpatient floor, or the critical care unit of the receiving facility. If inpatient critical care services are reported in the referring facility prior to transfer to the receiving hospital, use the critical care codes (99291, 99292).

The following services are included when performed during the pediatric patient transport by the physician providing critical care and may not be reported separately: routine monitoring evaluations (eg, heart rate, respiratory rate, blood pressure, and pulse oximetry), the interpretation of cardiac output measurements (93562), chest X-rays (71010, 71015, 71020), pulse oximetry (94760, 94761,

94762), blood gases and information data stored in computers (eg, ECGs, blood pressures, hematologic data) (99090), gastric intubation (43752, 43753), temporary transcutaneous pacing (92953), ventilatory management (94002, 94003, 94660, 94662) and vascular access procedures (36000, 36400, 36405, 36406, 36415, 36591, 36600). Any services performed which are not listed above should be reported separately.

Code 99466 is used to report the first 30 to 74 minutes of direct face-to-face time with the transport pediatric patient and should be reported only once on a given date. Code 99467 is used to report each additional 30 minutes provided on a given date. Face-to-face services of less than 30 minutes should not be reported with these codes.

▶(For total body cooling of neonates, see 0260T, 0261T)◀

 Rationale

Codes 0260T and 0261T have been established to report hypothermia procedures for neonates. To direct users to the appropriate codes to use to identify hypothermia procedures for neonates, a cross-reference has been placed within the guideline section of the existing Inpatient Neonatal Intensive Care Services and Pediatric and Neonatal Critical Care Services section directing users to the Category III code section for hypothermia services provided for neonates. For more information regarding the intended use for these codes, see the Rationale for Category III codes 0260T and 0261T.

99466   **Critical care** services delivered by a physician, face-to-face, during an interfacility transport of critically ill or critically injured pediatric patient, 24 months of age or younger; first 30-74 minutes of hands-on care during transport

Inpatient Neonatal and Pediatric Critical Care

The same definitions for critical care services apply for the adult, child, and neonate.

Codes 99468, 99469 are used . . .

The initial day neonatal critical care code . . .

Codes 99471-99476 are used to report services . . .

▶The pediatric and neonatal critical care codes include those procedures listed for the critical care codes (99291, 99292). In addition, the following procedures are also included (and are not separately reported by professionals, but may be reported by facilities) in the pediatric and neonatal critical care service codes (99468-99472, 99475, 99476) and the intensive care services codes (99477-99480;◀

▶Any services performed that are not included in these listings may be reported separately. Facilities may report the included services separately.◀

Invasive or non-invasive electronic monitoring of vital signs

Vascular access procedures

   Peripheral vessel catheterization (36000)

Other arterial catheters (36140, 36620)

Umbilical venous catheters (36510)

Central vessel catheterization (36555)

Vascular access procedures (36400, 36405, 36406)

Vascular punctures (36420, 36600)

Umbilical arterial catheters (36660)

Airway and ventilation management

Endotracheal intubation (31500)

Ventilatory management (94002-94004)

Bedside pulmonary function testing (94375)

Surfactant administration (94610)

Continuous positive airway pressure (CPAP) (94660)

Monitoring or interpretation of blood gases or oxygen saturation (94760-94762)

►Car Seat Evaluation (94780-94781)◄

Transfusion of blood components (36430, 36440)

Oral or nasogastric tube placement (43752)

Suprapubic bladder aspiration (51100)

Bladder catheterization (51701, 51702)

Lumbar puncture (62270)

Any services performed which are not listed above . . .

When a neonate or infant is not critically ill . . .

To report critical care services provided in the outpatient setting . . .

When critical care services are provided to neonates . . .

Critical care services to a pediatric patient . . .

Critical care services to a neonate or pediatric patient . . .

Critical care services provided by a second physician of a different specialty not reporting a 24-hour global code can be reported with the critical care codes 99291, 99292.

►When the critically ill neonate or pediatric patient improves and is transferred to a lower level of care, the transferring physician does not report a per day critical care service. Subsequent Hospital Care (99231-99233) or Critical Care Services (99291-99292) is reported, as appropriate based upon the condition of the neonate or child. The receiving physician reports a Subsequent Intensive Care (99478-99480) or Subsequent Hospital Care (99231-99233), as appropriate based upon the condition of the neonate or child.◄

No physician may report . . .

99468 **Initial inpatient neonatal critical care,** per day, for the evaluation and management of a critically ill neonate, 28 days of age or younger

✍ Rationale

The Inpatient Neonatal and Pediatric Critical Care guidelines have been revised for consistency with the current Critical Care guidelines for codes 99291-99292 to differentiate the inclusive provider services from the appropriate facility reporting of services frequently performed at the time of critical care.

Also, the inclusionary list of services included in these Inpatient Neonatal and Pediatric Critical Care guidelines applicable to codes 99468-99472, 99475, 99476, and 99477-99480 have been updated to include the new car seat evaluation codes 94780 and 94781.

New introductory language has also been added to the guidelines preceding code 99468 pertaining to the circumstance when the transfer of care of a sick neonate receiving intensive care services occurs from one physician to another physician in a different group, in which both providers will be providing intensive care services on the same date of service.

Initial and Continuing Intensive Care Services

Code 99477 represents the initial day . . .

▶When the neonate or infant improves after the initial day and is transferred to a lower level of care, the transferring physician does not report a per day intensive care service, Subsequent Hospital Care (99231-99233) is reported. When the neonate or infant becomes critically ill on a day when Initial or Subsequent Intensive Care Services have been performed and is transferred to a critical care level of care performed by a different physician, the transferring physician reports either the Critical Care Services performed (99291-99292) or the Intensive Care Service performed, but not both. The receiving physician reports Subsequent Inpatient Neonatal or Pediatric Critical Care (99469, 99472).◀

For the subsequent care of . . .

99477 **Initial hospital care**, per day, for the evaluation and management of the neonate, 28 days of age or younger, who requires intensive observation, frequent interventions, and other intensive care services;

✍ Rationale

New introductory language has been added to the Inpatient Neonatal Intensive Care Services and Pediatric and Neonatal Critical Care Services guidelines preceding code 99477 pertaining to the circumstance when the transfer of care of a sick neonate receiving intensive care services occurs from one physician to another physician in a different group, in which both providers will be providing intensive care services on the same date of service.

Surgery

Numerous changes have been made to the Surgery section, which include the addition of 60 codes, revision of 86 codes, and deletion of 48 codes.

Major changes have been made to the Integumentary System subsection including new guidelines to clarify the reporting of wound care management and skin substitutes. Comprehensive changes were made to the Skin Replacement Surgery subsection. This section was expanded to achieve greater granularity and consistency for these services.

A new series of codes for reporting application of multilayer compression systems have been added to the Application of Casts and Strapping subsection.

A large number of changes have been made to the Lungs and Pleura subsection, which include the development of new codes, deletion of codes that are obsolete, and revisions to existing codes to allow more specific identification of the types of procedures that are now performed. In addition, a number of language changes have been made to some of the guidelines and parenthetical notes. In some places, completely new guidelines and parenthetical notes have been developed to further exemplify the current surgical technologies that are available for lung procedures.

Many changes have been made to the codes and guidelines in the Cardiovascular System/Heart and Pericardium/Pacemaker or Pacing Cardioverter-Defibrillator section.

New guidelines for Diagnostic Studies of Arteriovenous (AV) Shunts for Dialysis and Interventions for Arteriovenous (AV) Shunts Created for Dialysis (AV Grafts and AV Fistula) have been added to the Vascular Injection Procedures subsection.

A number of changes have been implemented within the Spine and Spinal Cord section to identify the correct intent for identifying open versus percutaneous procedures for decompression procedures for the spine. The changes include additions, deletions, and revisions to guidelines, parenthetical notes, and code descriptors within this section.

Changes have been made to the neurostimulation codes throughout the CPT code set to provide language that is the same for these procedures as well as to more clearly portray the intended use for these procedures.

Surgery

Skin, Subcutaneous, and Accessory Structures

DEBRIDEMENT

▶Wound debridements (11042-11047) are reported by depth of tissue that is removed and by surface area of the wound. These services may be reported for injuries, infections, wounds and chronic ulcers. When performing debridement of a single wound, report depth using the deepest level of tissue removed. In multiple wounds, sum the surface area of those wounds that are at the same depth, but do not combine sums from different depths. For example: When bone is debrided from a 4 sq cm heel ulcer and from a 10 sq cm ischial ulcer, report the work with a single code, 11044. When subcutaneous tissue is debrided from a 16 sq cm dehisced abdominal wound and a 10 sq cm thigh wound, report the work with 11042 for the first 20 sq cm and 11045 for the second 6 sq cm. If all four wounds were debrided on the same day, use modifier 59 with either 11042, or 11044 as appropriate.◀

✎ Rationale

The example listed in the Debridement Guidelines has been editorially revised with the deletion of code 11045, as it is an add-on code reported in conjunction with code 11042 and wouldn't require the use of a modifier. The revised guideline now states to use modifier 59 with either code 11042 or 11044 as appropriate.

Introduction

11971   Removal of tissue expander(s) without insertion of prosthesis

▶(11975 has been deleted. To report insertion of non-biodegradable drug delivery implant for contraception, use 11981)◀

11976   Removal, implantable contraceptive capsules

▶(11977 has been deleted. To report removal of implantable contraceptive capsules with subsequent insertion of non-biodegradable drug delivery implant, use 11976 and 11981)◀

✎ Rationale

Implantable contraceptive capsule codes 11975 and 11977 have been deleted due to lack of utilization of this type of contraception. Parenthetical cross-reference notes have been added to direct users to the appropriate codes for insertion of nonbio-degradable drug delivery implant and for removal of implantable contraceptive capsules with subsequent insertion of nonbiodegradable drug delivery implant.

Repair (Closure)

Use the codes in this section to . . .

Definitions

The repair of wounds may be classified as . . .

Simple repair is used when the wound . . .

Intermediate repair includes the repair . . .

Complex repair includes the repair . . .

Instructions for listing services at time of wound repair:

1. The repaired wound(s) should be measured and recorded in centimeters, whether curved, angular, or stellate.

2. When multiple wounds are repaired, add together the lengths of those in the same classification (see above) and from all anatomic sites that are grouped together into the same code descriptor. For example, add together the lengths of intermediate repairs to the trunk and extremities. Do not add lengths of repairs from different groupings of anatomic sites (eg, face and extremities). Also, do not add together lengths of different classifications (eg, intermediate and complex repairs).

    ▶When more than one classification of wounds is repaired, list the more complicated as the primary procedure and the less complicated as the secondary procedure, using modifier 59.◀

3. Decontamination and/or debridement: Debridement is . . .

▶4. Involvement of nerves, blood vessels and tendons: Report under appropriate system (Nervous, Cardiovascular, Musculoskeletal) for repair of these structures. The repair of these associated wounds is included in the primary procedure unless it qualifies as a complex repair, in which case modifier 59 applies.◀

Simple ligation of vessels in an open wound is considered as part of any wound closure.

Simple "exploration" of nerves, blood vessels . . .

✍🏼 Rationale

In order to more appropriately describe the scenarios listed, modifier 59 has replaced modifier 51 in instructions number 2 and 4 of the repair guidelines.

▶SKIN REPLACEMENT SURGERY◀

▶Skin replacement surgery consists of surgical preparation and topical placement of an ***autograft*** (including tissue cultured autograft) or ***skin substitute graft*** (ie, homograft, allograft, xenograft). The graft is anchored using the provider's choice of fixation. When services are performed in the office, routine dressing supplies are not reported separately.

The following definition should be applied to those codes that reference "100 sq cm or 1% of body area of infants and children" when determining the involvement of body size: The measurement of 100 sq cm is applicable to adults and children 10 years of age and older; and percentages of body

---

surface area apply to infants and children younger than 10 years of age. The measurements apply to the size of the recipient area.

Procedures involving wrist and/or ankle are reported with codes that include arm or leg in the descriptor.

When a primary procedure requires a skin substitute or skin autograft for definitive skin closure (eg, orbitectomy, radical mastectomy, deep tumor removal), use 15100-15278 in conjunction with primary procedure.

For biological implant for soft tissue reinforcement, use 15777 in conjunction with primary procedure.

The supply of skin substitute graft(s) should be reported separately in conjunction with 15271-15278.◄

►**Definitions**◄

►Surgical preparation codes 15002-15005 for skin replacement surgery describe the initial services related to preparing a clean and viable wound surface for placement of an autograft, flap, skin substitute graft or for negative pressure wound therapy. In some cases, closure may be possible using adjacent tissue transfer (14000-14061) or complex repair (13100-13153). In all cases, appreciable nonviable tissue is removed to treat a burn, traumatic wound or a necrotizing infection. The clean wound bed may also be created by incisional release of a scar contracture resulting in a surface defect from separation of tissues. The intent is to heal the wound by primary intention, or by the use of negative pressure wound therapy. Patient conditions may require the closure or application of graft, flap, or skin substitute to be delayed, but in all cases the intent is to include these treatments or negative pressure wound therapy to heal the wound. Do not report 15002-15005 for removal of nonviable tissue/debris in a chronic wound (eg, venous or diabetic) when the wound is left to heal by secondary intention. See active wound management codes (97597, 97598) and debridement codes (11042-11047) for this service. For necrotizing soft tissue infections in specific anatomic locations, see 11004-11008.

Select the appropriate code from 15002-15005 based upon location and size of the resultant defect. For multiple wounds, sum the surface area of all wounds from all anatomic sites that are grouped together into the same code descriptor. For example, sum the surface area of all wounds on the trunk and arms. Do not sum wounds from different groupings of anatomic sites (eg, face and arms). Use 15002 or 15004, as appropriate, for excisions and incisional releases resulting in wounds up to and including 100 sq cm of surface area. Use 15003 or 15005 for each additional 100 sq cm or part thereof. For example: Surgical preparation of a 20 sq cm wound on the right hand and a 15 sq cm wound on the left hand would be reported with a single code, 15004. Surgical preparation of a 75 sq cm wound on the right thigh and a 75 sq cm wound on the left thigh would be reported with 15002 for the first 100 sq cm and 15003 for the second 50 sq cm. If all four wounds required surgical preparation on the same day, use modifier 59 with 15002, and 15004.

Autografts/tissue cultured autografts include the harvest and/or application of an autologous skin graft. Repair of donor site requiring skin graft or local flaps is reported separately. Removal of current graft and/or simple cleansing of the wound is included, when performed. Do not report 97602. Debridement is considered a separate procedure only when gross contamination requires prolonged cleansing, when appreciable amounts of devitalized or contaminated tissue are removed, or when debridement is carried out separately without immediate primary closure.

Select the appropriate code from 15040-15261 based upon type of autograft and location and size of the defect. The measurements apply to the size of the recipient area. For multiple wounds, sum the surface area of all wounds from all anatomic sites that are grouped together into the same code descriptor. For example, sum the surface area of all wounds on the trunk and arms. Do not sum wounds from different groupings of anatomic sites (eg, face and arms).

Skin substitute grafts include non-autologous human skin (dermal or epidermal, cellular and acellular) grafts (eg, homograft, allograft), non-human skin substitute grafts (ie, xenograft), and biological products that form a sheet scaffolding for skin growth. These codes are not to be reported for application of non-graft wound dressings (eg, gel, ointment, foam, liquid) or injected skin substitutes. Removal of current graft and/or simple cleansing of the wound is included, when performed. Do not report 97602. Debridement is considered a separate procedure only when gross contamination requires prolonged cleansing, when appreciable amounts of devitalized or contaminated tissue are removed, or when debridement is carried out separately without immediate primary closure.

Select the appropriate code from 15271-15278 based upon location and size of the defect. For multiple wounds, sum the surface area of all wounds from all anatomic sites that are grouped together into the same code descriptor. For example, sum the surface area of all wounds on the trunk and arms. Do not sum wounds from different groupings of anatomic sites (eg, face and arms). ◄

►Surgical Preparation◄

15002 Surgical preparation or creation of recipient site by excision of open wounds, burn eschar, or scar (including subcutaneous tissues), or incisional release of scar contracture, trunk, arms, legs; first 100 sq cm or 1% of body area of infants and children

(For linear scar revision, see 13100-13153)

+15003 each additional 100 sq cm, or part thereof, or each additional 1% of body area of infants and children (List separately in addition to code for primary procedure)

(Use 15003 in conjunction with 15002)

15004 Surgical preparation or creation of recipient site by excision of open wounds, burn eschar, or scar (including subcutaneous tissues), or incisional release of scar contracture, face, scalp, eyelids, mouth, neck, ears, orbits, genitalia, hands, feet and/or multiple digits; first 100 sq cm or 1% of body area of infants and children

+15005 each additional 100 sq cm, or part thereof, or each additional 1% of body area of infants and children (List separately in addition to code for primary procedure)

(Use 15005 in conjunction with 15004)

Autografts/Tissue Cultured Autograft

15040 Harvest of skin for tissue cultured skin autograft, 100 sq cm or less

15050 Pinch graft, single or multiple, to cover small ulcer, tip of digit, or other minimal open area (except on face), up to defect size 2 cm diameter

15100 Split-thickness autograft, trunk, arms, legs; first 100 sq cm or less, or 1% of body area of infants and children (except 15050)

+15101   each additional 100 sq cm, or each additional 1% of body area of infants and children, or part thereof (List separately in addition to code for primary procedure)

(Use 15101 in conjunction with 15100)

15110   Epidermal autograft, trunk, arms, legs; first 100 sq cm or less, or 1% of body area of infants and children

+15111   each additional 100 sq cm, or each additional 1% of body area of infants and children, or part thereof (List separately in addition to code for primary procedure)

(Use 15111 in conjunction with 15110)

15115   Epidermal autograft, face, scalp, eyelids, mouth, neck, ears, orbits, genitalia, hands, feet, and/or multiple digits; first 100 sq cm or less, or 1% of body area of infants and children

+15116   each additional 100 sq cm, or each additional 1% of body area of infants and children, or part thereof (List separately in addition to code for primary procedure)

(Use 15116 in conjunction with 15115)

15120   Split-thickness autograft, face, scalp, eyelids, mouth, neck, ears, orbits, genitalia, hands, feet, and/or multiple digits; first 100 sq cm or less, or 1% of body area of infants and children (except 15050)

+15121   each additional 100 sq cm, or each additional 1% of body area of infants and children, or part thereof (List separately in addition to code for primary procedure)

(Use 15121 in conjunction with 15120)

▶(For eyelids, see also 67961-67975)◀

15130   Dermal autograft, trunk, arms, legs; first 100 sq cm or less, or 1% of body area of infants and children

+15131   each additional 100 sq cm, or each additional 1% of body area of infants and children, or part thereof (List separately in addition to code for primary procedure)

(Use 15131 in conjunction with 15130)

15135   Dermal autograft, face, scalp, eyelids, mouth, neck, ears, orbits, genitalia, hands, feet, and/or multiple digits; first 100 sq cm or less, or 1% of body area of infants and children

+15136   each additional 100 sq cm, or each additional 1% of body area of infants and children, or part thereof (List separately in addition to code for primary procedure)

(Use 15136 in conjunction with 15135)

▲15150   Tissue cultured skin autograft, trunk, arms, legs; first 25 sq cm or less

+▲15151   additional 1 sq cm to 75 sq cm (List separately in addition to code for primary procedure)

(Do not report 15151 more than once per session)

(Use 15151 in conjunction with 15150)

+▲15152   each additional 100 sq cm, or each additional 1% of body area of infants and children, or part thereof (List separately in addition to code for primary procedure)

(Use 15152 in conjunction with 15151)

▲**15155**   Tissue cultured skin autograft, face, scalp, eyelids, mouth, neck, ears, orbits, genitalia, hands, feet, and/or multiple digits; first 25 sq cm or less

+▲**15156**   additional 1 sq cm to 75 sq cm (List separately in addition to code for primary procedure)

(Do not report 15156 more than once per session)

(Use 15156 in conjunction with 15155)

+▲**15157**   each additional 100 sq cm, or each additional 1% of body area of infants and children, or part thereof (List separately in addition to code for primary procedure)

(Use 15157 in conjunction with 15156)

▶(15170-15176 have been deleted. To report, see 15271-15278)◀

15200   Full thickness graft, free, including direct closure of donor site, trunk; 20 sq cm or less

+**15201**   each additional 20 sq cm, or part thereof (List separately in addition to code for primary procedure)

(Use 15201 in conjunction with 15200)

15220   Full thickness graft, free, including direct closure of donor site, scalp, arms, and/or legs; 20 sq cm or less

+**15221**   each additional 20 sq cm, or part thereof (List separately in addition to code for primary procedure)

(Use 15221 in conjunction with 15220)

15240   Full thickness graft, free, including direct closure of donor site, forehead, cheeks, chin, mouth, neck, axillae, genitalia, hands, and/or feet; 20 sq cm or less

(For finger tip graft, use 15050)

(For repair of syndactyly, fingers, see 26560-26562)

+**15241**   each additional 20 sq cm, or part thereof (List separately in addition to code for primary procedure)

(Use 15241 in conjunction with 15240)

15260   Full thickness graft, free, including direct closure of donor site, nose, ears, eyelids, and/or lips; 20 sq cm or less

+**15261**   each additional 20 sq cm, or part thereof (List separately in addition to code for primary procedure)

(Use 15261 in conjunction with 15260)

▶(For eyelids, see also 67961-67975)◀

▶(Repair of donor site requiring skin graft or local flaps is considered a separate procedure)◀

▶Skin Substitute Grafts◀

▶The supply of skin substitute graft(s) should be reported separately in conjunction with 15271-15278. For biologic implant for soft tissue reinforcement, use 15777 in conjunction with code for primary procedure.◀

●15271   Application of skin substitute graft to trunk, arms, legs, total wound surface area up to 100 sq cm; first 25 sq cm or less wound surface area

+●15272   each additional 25 sq cm wound surface area, or part thereof (List separately in addition to code for primary procedure)

▶(Use 15272 in conjunction with 15271)◀

▶(For total wound surface area greater than or equal to 100 sq cm, see 15273, 15274)◀

▶(Do not report 15271, 15272 in conjunction with 15273, 15274)◀

●15273   Application of skin substitute graft to trunk, arms, legs, total wound surface area greater than or equal to 100 sq cm; first 100 sq cm wound surface area, or 1% of body area of infants and children

+●15274   each additional 100 sq cm wound surface area, or part thereof, or each additional 1% of body area of infants and children, or part thereof (List separately in addition to code for primary procedure)

▶(Use 15274 in conjunction with 15273)◀

▶(For total wound surface area up to 100 sq cm, see 15271, 15272)◀

●15275   Application of skin substitute graft to face, scalp, eyelids, mouth, neck, ears, orbits, genitalia, hands, feet, and/or multiple digits, total wound surface area up to 100 sq cm; first 25 sq cm or less wound surface area

+●15276   each additional 25 sq cm wound surface area, or part thereof (List separately in addition to code for primary procedure)

▶(Use 15276 in conjunction with 15275)◀

▶(For total wound surface area greater than or equal to 100 sq cm, see 15277, 15278)◀

▶(Do not report 15275, 15276 in conjunction with 15277, 15278)◀

●15277   Application of skin substitute graft to face, scalp, eyelids, mouth, neck, ears, orbits, genitalia, hands, feet, and/or multiple digits, total wound surface area greater than or equal to 100 sq cm; first 100 sq cm wound surface area, or 1% of body area of infants and children

+●15278   each additional 100 sq cm wound surface area, or part thereof, or each additional 1% of body area of infants and children, or part thereof (List separately in addition to code for primary procedure)

▶(Use 15278 in conjunction with 15277)◀

▶(For total wound surface area up to 100 sq cm, see 15275, 15276)◀

▶(Do not report 15271-15278 in conjunction with 97602)◀

▶(15300, 15301 have been deleted. To report, see 15271-15274)◀

▶(15320, 15321 have been deleted. To report, see 15275-15278)◄

▶(15330, 15331 have been deleted. To report, see 15271-15274)◄

▶(15335, 15336 have been deleted. To report, see 15275-15278)◄

▶(15340, 15341 have been deleted. To report, see 15271-15278)◄

▶(15360, 15361 have been deleted. To report, see 15271-15274)◄

▶(15365, 15366 have been deleted. To report, see 15275-15278)◄

▶(15400, 15401 have been deleted. To report, see 15271-15274)◄

▶(15420, 15421 have been deleted. To report, see 15275-15278)◄

▶(15430, 15431 have been deleted. To report, see 15271-15278)◄

✍ Rationale

For CPT 2012, the Integumentary System subsection has been expanded to include new guidelines to clarify the reporting of wound care management and skin substitutes. Comprehensive changes were made to the Skin Replacement Surgery subsection (codes 15271-15278). Other changes include deletion of 24 codes, revision of six codes, and the addition of eight new codes and a number of new cross-references and instructional notes. This section was expanded to achieve greater granularity and consistency for these services.

The Skin Replacement Surgery subheading was revised, removing reference to "and skin substitutes" from the subheading as "Skin Substitutes Graft" warranted its own new subsection. The new skin replacement introductory guidelines were added to instruct that skin replacement surgery consists of the surgical preparation and topical placement of an autograft, which includes the tissue cultured auto-graft, or the skin substitute homograft, allograft, and xenograft. It instructs that the graft is anchored using the provider's choice of fixation, and when services are performed in the office, routine dressing supplies are not reported separately.

The guidelines also instruct how to report the skin replacement codes when referencing measurements of "100 sq cm or 1% of body area of infants and children" when determining the involvement of body size: the measurement of 100 sq cm is applicable to adults and children 10 years of age and older; and percentages of body surface area apply to infants and children younger than 10 years of age. When reporting these services, the measurements apply to the size of the recipient area. The guidelines also instruct when procedures involving wrist and/or ankle are reported with codes that include arm or leg in the descriptor.

The guidelines further instruct that when a primary procedure requires a skin substitute or skin autograft for definitive skin closure (eg, orbitectomy, radical mastectomy, deep tumor removal), use codes 15100-15278 in conjunction with the primary procedure. It is also appropriate to report code 15777 in conjunction with the primary procedure for biological implant for soft tissue reinforcement if applied. The supply of skin substitute graft(s) should be reported separately in conjunction with codes 15271-15278.

⊘=Modifier 51 Exempt   ⊙=Moderate Sedation   ✚=Add-on Code   𝒩=FDA approval pending

The "Surgical Preparation" subheading was moved to a more appropriate location and replaced with a "Definitions" subheading. The guidelines were revised to include definition of surgical preparation codes 15002-15005 for skin replacement surgery, which describes the initial services related to preparing a clean and viable wound surface for placement of an autograft, flap, skin substitute graft or for negative pressure wound therapy. The guidelines were further revised to provide an example that when performing surgical preparation of a 20 sq cm wound on the right hand and a 15 sq cm wound on the left hand to report a single code, 15004. Surgical preparation of a 75 sq cm wound on the right thigh and a 75 sq cm wound on the left thigh would be reported with code 15002 for the first 100 sq cm and 15003 for the second 50 sq cm. If all four wounds required surgical preparation on the same day, use modifier 59 with codes 15002 and 15004.

The guidelines also instruct that the autografts/tissue cultured autografts includes the harvest and/or application of an autologous skin graft. Repair of the donor site requiring skin graft or local flaps is reported separately. Removal of current graft and/or simple cleansing of the wound is included when performed. It would not be appropriate to report code 97602. Debridement is considered a separate procedure only when gross contamination requires prolonged cleansing, when appreciable amounts of devitalized or contaminated tissue are removed, or when debridement is carried out separately without immediate primary closure.

It is also appropriate to select the code from the range 15040-15261 based on the type of autograft and location and size of the defect. The measurements apply to the size of the recipient area. For multiple wounds, sum the surface area of all wounds from all anatomic sites that are grouped together into the same code descriptor. For example, sum the surface area of all wounds on the trunk and arms. It would not be appropriate to sum up the wounds from different groupings of anatomic sites (eg, face and arms).

The guidelines further instruct that the skin substitute grafts include non-autologous human skin (dermal or epidermal, cellular and acellular) grafts (eg, homograft, allograft), nonhuman skin substitute grafts (ie, xenograft) and biological products that form a sheet scaffolding for skin growth. These codes are not intended to be reported for the application of non-graft wound dressings (eg, gel, ointment, foam, liquid) or injected skin substitutes. Removal of current graft and/or simple cleansing of the wound is included when performed It would not be appropriate to report code 97602. Debridement is considered a separate procedure only when gross contamination requires prolonged cleansing, when appreciable amounts of devitalized or contaminated tissue are removed, or when debridement is carried out separately without immediate primary closure.

It is also appropriate to select the code from the range 15271-15278 based upon the location and size of the defect. For multiple wounds, sum the surface area of all wounds from all anatomic sites that are grouped together into the same code descriptor. For example, sum the surface area of all wounds on the trunk and arms. It would not be appropriate to sum up the wounds from different groupings of anatomic sites (eg, face and arms).

In support of the new guidelines and definitions for autografts and skin substitute grafts: (1) the surgical preparation subheading has been moved to precede the range of codes 15002-15005; (2) the application of skin replacement and skin substitutes heading and guidelines have been deleted to accommodate a new subsection entitled "skin substitute grafts" along with guidelines and eight new codes 15271-15278; (3) the autografts/tissue cultured autografts codes 15150-15157 have been editorially revised deleting the term "epidermal" and replacing it with the term "skin" autograft for consistency purposes; (4) the acellular dermal replacement subheading and codes 15170-15176 have been deleted; and (5) a cross-reference note has been added directing the user to report codes 15271-15278 for application of skin substitute graft.

To address changes in clinical practice, CPT 2012 has made comprehensive changes to the skin substitute section. A new subsection entitled "Skin Substitute Grafts" was added to accommodate the changes. New guidelines were written to instruct users that the supply of skin substitute graft(s) should be reported separately in conjunction with the application of skin substitute graft codes 15271-15278; and for biological implant for soft tissue reinforcement, use code 15777 in conjunction with the code for primary procedure.

A two-tier structure with eight new codes 15271-15278 have been established to report the application of skin substitute grafts, which are distinguished according to the anatomic location and surface area rather than by product description: (1) codes 15271, 15272, 15275, and 15276 describe the application for total wound surface area up to 100 sq cm; and (2) codes 15273, 15274, 15277, 15278 describe the application for total wound surface area greater than or equal to 100 sq cm; (3) code 15271 is intended to describe the application of skin substitute graft to the trunk, arms, legs, total wound surface area up to 100 sq cm; first 25 sq cm or less wound surface area; (4) add-on code 15272 is intended to describe each additional 25 sq cm wound surface area, or part thereof (List separately in addition to code for primary procedure); (5) code 15273 is intended to describe the application of skin substitute graft to the trunk, arms, legs, total wound surface area greater than or equal to 100 sq cm; first 100 sq cm wound surface area, or 1% of body area of infants and children; (6) add-on code 15274 is intended to describe each additional 100 sq cm wound surface area, or part thereof, or each additional 1% of body area of infants and children or part thereof (List separately in addition to code for primary procedure; (7) code 15275 is intended to describe the application of skin substitute graft to face, scalp, eyelids, mouth, neck, ears, orbits, genitalia, hands, feet, and/or multiple digits, total wound surface area up to 100 sq cm; first 25 sq cm or less wound surface area; (8) add-on code 15276 is intended to describe each additional 25 sq cm wound surface area, or part thereof (List separately in addition to code for primary procedure); (9) code 15277 is intended to describe the application of skin substitute graft to face, scalp, eyelids, mouth, neck, ears, orbits, genitalia, hands, feet, and/or multiple digits, total wound surface area greater than or equal to 100 sq cm; first 100 sq cm wound surface area, or 1% of body area of infants and children; and (10) add-on code 15278 is intended to describe each additional 100 sq cm wound surface area, or part thereof, or each additional 1%

of body area of infants and children, or part thereof (List separately in addition to code for primary procedure).

Furthermore, numerous parenthetical, instructional, and cross-reference notes have been added to support these changes.

In support of the establishment of codes 15271-15278, the allograft/tissue cultured allogeneic heading, guidelines and codes 15300-15366 have been deleted. Seven cross-reference notes have been added directing users to the appropriate codes 15271-15278 in lieu of the deleted codes 15300-15366.

In support of the establishment of codes 15271-15278, the xenograft heading, guidelines, and codes 15400-15431 have been deleted. Three cross-reference notes have been added directing users to the appropriate codes 15271-15278 in lieu of the deleted codes 15400-15431.

 ## Clinical Example (15271)

A 75-year-old female with chronic venous stasis disease presents with a 24 sq cm (4.0 x 6.0) clean, granulating, stalled, full-thickness, chronic ulceration of the medial lower leg. A recent culture is negative for bacteria. The wound has failed to respond to compression therapy and standard active wound care treatment. A skin substitute graft is applied.

Description of Procedure (15271)

Simple cleansing of the wound bed is performed and hemostasis achieved. The wound is measured and the appropriate sized skin substitute graft is prepared and applied to the prepared wound surface, including the wound margins, and secured in place.

 ## Clinical Example (15272)

A 75-year-old female with chronic venous stasis disease presents with a 48 sq cm (6.0 x 8.0) clean, granulating, stalled, full-thickness, chronic ulceration of the medial lower leg. A recent culture is negative for bacteria. The wound has failed to respond to compression therapy and standard active wound care treatment. After application of the first 25 sq cm of skin substitute graft (reported separately with code 15271), additional skin substitute graft is applied.

(Please note this is an add-on code.)

Description of Procedure (15272)

Additional simple cleansing of the wound and hemostasis is performed. Additional skin substitute graft material is prepared and applied to the prepared wound surface, including the wound margins, and secured in place.

Clinical Example (15273)

A mechanic was admitted to the burn center with burns on all four extremities and his lower back and abdomen, after his gasoline-saturated clothing was ignited from a spark. The burns involved 40% body surface area. Surgical excision of the burn tissue from the left lower leg beginning at the ankle and extending to the popliteal area was performed (reported separately). He now undergoes application of the first 100 sq cm of skin substitute graft on his left lower leg.

Description of Procedure (15273)
Under general anesthesia, hemostasis of the graft site with epinephrine soaked laparotomy pads and/or topical thrombin is accomplished. Skin substitute graft totaling 100 sq cm is prepared and applied to the prepared wound surface, including the wound margins, and secured in place.

Clinical Example (15274)
A mechanic was admitted to the burn center with burns on all four extremities and his lower back and abdomen, after his gasoline-saturated clothing was ignited from a spark. The burns involved 40% body surface area. Surgical excision of the burn tissue from the left lower leg beginning at the ankle and extending to the popliteal area was performed (reported separately). After application of the first 100 sq cm of skin substitute graft on his left lower leg (reported separately with code 15273), an additional 100 sq cm of skin substitute graft is applied to the same leg.

(Please note this is an add-on code.)

Description of Procedure (15274)
Additional hemostasis of the graft site with epinephrine soaked laparotomy pads and/or topical thrombin is accomplished. Additional skin substitute graft totaling 100 sq cm is applied to the leg and secured in place.

Clinical Example (15275)
A 68-year-old male with Type II diabetes presents with a 12.0 sq cm (3.0 x 4.0) clean, granulating, stalled, full-thickness, chronic ulceration of the plantar aspect of the right heel. A recent culture is negative for bacteria. The wound has failed to respond to standard active wound care treatment. A skin substitute graft is applied.

Description of Procedure (15275)
Simple cleansing of the wound bed is performed and hemostasis achieved. The wound is measured and the appropriate sized skin substitute graft is prepared and applied to the prepared wound surface, including the wound margins, and secured in place.

Clinical Example (15276)
A 68-year-old male with Type II diabetes presents with clean, granulating, full-thickness, chronic, stalled, ulcerations on the plantar aspect of his right and left heels. The ulcer on his left heel is 25 sq cm (5.0 x 5.0) and the ulceration on his right heel is 20 sq cm (4.0 x 5.0). A recent culture is negative for bacteria. The wounds have failed to respond to standard active wound care treatment. After application of the first 25 sq cm of skin substitute graft to the left heel (reported separately with code 15275), an additional 20 sq cm of skin substitute graft is applied to the right heel.

(Please note this is an add-on code.)

Description of Procedure (15276)

Additional simple cleansing of the wound and hemostasis is performed. Additional skin substitute graft material is prepared and applied to the prepared wound surface, including the wound margins, and secured in place.

 Clinical Example (15277)

A mechanic was admitted to the burn center with burns on all four extremities and his lower back and abdomen, after his gasoline-saturated clothing was ignited from a spark. The burns involved 40% body surface area. Surgical excision of the burn tissue from his right hand beginning at the wrist was performed (reported separately). He now undergoes application of the first 100 sq cm of skin substitute graft on his right hand and fingers.

Description of Procedure (15277)

Under general anesthesia, hemostasis of the graft site with epinephrine soaked laparotomy pads and/or topical thrombin is accomplished. Skin substitute graft totaling 100 sq cm is prepared and applied to the prepared wound surface, including the wound margins, and secured in place.

Clinical Example (15278)

A mechanic was admitted to the burn center with burns on all four extremities and his lower back and abdomen, after his gasoline-saturated clothing was ignited from a spark. The burns involved 40% body surface area. Surgical excision of the burn tissue from his right hand beginning at the wrist was performed (reported separately). After application of the first 100 sq cm of skin substitute graft to the right hand and fingers (reported separately with code 15277), an additional 100 sq cm of skin substitute graft is applied to his left hand and fingers.

(Please note this is an add-on code.)

Description of Procedure (15278)

Additional hemostasis of the graft site with epinephrine soaked laparotomy pads and/or topical thrombin is accomplished. Additional skin substitute graft totaling 100 sq cm is applied to the leg and secured in place.

OTHER FLAPS AND GRAFTS

15775   Punch graft for hair transplant; 1 to 15 punch grafts

15776   more than 15 punch grafts

(For strip transplant, use 15220)

+●15777   Implantation of biologic implant (eg, acellular dermal matrix) for soft tissue reinforcement (eg, breast, trunk) (List separately in addition to code for primary procedure)

▶(For bilateral breast procedure, report 15777 with modifier 50)◀

▶(For implantation of mesh or other prosthesis for open incisional or ventral hernia repair, use 49568 in conjunction with 49560-49566)◀

►(For insertion of mesh or other prosthesis for closure of a necrotizing soft tissue infection wound, use 49568 in conjunction with 11004-11006)◄

►(For topical application of skin substitute graft to a wound surface, see 15271-15278)◄

►(For repair of anorectal fistula with plug (eg, porcine small intestine submucosa [SIS]), use 46707)◄

►(For insertion of mesh or other prosthesis for repair of pelvic floor defect, use 57267)◄

►(The supply of biologic implant should be reported separately in conjunction with 15777)◄

 ## Rationale

A new add-on code 15777 has been established to report the implantation of biologic implant (eg, acellular dermal matrix) for soft tissue reinforcement (eg, breast, trunk) in addition to the primary procedure. This is in contrast to codes 15271-15278, which are intended for reporting topical application of skin substitute grafts. Seven cross-reference notes have been added instructing the user to select the appropriate code for skin substitute services and other services.

Clinical Example (15777)

A 50-year-old female proceeds with immediate unilateral breast reconstruction with a separately reported tissue expander following a mastectomy and sentinel lymph node dissection. A 140 sq cm piece of acellular dermal matrix is sutured to the subpectoral pocket rim before the skin flaps are brought together. The skin is closed primarily.

(Please note this is an add-on code.)

Description of Procedure (15777)

Following a separately reported mastectomy and sentinel node dissection, the plastic surgeon elevates the pectoralis muscle as part of a separately reported insertion of a tissue expander. Prior to the expander placement, the plastic surgeon confirms that a biologic tissue substitute is required, identifies the correct substitute, and prepares it on the sterile field according to package directions. At the lateral border of the elevated pectoralis a 140 sq cm piece of acellular dermal matrix is trimmed to shape the curve of the breast and sutured to the entire inferior and lateral border of the pectoralis major muscle. A separately reported tissue expander is then placed, and the remaining edges of the acellular dermal matrix are sutured to the chest wall. The pocket is irrigated with saline and antibiotic solution.

BURNS, LOCAL TREATMENT

►Procedures 16000-16036 refer to local treatment of burned surface only. Codes 16020-16030 include the application of materials (eg, dressings) not described in codes 15100-15278.◄

List percentage of body surface involved and depth of burn.

For necessary related medical services (eg, hospital visits, detention) in management of burned patients, see appropriate services in **Evaluation and Management** and **Medicine** sections.

For the application of skin grafts or skin substitutes, see codes 15100-15650.

16000   Initial treatment, first degree burn, when no more than local treatment is required

 Rationale

In support of the establishment of codes 15271-15278, the Burn, Local Treatment guidelines have been revised to expand the range of codes for the reporting of skin replacement graft(s).

Breast

REPAIR AND/OR RECONSTRUCTION

(To report bilateral procedure, report modifier 50 with the procedure code)

▶(For biologic implant for soft tissue reinforcement, use 15777 in conjunction with primary procedure)◀

19316   Mastopexy

 Rationale

In support of the establishment of code 15777, a cross-reference note has been added preceding code 19316 directing users to report code 15777 for biologic implant for soft tissue reinforcement, in conjunction with the primary procedure.

Musculoskeletal System

General

INTRODUCTION OR REMOVAL

20526   Injection, therapeutic (eg, local anesthetic, corticosteroid), carpal tunnel

●**20527**   Injection, enzyme (eg, collagenase), palmar fascial cord (ie, Dupuytren's contracture)

▶(For manipulation of palmar fascial cord (ie, Dupuytren's cord) post enzyme injection (eg, collagenase), use 26341)◀

 Rationale

Two new codes have been established for the treatment of Dupuytren's contracture. Code 20527 is for the injection of an enzyme (eg, collagenase) into the palmar fascial cord (ie, Dupuytren's cord), and code 26341 is for the manipulation of the palmar fascial cord performed on a subsequent day with some follow-up care included (eg, wound check). Cross-references following each code were added to reference the new codes.

🩺 **Clinical Example (20527)**

A 60-year-old male with Dupuytren's contracture presents with a cord resulting in a fixed flexion contracture of the metacarpophalangeal or proximal interphalangeal joint. The patient undergoes enzyme (eg, collagenase) injection into the cord. Note: Manipulation of palmar fascial cord is reported separately.

Description of Procedure (20527)

The contracted fascial cord is injected in three separate but proximate locations with enzyme. During the course of the injection, appropriate needle placement is confirmed by assessing neural function and tendon flexion. Great care is taken to avoid injection into the adjacent neurovascular bundles and flexor tendons.

Spine (Vertebral Column)

Cervical, thoracic, and lumbar spine.

Within the spine section, bone grafting . . .

To report bone grafts performed after arthrodesis . . .

Example:

Posterior arthrodesis of L5-S1 for degenerative . . .

Within the spine section, instrumentation . . .

Example:

Posterior arthrodesis of L4-S1, utilizing morselized . . .

Vertebral procedures are sometimes . . .

When arthrodesis is performed in addition . . .

Example:

Treatment of a burst fracture of L2 by . . .

When two surgeons work together as primary . . .

Example:

A 42-year-old male with a history of posttraumatic . . .

(Do not append modifier 62 to bone graft code 20931) (For injection procedure for myelography, use 62284)

(For injection procedure for discography, see 62290, 62291)

(For injection procedure, chemonucleolysis, single or multiple levels, use 62292)

▶(For injection procedure for facet joints, see 64490-64495, 64633-64636)◀

(For needle or trocar biopsy, see 20220-20225)

🖎 Rationale

In support of the changes to the destruction of paravertebral facet joint nerve by neurolytic agent codes, the parenthetical note in the Musculoskeletal System/ Spine (Vertebral Column) that directs users to the injection procedure for facet joint codes has been revised to reflect this change. See the Nervous System/ Extracranial Nerves, Peripheral Nerves, and Autonomic Nervous System/ Destruction by Neurolytic Agent (eg, Chemical, Thermal, Electrical, or Radiofrequency) section of this book for an explanation of deleted codes 64622, 64623, 64626, and 64627 and codes 64633-64636.

VERTEBRAL BODY, EMBOLIZATION OR INJECTION

⊙▲22520   Percutaneous vertebroplasty (bone biopsy included when performed), 1 vertebral body, unilateral or bilateral injection; thoracic

⊙▲22521   lumbar

+▲22522   each additional thoracic or lumbar vertebral body (List separately in addition to code for primary procedure)

        ▶(Do not report 22520-22522 in conjunction with 20225, 22310-22315, 22325, 22327 when performed at the same level as 22520-22522)◀

        (Use 22522 in conjunction with 22520, 22521 as appropriate)

        (For radiological supervision and interpretation, see 72291, 72292)

22523   Percutaneous vertebral augmentation, including cavity creation (fracture reduction and bone biopsy included when performed) using mechanical device, 1 vertebral body, unilateral or bilateral cannulation (eg, kyphoplasty); thoracic

22524   lumbar

+22525   each additional thoracic or lumbar vertebral body (List separately in addition to code for primary procedure)

        ▶(Do not report 22523-22525 in conjunction with 20225, 22310-22315, 22325, 22327 when performed at the same level as 22523-22525)◀

        (Use 22525 in conjunction with 22523, 22524)

        (For radiological supervision and interpretation, see 72291, 72292)

✎ Rationale

An exclusionary parenthetical following codes 22520-22522 has been added, and the exclusionary parenthetical following the codes 22523-22525 has been revised to preclude the reporting of fracture reduction and bone biopsy procedures in conjunction with the vertebroplasty/kyphoplasty codes. In addition, the phrase "bone biopsy included when performed" has been added to the vertebroplasty codes for consistency with the kyphoplasty codes.

ARTHRODESIS

Posterior, Posterolateral or Lateral Transverse Process Technique

22600   Arthrodesis, posterior or posterolateral technique, single level; cervical below C2 segment

▲ **22610**   thoracic (with lateral transverse technique, when performed)

▲ **22612**   lumbar (with lateral transverse technique, when performed)

▶(Do not report 22612 in conjunction with 22630 for the same interspace and segment, use 22633)◀

+ 22614   each additional vertebral segment (List separately in addition to code for primary procedure)

▶(Use 22614 in conjunction with 22600, 22610, 22612, 22630 or 22633 when performed at a different level. When performing a posterior or posterolateral technique for fusion/arthrodesis at an additional level, use 22614. When performing a posterior interbody fusion arthrodesis at an additional level, use 22632. When performing a combined posterior or posterolateral technique with posterior interbody arthrodesis at an additional level, use 22634)◀

▶(For facet joint fusion, see 0219T-0222T)◀

(For placement of a posterior intrafacet implant, see 0219T-0222T)

22630   Arthrodesis, posterior interbody technique, including laminectomy and/or discectomy to prepare interspace (other than for decompression), single interspace; lumbar

▶(Do not report 22630 in conjunction with 22612 for the same interspace and segment, use 22633)◀

+ 22632   each additional interspace (List separately in addition to code for primary procedure)

▶(Use 22632 in conjunction with 22612, 22630, or 22633 when performed at a different level. When performing a posterior interbody fusion arthrodesis at an additional level, use 22632. When performing a posterior or posterolateral technique for fusion/arthrodesis at an additional level, use 22614. When performing a combined posterior or posterolateral technique with posterior interbody arthrodesis at an additional level, use 22634)◀

● **22633**   Arthrodesis, combined posterior or posterolateral technique with posterior interbody technique including laminectomy and/or discectomy sufficient to prepare interspace (other than for decompression), single interspace and segment; lumbar

▶(Do not report with 22612 or 22630 at the same level)◀

+● 22634   each additional interspace and segment (List separately in addition to code for primary procedure)

▶(Use 22634 in conjunction with 22633)◀

✍ Rationale

In response to the AMA RUC Five-Year Review Identification Workgroup analyses to combine codes that are frequently reported together, the arthrodesis family of codes has been revised and expanded to include two new lumbar arthrodesis codes, 22633 and 22634. Existing arthrodesis codes 22610 (thoracic) and 22612 (lumbar) have been revised, and several parenthetical notes have been added throughout this section to provide additional instructions for the appropriate reporting of these codes.

Codes 22633 and 22634 have been established to report lumbar arthrodesis utilizing a combined posterior or posterolateral technique with a posterior interbody technique including laminectomy and/or discectomy sufficient to prepare interspace (other than for decompression) for each interspace and segment. Codes

22612 or 22630 should not be reported at the same level. A note has been added following code 22633 to indicate that instruction. Also, code 22634 should not be reported with code 22633. An exclusionary note following code 22634 indicates that instruction.

Codes 22610 (thoracic) and 22612 (lumbar) have been revised by replacing the phrase, "or without" with "when performed."

An instructional note has been added following code 22612 to indicate that code 22612 should not be reported in conjunction with code 22630 for the same interspace and segment. Instead, code 22633 should be reported in these instances.

The parenthetical note following code 22614 has been updated to clarify that: (1) code 22614 should be reported with codes 22600, 22610, 22612, 22630, or 22633 when performed at a different level; (2) when performing a posterior or posterolateral technique for fusion/arthrodesis at an additional level, code 22614 should be reported; (3) code 22632 should be reported when performing a posterior interbody fusion arthrodesis at an additional level; and (4) code 22634 should be reported when performing a combined posterior or posterolateral technique with posterior interbody arthrodesis at an additional level.

An instructional note has been added following code 22630 to indicate that code 22630 should not be reported in conjunction with code 22612 for the same interspace and segment. Instead, code 22633 should be reported in these instances.

The parenthetical note following code 22632 has been updated to clarify its intended use with codes 22612, 22614, 22630, 22633, and 22634. Code 22632 should be reported in conjunction with codes 22612, 22630, and 22633 when performed at different levels. In addition, code 22632 should be reported when posterior interbody fusion arthrodesis is performed at an additional level. Code 22614 should be reported when posterior or posterolateral technique for fusion/arthrodesis is performed at an additional level. When performing a combined posterior or posterolateral technique with posterior interbody arthrodesis at an additional level, code 22634 should be reported.

A second cross-reference note was added following code 22614 instructing users to see codes 0219T-0222T for facet joint fusion.

Clinical Example (22633)

A 68-year-old female presents with a degenerative spondylolisthesis of L4-5 causing mechanical low back pain. Nonoperative treatments have failed to control her symptoms.

Description of Procedure (22633)

The midline skin incision is made, the subcutaneous and muscular tissues are incised and reflected, and the dorsal aspects of the relevant spinal segments are exposed. The surgical segments are identified and the posterolateral elements of the spine (eg, facet joint[s], lamina, and/or transverse process[es])are exposed. The necessary portion of the facet joint is removed along with the lateral aspect of the lamina are removed to expose the disc space. Additional decompression (eg, lumbar disc herniation or lumbar stenosis), if required, is reported separately. The thecal sac and nerve root(s) are identified, dissected, and retracted. The disc space is identified and the posterior annulus is incised, followed by removal of disc material sufficient to allow creation of a bone graft recipient bed. Following this, the intervertebral fusion graft material(s) (eg, allograft, autograft, intervertebral cage[s] are reported separately) are placed unilaterally or bilaterally as determined by the spinal pathology. Following placement of the intervertebral graft, the transverse process, and/or facet are decorticated and graft material (reported separately) is placed posterolaterally for a fusion. If used, spinal instrumentation is placed (reported separately) as an adjunct to fusion. The wound is irrigated and closed in layers with application of a sterile dressing.

Clinical Example (22634)

A 68-year-old female presents with severe disc degeneration with lateral listhesis at L4-5 above a L5-S1 lytic or isthmic spondylolisthesis. She has significant low back pain that has not responded to nonoperative treatment and undergoes fusion at L4-5 and L5-S1.

(Please note this is an add-on code.)

Description of Procedure (22634)

The exposed spinal segments are identified and the posterolateral elements of the spine (eg, facet joint[s], lamina, and/or transverse process[es]) are exposed. The necessary portion of the facet joint is removed along with the lateral aspect of the lamina to expose the disc space. Additional decompression (eg,lumbar disc herniation or lumbar stenosis), if required, is reported separately. The thecal sac and nerve root(s) are identified, dissected, and retracted. The disc space is identified and the posterior annulus is incised, followed by removal of disc material sufficient to allow creation of a bone graft recipient bed. Following this, the intervertebral fusion graft material(s) (eg, allograft, autograft, intervertebral cage[s] are reported separately) are placed unilaterally or bilaterally as determined by the spinal pathology. Following placement of the intervertebral graft, the transverse process, and/or facet are decorticated and graft material (reported separately) is placed posterolaterally for a fusion. If used, spinal instrumentation is placed (reported separately) as an adjunct to fusion.

SPINAL INSTRUMENTATION

Segmental instrumentation is defined as . . .

Non-segmental instrumentation is defined as . . .

Insertion of spinal instrumentation is reported . . .

To report bone graft procedures, see . . .

A vertebral segment describes the basic . . .

▶Codes 22849, 22850, 22852, and 22855 are subject to modifier 51 if reported with other definitive procedure(s), including arthrodesis, decompression, and exploration of fusion. Code 22849 should not be reported in conjunction with 22850, 22852, and 22855 at the same spinal levels. Only the appropriate insertion code (22840-22848) should be reported when previously placed spinal instrumentation is being removed or revised during the same session where new instrumentation is inserted at levels including all or part of the previously instrumented segments. Do not report the reinsertion (22849) or removal (22850, 22852, 22855) procedures in addition to the insertion of the new instrumentation (22840-22848).◄

+22840   Posterior non-segmental instrumentation (eg, Harrington rod technique, pedicle fixation across 1 interspace, atlantoaxial transarticular screw fixation, sublaminar wiring at C1, facet screw fixation) (List separately in addition to code for primary procedure)

✍ Rationale

The spinal instrumentation introductory guidelines have been revised to more accurately reflect the intended use of codes in this section when used to identify reinsertion of spinal instrumentation. New instructions have now been added that note that the appropriate spinal instrumentation insertion code is the only code that should be used when a previously placed spinal instrumentation device is being removed or changed during the same session as new instrumentation even if the insertion includes new levels and/or part of the previously instrumented segments. The guidelines also specify that reinsertion (22849) and/or removal (22850) should not be additionally reported with insertion of new instrumentation (22840-22848). Instead, the intent is that when insertion of instrumentation is performed that involves the original levels as well as new levels, only the appropriate code for the type of instrumentation (anterior or posterior) should be used according to the level(s) of instrumentation performed for the procedure.

Hand and Fingers

INCISION

26040   Fasciotomy, palmar (eg, Dupuytren's contracture); percutaneous

26045   open, partial

►(For palmar fasciotomy by enzyme injection (eg, collagenase), see 20527, 26341)◄

(For fasciectomy, see 26121-26125)

EXCISION

26123   Fasciectomy, partial palmar with release of single digit including proximal interphalangeal joint, with or without Z-plasty, other local tissue rearrangement, or skin grafting (includes obtaining graft);

+26125   each additional digit (List separately in addition to code for primary procedure)

(Use 26125 in conjunction with 26123)

►(For palmar fasciotomy by enzyme injection (eg, collagenase), see 20527, 26341)◄

(For fasciotomy, see 26040, 26045)

REPAIR, REVISION, AND/OR RECONSTRUCTION

26340   Manipulation, finger joint, under anesthesia, each joint

(For application of external fixation, see 20690 or 20692)

●**26341**   Manipulation, palmar fascial cord (ie, Dupuytren's cord), post enzyme injection (eg, collagenase), single cord

▶(For enzyme injection (eg, collagenase), palmar fascial cord (eg, Dupuytren's contracture), use 20527)◀

▶(Report custom orthotic fabrication/application separately)◀

Rationale

A code for the manipulation of the palmar fascial cord performed on a subsequent day with some follow-up care included (eg, wound check) was established in conjunction with a new code, 20527, for the treatment of Dupuytren's contracture by injection of an enzyme (eg, collagenase) into the palmar fascial cord (ie, Dupuytren's cord). Cross-references were added following codes 26125 and 26341 to direct the user to the new codes, and an instructional note was added to instruct the use of an additional code for orthotic fabrication/application.

Clinical Example (26341)

A 60-year-old male with Dupuytren's contracture who underwent enzyme (eg, collagenase) injection into a palmar fascial cord (separately reported) the previous day presents for manipulation of the contracted finger. (Note that fabrication and application of an orthosis would be reported separately.)

Description of Procedure (26341)

The wrist is held in flexion while gentle but firm traction is placed across the contracted finger until the rupture of the fascial cord is felt and the digit fully extends. This process can be repeated two more times at 10-minute intervals if full extension is not initially achieved. Once the digit is fully extended, the tendon function is evaluated.

Pelvis and Hip Joint

INTRODUCTION OR REMOVAL

▲**27096**   Injection procedure for sacroiliac joint, anesthetic/steroid, with image guidance (fluoroscopy or CT) including arthrography when performed

▶(27096 is to be used only with CT or fluoroscopic imaging confirmation of intra-articular needle positioning)◀

▶(If CT or fluoroscopy imaging is not performed, use 20552)◀

(Code 27096 is a unilateral procedure. For bilateral procedure, use modifier 50)

✍ Rationale

Injection code 27096 has been revised to include image guidance (fluoroscopy or CT) and arthrogrphy when performed. The first parenthetical note following code 27096 has been updated to indicate that code 27096 is to be used only with CT or fluoroscopy imaging confirmation of intra-articular needle positioning. An instructional note has been added to indicate that code 20552 should be reported if CT or fluoroscopy imaging is not performed. In support of these changes, the second and third cross-reference notes following code 27096 have been deleted from CPT 2012 and several changes were made to the Radiological section.

🩺 Clinical Example (27096)

A 37-year-old female presents with a 2-month history of pain rated 6-9/10 in the area of the sacroiliac joint. She has been treating her pain with NSAID's and physical therapy without any significant relief. Her pain is exacerbated with sitting, standing, or walking and relieved by lying down. Her physical examination is notable for tenderness to palpation of the left sacroiliac joint and reproduction of her pain with provacative sacroiliac stress tests. Her history and physicial examination are consistant with sacroiliac joint pain and she is subsequently scheduled for a diagnostic and therapeutic sacroiliac joint injection with local anesthetic and steroid.

Description of Procedure (27096)

The area overlying the sacroiliac joint is prepped with betadine and draped. Utilizing intermittent fluoroscopic guidance, the fluoroscopy machine is rotated until the sacroiliac joint is visualized. The skin and subcutaneous tissues are anesthetized with 4 cc of 1% lidocaine. A 25-gauge needle is carefully advanced into the joint and verified with various fluoroscopic views and injection of contrast to confirm placement into the joint and tissues. A-P, lateral, and oblique spot films are taken and saved. A mixture of local anesthetic and steroid is then injected into the joint and/or periarticular tissues. The needle is removed and the patient is transported to the recovery room for further monitoring and assessment of any pain relief.

Application of Casts and Strapping

LOWER EXTREMITY

Strapping—Any Age

29520	Strapping; hip
29530	knee
29540	ankle and/or foot
	▶(Do not report 29540 in conjunction with 29581, 29582)◀
29550	toes
29580	Unna boot

►(Do not report 29580 in conjunction with 29581, 29582)◄

▲ 29581   Application of multi-layer compression system; leg (below knee), including ankle and foot

►(Do not report 29581 in conjunction with 29540, 29580, 29582, 36475, 36478, 97140)◄

● 29582   thigh and leg, including ankle and foot, when performed

►(Do not report 29582 in conjunction with 29540, 29580, 29581, 36475, 36478, 97140)◄

● 29583   upper arm and forearm

►(Do not report 29583 in conjunction with 29584, 97140)◄

● 29584   upper arm, forearm, hand, and fingers

►(Do not report 29584 in conjunction with 29583, 97140)◄

✍ Rationale

A new series of codes for reporting application of multilayer compression systems to the thigh, leg, ankle, foot, upper arm, forearm, hand, and fingers have been added to CPT 2012.

In support of the addition of codes 29582-29584, and to create consistency in this series of codes, existing multilayer compression system code 29581 has been editorially revised to eliminate reference to diagnostic terms, and include reference to anatomic regions.

Revised code 29581 is intended for reporting application of multilayer compression systems to the leg (below knee), including ankle and foot. Code 29582 is intended for reporting application of multilayer compression systems to the thigh and leg, including ankle and foot when performed. Code 29583 is intended for reporting application of multilayer compression systems to the upper arm and forearm. Finally, code 29584 is intended for reporting application of multilayer compression systems to the upper arm, forearm, hand, and fingers.

Several parenthetical notes and cross-references in the CPT code set have been created and updated in response to the revision of code 29581 and the establishment of codes 29582, 29583, and 29584. The exclusionary parenthetical notes following strapping codes 29540, 29580, and 29581 have been updated to limit reporting these services in conjunction with other services.

Three new parenthetical notes have been added following codes 29582, 29583, and 29584 to indicate which services should not be reported in conjunction with these procedures.

⚕ Clinical Example (29582)

The patient is a 43-year-old female with a long history of venous insufficiency due to severe venous incompetence with reflux of the truncal and greater saphenous veins. The patient is obese and lives alone. Postoperative high compression is required for 1 to 2 weeks and is usually provided by wearing a class II compression stocking. Therapeutic, full leg compression is required to reduce the potential risk of venous thromboembolism, prevent refilling of the ablated veins, and to reduce postoperative bruising and tenderness. During pre-op education, the surgeon has noticed that the patient has mobility limitations due to her obesity and has recommended the use of postop multilayer compression system rather than high compression stockings.

Description of Procedure (29582)

With the foot in a 90-degree dorsiflexed position, the foot and ankle were bandaged, and the process continued up the leg, covering the skin with no gaps, to the groin. A figure of eight wrapping technique was used around the knee. An additional layer was applied with a 50% overlap and full stretch from the foot to the groin.

 Clinical Example (29583)

The patient is a 45-year-old female 9 months status post-right mastectomy, radiation, and chemotherapy. She presents to her oncologist with heaviness, tightness, and swelling of her right arm and reports that her arm has been getting progressively uncomfortable, which is beginning to interfere with her responsibilities at work. On examination, the right hand is swollen, the arm tissue is firm with 3+ pitting, and the circumference is 5 cm larger than the left arm. Range of motion is limited. Diagnosis of moderate (Grade 2) edema is made and the patient is referred to the Physical Therapy Lymphedema Program for application of multilayer compression system.

Description of Procedure (29583)

The arm was positioned with the elbow in slight flexion (135 degrees) and the fingers spread wide, with the hand position palm down. The first bandage layer was applied from the palm to the top of the arm. A figure eight technique was used at the elbow. An additional layer was applied with 50% overlap and full stretch from the palm to the top of the arm.

Clinical Example (29584)

The patient is a 52-year-old female 12 months status post bi-lateral mastectomy, radiation, and chemotherapy. She presents to her oncologist with heaviness, tightness, and swelling of her left arm, hand, and fingers and reports that the swelling has been getting progressively uncomfortable, which is beginning to interfere with her responsibilities at work. On examination, the left hand and fingers are swollen, the arm tissue is firm with 3+ pitting, and the circumference is 5 cm larger than the right arm. Range of motion is limited. Diagnosis of moderate (Grade 2) edema is made and the patient is referred to the Physical Therapy Lymphedema Program for application of multilayer compression system.

Description of Procedure (29584)

The left arm was positioned with the elbow in slight flextion (135 degrees) and the fingers spread wide, with the hand position palm down. The fingers, hand, and arm are bandaged with a tubular guaze sleeve; soft roll gauze was used for the fingers, followed by padding materials. The fingers were all individually wrapped. After securing the gauze and padding materials, the first compression bandage layer was applied to the fingers, palm, and up to the top of the arm. A figure-of-eight technique was used at the elbow. An additional layer was applied with 50% overlap and full stretch from the palm to the top of the arm.

29806   Arthroscopy, shoulder, surgical; capsulorrhaphy

29826   decompression of subacromial space with partial acromioplasty, with coracoacromial ligament (ie, arch) release, when performed (List separately in addition to code for primary procedure)

(For open procedure, use 23130 or 23415)

▶(Use 29826 in conjunction with 29806-29825, 29827, 29828)◀

Rationale

To address the concerns of the AMA/Specialty Society RVS Update Committee (RUC) related to screening of codes that are performed together more than 75% of the time, code 29826 for reporting arthroscopy, shoulder, surgical; decompression of subacromial space with partial acromioplasty, with or without coracoacromial release was converted to an add-on code. Code 29826 is billed more than 95% of the time with other arthroscopic repair of the shoulder codes. Therefore, it was decided that instead of relying on multiple procedure reduction rules, it would be better to convert 29826 to an add-on code. The codes that may be reported in conjuction with code 29826 are 29806, 29807, 29819, 29820, 29821, 29822, 29823, 29824, 29825, 29827, and 29828. In addition, code 29826 was revised to more specifically delineate the structure involved "coraco-acromial ligament (ie, arch)," and the preferred term "when performed" was substituted in place of "with or without."

Clinical Example (29826)

A 40-year-old female tennis player presents with a 4-month history of shoulder pain. The symptoms are worse at night, with overhead activity, and are affecting her daily activities. On physical exam she has pain on palpation of the greater tuberosity, restricted range of motion and weakness on muscle testing. An impingement test is positive. X rays are normal and an MRI reveals rotator cuff tendinosis. A subacromial corticosteroid injection and physical therapy afford transient relief. She undergoes arthroscopic subacromial decompression with partial acromioplasty, in addition to other reconstructive procedure(s). (Please note this is an add-on code.)

Description of Procedure (29826)

The subacromial bursa is accessed via the posterior portal which reveals some fraying of the coracoacromial ligament accompanied by a bursal-side partial thickness rotator cuff tear. A lateral arthroscopic portal is developed and bursal tissue and the bursal side cuff are debrided for visualization. The coracoacromial ligament is released with a radiofrequency device. The arthroscope is placed in the lateral portal and an acromioplasty is performed using a bone-block technique from posterior to anterior with a motorized bone-cutting shaver. Hemostasis is obtained with a radiofrequency device.

29871	Arthroscopy, knee, surgical; for infection, lavage and drainage
	(For implantation of osteochondral graft for treatment of articular surface defect, see 27412, 27415, 29866, 29867)
29873	with lateral release
29877	debridement/shaving of articular cartilage (chondroplasty)
	▶(When performed with arthroscopic meniscectomy, see 29880 or 29881)◀
▲**29880**	with meniscectomy (medial AND lateral, including any meniscal shaving) including debridement/shaving of articular cartilage (chondroplasty), same or separate compartment(s), when performed
▲**29881**	with meniscectomy (medial OR lateral, including any meniscal shaving) including debridement/shaving of articular cartilage (chondroplasty), same or separate compartment(s), when performed

✍ Rationale

As part of the AMA/Specialty Society RVS Update Committee (RUC) analysis of codes, the RUC concurred that codes 29880 and 29881 for reporting knee arthroscopy with meniscectomy are typically performed with 29877 for reporting arthroscopy of the knee requiring a chondroplasty (debridement/shaving of articular cartilage). To address the RUC recommendation that the three codes, 29880, 29881 and 29877 be bundled, codes 29880 and 29881 were revised to include chondroplasty when performed and a cross-reference was added to direct users to codes 29880 and 29881 when arthroscopic chondroplasty is performed in conjunction with arthroscopic meniscectomy.

🩺 Clinical Example (29880)

A 60-year-old female presents with a 2-month history of pain and swelling of her right knee. She cannot recall any specific trauma. On physical examination she walks with a limp. There is an effusion with medial and lateral joint line tenderness. Flexion of the knee is restricted and produces pain. X rays show medial joint space narrowing and an MRI reveals medial and lateral meniscal tears. Despite rest and anti-inflammatory medication the pain and disability persist, affecting daily living activities. A corticosteroid injection and physical therapy afford only transient relief. She undergoes arthroscopic medial and lateral meniscectomies with chondral debridement of the patella, trochlea, and medial and lateral femoral condyles.

Description of Procedure (29880)

Under anesthesia, anteromedial and anterolateral portals are introduced and a diagnostic arthroscopy reveals knee synovitis. A limited synovectomy is performed for visualization. There are chondral changes on patella, trochlea, and the medial femoral condyle with a complex tear of the medial meniscus. The cruciate ligaments are normal and the lateral joint line shows degenerative changes with a horizontal tear of the lateral meniscus. The meniscal tears are probed and then removed with basket forceps and a motorized shaver back to a rim of stable tissue. The chondral lesions are then debrided to stable cartilage. The instrumentation is removed, tourniquet let down, and the wounds are closed.

Clinical Example (29881)

A 60-year-old male presents with pain and swelling of the left knee after stepping in a hole while playing golf. On physical examination, he walks with a limp. There is an effusion in the knee with medial joint line tenderness. Flexion of the knee is restricted and produces pain. Weight bearing X rays show medial joint space narrowing and subchondral sclerosis. An MRI reveals a medial meniscal tear. Despite rest, anti-inflammatory medication, and physical therapy, the pain and disability persist, affecting daily living activities. He undergoes arthroscopic medial meniscectomy with chondral debridement of the patella, trochlea, and medial femoral condyle.

Description of Procedure (29881)

Under anesthesia, anteromedial and anterolateral portals are introduced and a diagnostic arthroscopy reveals knee synovitis. A limited synovectomy is performed for visualization. There are chondral changes on the patella, trochlea, and medial femoral condyle with a flap tear of the medial meniscus. The cruciate ligaments and lateral joint line are normal. The meniscal tear is probed and then removed with basket forceps and a motorized shaver back to a rim of stable tissue. The chondral lesions are debrided back to stable cartilage. The instrumentation is removed, tourniquet let down, and the wounds are closed.

Respiratory System

Lungs and Pleura

▶Pleural cavity or lung biopsy procedures may be accomplished using a percutaneous, thoracoscopic (Video-Assisted Thoracoscopic Surgery [VATS]), or thoracotomy approach. They involve the removal of differing amounts of tissue for diagnosis. A biopsy may be performed using different techniques such as incision or wedge. Lung resection procedures include diagnostic and therapeutic procedures, including the removal of blebs, bullae, cysts, and benign or malignant tumors or lesions. These procedures may involve the removal of small portions of the lung or even an entire lung. Additionally, lung resection procedures may require the removal of adjacent structures. Both diagnostic lung biopsies and therapeutic lung resections can be performed utilizing a wedge technique. However, a diagnostic biopsy of a lung nodule using a wedge technique requires only that a tissue sample be obtained without particular attention to resection margins. A therapeutic wedge resection requires attention to margins and complete resection even when the wedge resection is ultimately followed by a more extensive resection. In the case of a wedge resection where intraoperative pathology consultation determines that a more extensive resection is required in the same anatomic location, it becomes classified as a diagnostic wedge resection (32507, 32668). When no more extensive resection is required, the same procedure is a therapeutic wedge resection (32505, 32666).

Pleural or lung biopsies or diagnostic wedge resections should be reported using codes 32096, 32097, 32098, 32400, 32405, 32507, 32607, 32608, 32609 or 32668. The open or thoracoscopic (VATS) therapeutic resection of lung mass or nodules via a wedge resection is reported using codes 32505, 32506, 32666, and 32667. More extensive anatomic lung resection procedures, which can be performed with either thoracotomy or thoracoscopic (VATS) approaches, include: segmentectomy, lobectomy, bilobectomy, and pneumonectomy.

When diagnostic biopsy(ies) of the lung are performed, regardless of the approach (ie, open or thoracoscopic [VATS]), or technique (eg, incisional resection, cautery resection, or stapled wedge), and the specimen is sent for intraoperative pathology consultation, and during that same operative session the surgeon uses these results to determine the extent of the necessary surgical resection that includes the anatomical location biopsied, only the most extensive procedure performed (eg, segmentectomy, lobectomy, thoracoscopic [VATS] lobectomy) should be reported.

The therapeutic wedge resection codes (32505, 32506, 32666, or 32667) should not be reported in addition to the more extensive lung procedure (eg, lobectomy) unless the therapeutic wedge resection was performed on a different lobe or on the contralateral lung, whether or not an intraoperative pathology consultation is used to determine the extent of lung resection. When a diagnostic wedge resection is followed by a more extensive procedure in the same anatomical location, report add-on codes 32507 or 32668 with the more extensive procedure(s). When a therapeutic wedge resection (32505, 32506, 32666, or 32667) is performed in a different lobe than the more extensive lung resection (eg, lobectomy), report the therapeutic wedge resection with modifier 59.◀

✎ Rationale

A large number of changes have been made to the Lungs and Pleura section of the CPT code set. These changes have been made to reflect current medical practice by differentiating procedures that were originally identified by single codes. This includes the development of new codes, deletion of codes that are obsolete, and revisions to existing codes to allow more specific identification of the types of procedures that are now performed. In addition, a number of language changes have been made to some of the guidelines and parenthetical notes. In some places, completely new guidelines and parenthetical notes have been developed to further exemplify the current surgical technologies that are available for lung procedures.

The general section headings have been retained for the Lungs and Pleura section because the categories of lung procedures remain the same. However, a new section has been added to identify Video-Assisted Thoracoscopic Surgery (VATS). This is a more descriptive term identifying current technology for thoracoscopic surgery of the lungs. The new heading, Thoracoscopy (VATS), follows code 32562.

New guidelines have been developed for the Lungs and Pleura section. The new guidelines provide definitions and instructions regarding the different types of procedures that may be used within this section. This includes a description of the types of approaches that may be used for lung procedures (percutaneous, VATS, or thoracotomy approaches), the amount and type of tissue(s) that may be removed, whether the procedure is considered to be therapeutic or diagnostic, and the ways in which these removals may be performed. In addition, wedge resections are now more distinctly identified, as these procedures may involve either diagnostic or therapeutic removals. The guidelines also provide instructions regarding when it is appropriate to report more extensive procedures noting that "wedge resections that are followed by more extensive resections . . . of the same anatomic location . . . become classified as diagnostic wedge resection." Other lesser resections are considered to be therapeutic and are identified by other, more appropriate codes (such as codes 32505, 32666).

To ensure proper use of these codes, the guidelines list the specific codes that should be used for pleural or lung biopsies or diagnostic wedge resections (32096, 32097, 32098, 32400, 32405, 32507, 32607, 32608, 32609, or 32668) and open or thoracoscopic therapeutic resections performed via wedge resection (32505, 32506, 32666, and 32667). Direction is also provided regarding procedures that are considered as more extensive (segmentectomy, lobectomy, bilobectomy, and pneumonectomy). These procedures have separate codes that are used to identify that specific type of resection procedure.

The guidelines also provide specific instructions when the services of intraoperative pathology are used. In these circumstances, if a more extensive procedure is required due to the results, then only the most extensive procedure is reported.

Further instructions are also noted regarding the use of therapeutic wedge resection procedures (codes 32505, 32506, 32666, or 32667). The guidelines specifically prohibit use of these codes in addition to more extensive lung procedure codes (such as lobectomies) unless the procedures were performed on different lobes or contralateral lung, whether the procedure was provided with the intraoperative pathologic consultation. When a diagnostic wedge resection is followed by a more extensive procedure in the same anatomical location, the guidelines specify that an appropriate add-on code should be reported in addition to the extensive procedure.

INCISION

(32000 has been deleted. To report, use 32421)

(32002 has been deleted. To report, use 32422)

(32005 has been deleted. To report, use 32560)

(32019 has been deleted. To report, use 32550)

(32020 has been deleted. To report, use 32551)

▶(To report wound exploration due to penetrating trauma without thoracotomy, use 20101)◀

32035 Thoracostomy; with rib resection for empyema

32036 with open flap drainage for empyema

▶(To report wound exploration due to penetrating trauma without thoracotomy, use 20101)◀

▶(32095 has been deleted. To report, see 32096, 32097, 32098 for thoracotomy with biopsy of the lung or pleura)◀

●**32096** Thoracotomy, with diagnostic biopsy(ies) of lung infiltrate(s) (eg, wedge, incisional), unilateral

▶(Do not report 32096 more than once per lung)◀

▶(Do not report 32096 in conjunction with 32440, 32442, 32445, 32488)◀

●**32097** Thoracotomy, with diagnostic biopsy(ies) of lung nodule(s) or mass(es) (eg, wedge, incisional), unilateral

►(Do not report 32097 more than once per lung)◄

►(Do not report 32097 in conjunction with 32440, 32442, 32445, 32488)◄

●**32098**   Thoracotomy, with biopsy(ies) of pleura

►(To report wound exploration due to penetrating trauma without thoractomy, use 20101)◄

Rationale

A parenthetical cross-reference has been placed in several locations to direct users to the appropriate code to report exploration of the chest without a thoracotomy.

Three separate codes have been added to the Incision section to identify the different types of incisional (thoracotomy) biopsy procedures that may be provided for the lungs. These include: (1) diagnostic biopsy(ies) of lung infiltrates; (2) diagnostic biopsy(ies) of the of lung nodules or masses; and (3) biopsy(ies) of the pleura. To accommodate the new codes, code 32095 has been deleted, as this code generically identified biopsy procedures provided for the lungs or pleura via thoracotomy. Exclusionary parenthetical notes have also been listed following codes 32096 and 32097 to restrict use of these codes: (1) more than once per lung; and (2) from use with other, more extensive procedures. This is in conjunction with the guidelines previously noted that direct users to report the most extensive procedure alone when a more extensive lung resection procedure is provided.

Clinical Example (32096)

A 56-year-old female intubated patient has worsening hypoxia. Bilateral diffuse pulmonary infiltrates progressively worsen. Bronchoscopy and bronchoalveolar lavage are nondiagnostic. Microbiologic cultures show usual flora. Patient continues to deteriorate from a respiratory standpoint. Open lung biopsy for diagnosis is necessary.

Description of Procedure (32096)

An anterolateral thoracotomy incision is made, and utilizing electrocautery the chest is carefully entered. It may be necessary to remove a segment of rib to prevent trauma when spreading of the ribs for exposure. Adhesions between the lung and chest wall are freed. Pleural fluid if present and if appropriate is sent for cytology and microbiology. The chest and lung are explored, which includes both visual inspection and palpation of the parietal pleura, visceral pleura, and lung. Abnormalities of the visceral pleura and lung are noted. It is confirmed that a diffuse infiltrative nonlocalized process is involving the lung. Both abnormal and normal regions of lung are identified and their relationship to the pulmonary vasculature and bronchial tree assessed to determine that biopsy is feasible. If possible, single lung ventilation of the contralateral lung is instituted to facilitate exposure. The lung is mobilized as needed for assistance in exposing the areas to be biopsied. Using multiple firings of tissue staplers, a wedge resection of the lung is performed removing a portion of lung that contains both abnormal and normal lung tissue. Typically, a second wedge resection from a separate portion of the ipsilateral lung is performed in the same manner. Sterile portions of the resected lung tissue are prepared and sent for appropriate microbiologic testing. The remaining portions of resected lung are typically sent for frozen section pathologic evaluation to ensure that adequate biopsy material has been obtained. If not, additional biopsies are taken. As needed, hemostasis is secured with electrocautery and if necessary the staple lines reinforced with suture. The anesthetist is asked to inflate the operated lung and it is assessed for both hemostasis and air leakage. The chest cavity is irrigated. A chest tube(s) is inserted through a separate interspace incision(s) to provide evacuation of air and fluid from the chest. A surgical pause is conducted while an instrument, needle, and sponge count is completed and confirmed by the surgeon. The ribs are reapproximated with care to avoid injury to the intercostal neurovascular bundles and the chest wall musculature closed in layers with running suture. The subcutaneous tissue and skin are approximated.

Clinical Example (32097)

A 72-year-old male with a history of smoking presents with a newly discovered lung nodule. The nodule location is not amenable to either transthoracic needle aspiration or bronchoscopic biopsy. Lung cancer is suspected. At thoracotomy, multiple other small nodules are found throughout both lungs, worrisome for metastatic disease.

Description of Procedure (32097)

A thoracotomy incision is made, and utilizing electrocautery the chest is carefully entered over the top of the sixth rib. It may be necessary to remove a segment of rib to prevent trauma when spreading the ribs for exposure. Adhesions between the lung and chest wall are freed. Pleural fluid, if present and if appropriate, is sent for cytology and, if appropriate, microbiologic testing. The chest cavity and lung are explored which includes both visual inspection and palpation of the parietal and visceral pleura, diaphragm, mediastinum, and each lung lobe. If possible, single lung ventilation of the contralateral lung is instituted to facilitate exposure. Abnormalities are noted including the presence of multiple small nodules present throughout all of the lung lobes. The small nodules are worrisome for metastatic cancer. The lung is mobilized as needed for assistance in exposing the areas to be biopsied. Using electrocautery a nodule(s) is removed. As necessary, hemostasis is secured with electrocautery and if needed the lung parenchymal defect closed with suture. Sterile portions of the resected nodule(s) are prepared and saved for appropriate microbiologic testing. The remaining portions of the resected lung nodule(s) are sent for frozen section evaluation to obtain a histopathologic diagnosis. Metastatic lung cancer is confirmed. Based upon the number of metastatic nodules observed, the primary tumor is deemed unresectable. The anesthetist is asked to inflate the operated lung and it is assessed for both hemostasis and air leakage. The chest cavity is irrigated. A chest tube(s) is inserted through a separate interspace incision(s) to provide evacuation of air and fluid from the chest. A surgical pause is conducted while an instrument, needle, and sponge count is completed and confirmed by the surgeon. The ribs are reapproximated with care to avoid injury to the intercostal neurovascular bundles and the chest wall musculature closed in layers with running suture. The subcutaneous tissue and skin are approximated.

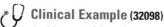

Clinical Example (32098)

A 60-year-old male presents with chest pain and diffuse pleural thickening.

Description of Procedure (32098)

A thoracotomy incision is made, and utilizing electrocautery, the chest is carefully entered. It may be necessary to remove a segment of rib for exposure. Adhesions between the lung and chest wall are freed. Pleural fluid if present and if appropriate is sent for cytology and if appropriate microbiologic testing. The chest cavity and lung are explored which includes both visual inspection and palpation of the parietal and visceral pleura, diaphragm, mediastinum, and each lung lobe. If possible, single lung ventilation of the contralateral lung is instituted to facilitate exposure. Pleural abnormalities are noted. The lung is retracted as needed for assistance in exposing the areas to be biopsied. The worrisome portions of the pleura are assessed for feasibility of biopsy. Using biopsy forceps or scalpel, pleural biopsies are performed, removing at least 1 cm portions of pleura. As necessary, hemostasis is secured with electrocautery. Sterile portions of the resected pleura are prepared and saved for appropriate microbiologic testing. The remaining portions of resected pleura are sent for frozen section evaluation to ensure adequate tissue has been obtained, and if possible to obtain histopathologic diagnosis. The anesthetist is asked to inflate the operated lung and it is assessed for both hemostasis and air leakage. The chest cavity is irrigated. A chest tube(s) is inserted through a separate interspace incision(s) to provide evacuation of air and fluid from the chest. A surgical pause is conducted while an instrument, needle, and sponge count is completed and confirmed by the surgeon. The ribs are reapproximated with care to avoid injury to the intercostal neurovascular bundles and the chest wall musculature closed in layers with running suture. The subcutaneous tissue and skin are approximated.

▲ 32100   Thoracotomy; with exploration

▲ 32110   with control of traumatic hemorrhage and/or repair of lung tear

▲ 32120   for postoperative complications

▲ 32124   with open intrapleural pneumonolysis

▲ 32140   with cyst(s) removal, includes pleural procedure when performed

▲ 32141   with resection-plication of bullae, includes any pleural procedure when performed

(For lung volume reduction, use 32491)

▲ 32150   with removal of intrapleural foreign body or fibrin deposit

▲ 32151   with removal of intrapulmonary foreign body

▲ 32160   with cardiac massage

(For segmental or other resections of lung, see 32480-32504)

✍️ Rationale

To accommodate the use of more granular coding, the parent portion of the 32100 series of codes has been revised, removing references to "biopsy" and "major" as other codes have been developed to separately identify biopsy and excision procedures according to the type of excision provided. In addition, changes have been made to codes 32140 and 32141 to reflect current CPT coding convention for services that are inherently included with these procedures when they are performed.

🩺 Clinical Example (32100)

A 65-year-old female with biopsy proven hilar lung cancer and limited lung function who would not tolerate pneumonectomy is explored through a thoracotomy. There is no evidence of pleural or mediastinal nodal metastases. The tumor is found to involve both the superior and inferior pulmonary veins and can only be resected completely if pneumonectomy is performed, therefore the patient is unfortunately deemed unresectable and the thoracotomy is closed.

Description of Procedure (32100)

A thoracotomy incision is made, and utilizing electrocautery, the chest is carefully entered over the top of the sixth rib. It may be necessary to remove a segment of rib to prevent trauma when spreading the ribs for exposure. Adhesions between the lung and chest wall are freed. Pleural fluid if present and if appropriate is sent for cytology and if appropriate microbiologic testing. The chest cavity and lung are explored which includes both visual inspection and palpation of the parietal and visceral pleura, diaphragm, mediastinum, and each lung lobe. If possible, single lung ventilation of the contralateral lung is instituted to facilitate exposure. Abnormalities are noted but no biopsies are performed. Prior to dissecting out the lobar vessels, the main pulmonary artery is dissected out and encircled with vascular tapes in anticipation of performing a difficult lobar dissection. In addition, the appropriate pulmonary vein is dissected out, encircled with vascular tapes. The major fissure is dissected out and the fissure is divided with several applications of the stapling device. The interlobar pulmonary artery branches are dissected out and encircled with vascular tapes. Unfortunately, the tumor is found to involve the main interlobar pulmonary artery and the patient is deemed unresectable, given the patient's limited lung function. The chest cavity is irrigated. A chest tube(s) is inserted through a separate interspace incision(s) to provide evacuation of air and fluid from the chest. A surgical pause is conducted while an instrument, needle, and sponge count is completed and confirmed by the surgeon. The ribs are reapproximated with care to avoid injury to the intercostal neurovascular bundles and the chest wall musculature closed in layers with running suture. The subcutaneous tissue and skin are approximated.

▶EXCISION/RESECTION◀

32310	Pleurectomy, parietal (separate procedure)
32320	Decortication and parietal pleurectomy
32400	Biopsy, pleura; percutaneous needle

⊘=Modifier 51 Exempt   ⊙=Moderate Sedation   ✚=Add-on Code   𝒩=FDA approval pending

(If imaging guidance is performed, see 76942, 77002, 77012, 77021)

(For fine needle aspiration, use 10021 or 10022)

▶(32402 has been deleted. To report open biopsy of pleura, use 32098)◀

⊙▲**32405**   Biopsy, lung or mediastinum, percutaneous needle

▶(For open biopsy of lung, see 32096, 32097. For open biopsy of mediastinum, see 39000 or 39010. For thoracoscopic [VATS] biopsy of lung, pleura, pericardium or mediastinal space structure, see 32604, 32606, 32607, 32608, 32609)◀

🖎 Rationale

Several changes have been made to the Excision section beginning with the revision to the heading, which has been revised to state Excision/Resection to more accurately describe the procedures included in the subsection. Code 32402 has been deleted to accommodate the development of code 32098. As a result, a parenthetical note has been included directing users to report this new code for open biopsy of the pleura. Code 32405 has been revised—added conscious sedation symbol—to note that moderate sedation is inherently included as part of this procedure. A parenthetical cross-reference has been developed to direct users to the appropriate codes for various biopsy procedures. This includes the use of codes 32096-32097 for open biopsy of the lung, code 39000 or 39010 for open biopsy of the mediastinum, and the use of code 32604, 32606, 32607, 32608, or 32609 to report VATS biopsy of the lung, pleura, pericardium, or mediastinal space.

REMOVAL

32420   Pneumocentesis, puncture of lung for aspiration

32421   Thoracentesis, puncture of pleural cavity for aspiration, initial or subsequent

(If imaging guidance is performed, see 76942, 77002, 77012)

32422   Thoracentesis with insertion of tube, includes water seal (eg, for pneumothorax), when performed (separate procedure)

▲**32440**   Removal of lung, pneumonectomy;

▲**32442**   with resection of segment of trachea followed by broncho-tracheal anastomosis (sleeve pneumonectomy)

▲**32445**   extrapleural

(For extrapleural pneumonectomy, with empyemectomy, use 32445 and 32540)

▶(If lung resection is performed with chest wall tumor resection, report the appropriate chest wall tumor resection 19260-19272, in addition to lung resection 32440-32445)◀

▲**32480**   Removal of lung, other than pneumonectomy; single lobe (lobectomy)

▲**32482**   2 lobes (bilobectomy)

▲**32484**   single segment (segmentectomy)

(For removal of lung with bronchoplasty, use 32501)

▲**32486**   with circumferential resection of segment of bronchus followed by broncho-bronchial
anastomosis (sleeve lobectomy)

▲**32488**   with all remaining lung following previous removal of a portion of lung
(completion pneumonectomy)

►(For lobectomy or segmentectomy, with concomitant decortication, use 32320 and the appropriate
removal of lung code)◄

▲**32491**   with resection-plication of emphysematous lung(s) (bullous or non-bullous) for lung
volume reduction, sternal split or transthoracic approach, includes any pleural procedure,
when performed

►(32500 has been deleted. To report open wedge resection of lung see 32505, 32506, 32507)◄

►(If lung resection is performed with chest wall tumor resection, report the appropriate chest wall
tumor resection 19260-19272, in addition to lung resection 32480, 32482, 32484, 32486, 32488,
32505, 32506, 32507)◄

●**32505** Thoracotomy; with therapeutic wedge resection (eg, mass, nodule), initial

►(Do not report 32505 in conjunction with 32440, 32442, 32445, 32488)◄

✚●**32506**   with therapeutic wedge resection (eg, mass or nodule), each additional resection, ipsilateral (List
separately in addition to code for primary procedure)

►(Report 32506 only in conjunction with 32505)◄

►(If lung resection is performed with chest wall tumor resection, report the appropriate chest wall
tumor resection 19260-19272, in addition to lung resection 32480, 32482, 32484, 32486, 32488,
32505, 32506, 32507)◄

✚●**32507**   with diagnostic wedge resection followed by anatomic lung resection (List separately in addition
to code for primary procedure)

►(Report 32507 in conjunction with 32440, 32442, 32445, 32480, 32482, 32484, 32486, 32488, 32503,
32504)◄

✐ Rationale

The Removal section also includes many changes. Code ranges 32440-32445 and
32480-32491 have been revised by removing the term "total" to accommodate the
new codes that have been added, which specifically identify more extensive lung
excision procedures. This includes the addition of codes that identify diagnostic
and therapeutic lung resection procedures by various approaches (eg, open or thoracoscopically [Video-Assisted Thoracoscopic Surgery]). Also listed after both code
ranges are parenthetical notes directing users to the appropriate codes to use to
identify lung resection performed with chest wall tumor resection.

A number of editorial revisions have also been included with codes 32488 and
32491, using language that is more appropriate for CPT coding convention.

In addition, to accommodate the use of new codes that specifically identify wedge
resections, code 32500 has been deleted. A parenthetical note has been added to

note that code 32500 has been deleted and to direct users to appropriate codes to identify the specific type of open wedge resection procedure of the lung that was provided.

Three new codes have been included to identify wedge resection completed via thoracotomy. Code 32505 is used to report the initial wedge resection performed via thoracotomy. Code 32506 is used to identify additional wedge resections. Code 32507 identifies diagnostic wedge resection for thoracotomy that is followed by an anatomic lung resection. The services identified by codes 32506 and 32507 are both *add-on* procedures. As a result, they are not independently reported. Instead, these codes are reported in addition to certain procedures. Code 32506 is reported only in addition to code 32505, while code 32507 is reported in addition to a number of other services, which include removal of lung via pneumonectomy (identified by codes 32440, 32442, and 32445), lung removal by single lobectomy (32480), bilobectomy (32482), segementectomy (32484), sleeve lobectomy (32846), or completion pneumonectomy (32488). Both codes 32506 and 32507 include parenthetical notes that direct users regarding the appropriate codes to report these add-on procedures. In addition, an instructional parenthetical has been included following code 32506 to direct users to use codes 19260-19272 to report chest wall tumor resections that are performed in addition to lung resections (32480, 32482, 32484, 32486, 32488, 32505-32507).

An exclusionary parenthetical note has also been placed following code 32505. This note restricts the use of this thoracotomy-wedge-resection-procedure code from being reported with other pneumonectomy removal of lung procedures (32440, 32442, 32445), as well a specific nonpneumonectomy lung removal procedure (32488).

 Clinical Example (32505)

A 62-year-old male nonsmoker with a history of resected colon cancer and adjuvant chemotherapy is found to have a growing right pulmonary nodule. There is no evidence of locally recurrent colon cancer or intra-abdominal metastatic disease. There is no mediastinal lymphadenopathy or evidence of other pulmonary nodules. Pulmonary function is normal. Metastatic colon cancer to the right lung is suspected.

Description of Procedure (32505)

A thoracotomy incision is made, and utilizing electrocautery, the chest is carefully entered over the top of the sixth rib. It may be necessary to remove a segment of rib to prevent trauma when spreading the ribs for exposure. Adhesions between the lung and chest wall are freed. Pleural fluid, if present and if appropriate, is sent for cytology and, if appropriate, microbiologic testing.

The chest cavity and lung are explored which includes both visual inspection and palpation of the parietal and visceral pleura, diaphragm, mediastinum, and each lung lobe. If possible, single lung ventilation of the contralateral lung is instituted to facilitate exposure. Abnormalities are noted. The worrisome lung nodule is located and its relationship to the pulmonary vasculature and bronchial tree assessed to determine if resection is feasible. The lung is mobilized as necessary for assistance in exposing the nodule. Using multiple firings of tissue staplers a wedge resection of the nodule is performed, removing the nodule with at least a 1- to 2 cm free margin of normal lung parenchyma. As necessary hemostasis is secured with electrocautery and if needed the staple lines reinforced with suture. Sterile portions of the resected nodule are prepared and sent for, if appropriate, microbiologic testing. The remaining portions of resected lung are sent for frozen section evaluation to obtain a histopathologic diagnosis and confirm a clean margin. If cancer is confirmed, then thoracic lymphadenectomy may be indicated. The anesthetist is asked to inflate the operated lung and it is assessed for both hemostasis and air leakage. The chest cavity is irrigated. A chest tube(s) is inserted through a separate interspace incision(s) to provide evacuation of air and fluid from the chest. A surgical pause is conducted while an instrument, needle, and sponge count is completed and confirmed by the surgeon. The ribs are reapproximated with care to avoid injury to the intercostal neurovascular bundles and the chest wall musculature closed in layers with running suture. The subcutaneous tissue and skin are approximated.

Clinical Example (32506)

A 62-year-old male nonsmoker with a history of resected colon cancer and adjuvant chemotherapy is found to have a growing right upper lobe pulmonary nodule. There is no evidence of locally recurrent colon cancer or intra-abdominal metastatic disease. There is no mediastinal lymphadenopathy but an additional pulmonary nodule within the lower lobe is found. Pulmonary function is normal. Metastatic colon cancer to the right lung is suspected. The patient has a right thoracotomy with wedge resection of the right upper lobe nodule (separately reported). Frozen section pathology reveals grade 2 adenocarcinoma consistent with a colon primary. A separate wedge resection of the right lower lobe nodule is performed also showing metastatic colon cancer.

(Please note this is an add-on code.)

Description of Procedure (32506)

If there is more than one lung nodule present, then after the first wedge resection is performed and histopathologic diagnosis confirmed, wedge resection of the additional nodule(s) may be indicated. This entails performing the additional necessary wedge resection(s) in the same fashion as the initial wedge resection utilizing multiple firings of the tissue staplers ensuring clean margins. Some nodules may require electrocautery resection with suture closure of the lung parenchymal defect. Each of the resected nodules should be sent for histopathologic examination. The anesthetist is asked to inflate the operated lung and all resection sites are assessed for both hemostasis and air leakage. Additional suture reinforcement of staple (suture) lines is done as needed.

Clinical Example (32507)

A 62-year-old male smoker is found to have a growing left spiculated pulmonary nodule now measuring 3 cm in size. There is no evidence of metastatic disease. Pulmonary function is normal. Resection is indicated.

⊘=Modifier 51 Exempt   ⊙=Moderate Sedation   ✚=Add-on Code   ⊿=FDA approval pending

The patient undergoes a diagnostic wedge resection to be followed by an appropriate more extensive resection (reported separately) based upon intraoperative pathology findings. This service represents only the additional services of the diagnostic wedge resection in a patient who goes on to have a more extensive lung resection procedure based upon the intraoperative pathology findings.

(Please note this is an add-on code.)

Description of Procedure (32507)

A thoracotomy incision is made, and utilizing electrocautery the chest is carefully entered over the top of the sixth rib. It may be necessary to remove a segment of rib to prevent trauma when spreading the ribs for exposure. Adhesions between the lung and chest wall are freed. Pleural fluid if present and if appropriate is sent for cytology and if appropriate microbiologic testing. The chest cavity and lung are explored, which includes both visual inspection and palpation of the parietal and visceral pleura, diaphragm, mediastinum, and each lung lobe. Abnormalities are noted. The worrisome lung nodule is located and its relationship to the pulmonary vasculature and bronchial tree assessed to determine that biopsy is feasible. If possible, single lung ventilation of the contralateral lung is instituted to facilitate exposure. The lung is mobilized as needed for assistance in exposing the nodule. Using multiple firings of tissue staplers a wedge resection of the nodule is performed removing the nodule with at least a 1 to 2 cm margin of normal lung parenchyma. As necessary, hemostasis is secured with electrocautery and if needed the staple lines reinforced with suture. Sterile portions of the resected nodule are saved for appropriate microbiologic testing if indicated. The remaining portions of resected lung are sent for frozen section evaluation to obtain a histopathologic diagnosis. If lung cancer is confirmed, then anatomic resection (eg, segmentectomy, lobectomy, pneumonectomy) (separately reported) may be indicated.

►THORACOSCOPY (VIDEO-ASSISTED THORACIC SURGERY [VATS])◄

►Surgical thoracoscopy (video-assisted thoracic surgery [VATS]) always includes diagnostic thoracoscopy.◄

▲**32601**   Thoracoscopy, diagnostic (separate procedure); lungs, pericardial sac, mediastinal or pleural space, without biopsy

►(32602 has been deleted. To report lung or pleural space biopsy(ies), see 32607, 32608, 32609)◄

►(32603 has been deleted. To report diagnostic thoracoscopy, pericardial sac, without biopsy use 32601)◄

32604   pericardial sac, with biopsy

►(32605 has been deleted. To report diagnostic thoracoscopy within the mediastinal space, use 32601)◄

►(For open pericardial biopsy, use 39010)◄

●**32607**   Thoracoscopy; with diagnostic biopsy(ies) of lung infiltrate(s) (eg, wedge, incisional), unilateral

►(Do not report 32607 more than once per lung)◄

▶(Do not report 32607 in conjunction with 32440, 32442, 32445, 32488, 32671)◀

●**32608**   with diagnostic biopsy(ies) of lung nodule(s) or mass(es) (eg, wedge, incisional), unilateral

▶(Do not report 32608 more than once per lung)◀

▶(Do not report 32608 in conjunction with 32440, 32442, 32445, 32488, 32671)◀

●**32609**   with biopsy(ies) of pleura

32650   Thoracoscopy, surgical; with pleurodesis (eg, mechanical or chemical)

▲**32655**   with resection-plication of bullae, includes any pleural procedure when performed

▶(For thoracoscopic [VATS] lung volume reduction surgery, use 32672)◀

32656   with parietal pleurectomy

▶(32657 has been deleted. To report thoracoscopic [VATS] wedge resection of lung, see 32666, 32667, 32668)◀

32658   with removal of clot or foreign body from pericardial sac

32659   with creation of pericardial window or partial resection of pericardial sac for drainage

▶(32660 has been deleted)◀

32661   with excision of pericardial cyst, tumor, or mass

32662   with excision of mediastinal cyst, tumor, or mass

▲**32663**   with lobectomy (single lobe)

▶(For thoracoscopic [VATS] segmentectomy, use 32669)◀

32664   with thoracic sympathectomy

32665   with esophagomyotomy (Heller type)

▶(For exploratory thoracoscopy, and exploratory thoracoscopy with biopsy, see 32601-32609)◀

●**32666**   with therapeutic wedge resection (eg, mass, nodule), initial unilateral

▶(To report bilateral procedure, report 32666 with modifier 50)◀

▶(Do not report 32666, in conjunction with 32440, 32442, 32445, 32488, 32671)◀

+●**32667**   with therapeutic wedge resection (eg, mass or nodule), each additional resection, ipsilateral (List separately in addition to code for primary procedure)

▶(Report 32667 only in conjunction with 32666)◀

▶(Do not report 32667 in conjunction with 32440, 32442, 32445, 32488, 32671)◀

+●**32668**   with diagnostic wedge resection followed by anatomic lung resection (List separately in addition to code for primary procedure)

▶(Report 32668 in conjunction with 32440, 32442, 32445, 32480, 32482, 32484, 32486, 32488, 32503, 32504, 32663, 32669, 32670, 32671)◀

●**32669**   with removal of a single lung segment (segmentectomy)

            ⊘=Modifier 51 Exempt   ⊙=Moderate Sedation   **+**=Add-on Code   ✔=FDA approval pending

●32670	with removal of two lobes (bilobectomy)
●32671	with removal of lung (pneumonectomy)
●32672	with resection-plication for emphysematous lung (bullous or non-bullous) for lung volume reduction (LVRS), unilateral includes any pleural procedure, when performed
●32673	with resection of thymus, unilateral or bilateral

▶(For open thymectomy see 60520, 60521, 60522)◀

▶(For open excision mediastinal cyst see 39200, for open excision mediastinal tumor use 39220)◀

▶(For exploratory thoracoscopy, and exploratory thoracoscopy with biopsy, see 32601-32609)◀

| +●32674 | with mediastinal and regional lymphadenectomy (List separately in addition to code for primary procedure) |

▶(On the right, mediastinal lymph nodes include the paratracheal, subcarinal, paraesophageal, and inferior pulmonary ligament)◀

▶(On the left, mediastinal lymph nodes include the aortopulmonary window, subcarinal, paraesophageal, and inferior pulmonary ligament)◀

▶(Report 32674 in conjunction with 32440, 32442, 32445, 32480, 32482, 32484, 32486, 32488, 32503, 32504, 32505, 32663, 32666, 32667, 32669, 32670, 32671)◀

▶(To report mediastinal and regional lymphadenectomy via thoracotomy, use 38746)◀

✍ Rationale

The heading for this section has been revised to note the more specific terminology that is now used to identify thoracoscopic lung procedures (Video-Assisted Thoracoscopic Surgery [VATS]). The guideline listed following the title has also been revised to reflect the more conventional term.

Code 32601 has been revised to include "pericardial sac" and "mediastinal" because this service is intended to include these anatomic areas as part of the diagnostic procedure.

Codes 32602, 36203, and 36205 have been deleted to accommodate the new codes to identify biopsy procedures. Parenthetical notes have been developed to direct users to the appropriate codes to use to identify performance of these biopsy procedures.

New codes 32607, 32608, and 32609 are used to identify thoracoscopic biopsy procedures. As indicated in the heading of this section, the term "thoracoscopy" has been revised to "Video-Assisted Thoracoscopic Surgery." The intent is to note updated terminology for these thoracoscopic procedures. As was noted in previous sections, the codes used to identify thoracoscopic biopsies identify different techniques. Code 32607 identifies diagnostic biopsy of lung infiltrates, code 32608 identifies diagnostic biopsy of lung nodules or masses, and code 32609 identifies thoracoscopic biopsy of the pleural. Parenthetical notes have been placed after codes 32607 and 32608 to direct users regarding usage intent: (1) restricting use of each code more than once per lung and (2) restricting use of these codes with more extensive surgical procedures.

Code 32655 has been editorially revised to reflect "resection" or plication of bullae. In addition, the descriptor has been revised to indicate that this includes any type of pleural procedure when performed. A parenthetical note has also been placed to direct users to the appropriate code to use for VATS lung volume surgery.

Codes 32657 and 32660 have been deleted. A parenthetical note has been placed following code 32657 to direct users to the appropriate codes to use to identify VATS wedge resection of the lung. Code 32660 has been deleted, as this procedure is no longer performed.

Code 32663 has been revised by deleting the language that notes "total" from the descriptor. As was true for other codes used to identify resection procedures, this change has been made to allow more granular identification of thoracoscopic lung removal procedures.

Codes 32666 through 32674 represent different levels of thoracoscopic excision of lung. Each procedure represents a certain level of removal according to the type and amount of tissue that is being excised.

Code 32666 identifies an initial therapeutic wedge resection using VATS. If performed bilaterally, modifier 50 may be appended to the code to note provision of the service on the other side. This is noted by placement of a parenthetical note that directs users regarding this intent. An additional note also restricts the use of the code, ie, from being used in conjunction with codes 32440, 32442, 32445, 32488, and 32671.

Code 32667 is used to report additional thoracoscopic therapeutic wedge resections. It is an add-on code, and is therefore, only reported in addition to code 32666. Parenthetical notes have been added following this code to: (1) restrict its use with code 32666 and (2) remind users that other, more extensive procedures should not be reported in conjunction with this code.

Code 32668 is used to report diagnostic wedge resection that is followed by anatomic lung resection. This is also an add-on code. As a result, a parenthetical note is included listing the primary procedures that 32668 is reported in conjunction with.

Codes 32669-32674 are used to report VATS removal procedures that vary according to the amount of tissue removed, the type of tissue removed, or in the difficulty of removal. Parenthetical notes included in this section provide a number of instructions for users. These include: (1) appropriate codes to use for open thymectomy; (2) appropriate codes to use for open excision of mediastinal cyst or tumors; (3) codes that should be used for exploratory thoracoscopy (including exploration that includes biopsy); (4) codes that should be reported for mediastinal and regional lymphadenectomy performed via thoracotomy; and (5) codes that may be reported in conjunction with add-on code 32674. There are also parentheticals that direct users regarding lymph nodes that should be included with identifying right- and left-sided mediastinal lymph node removals.

Clinical Example (32601)

A 72-year-old male presents with a 4-week history of progressive shortness of breath. Chest x-ray shows blunting of the costophrenic angles on the right. Thoracentesis is nondiagnostic.

Description of Procedure (32601)

The site for the initial trocar placement is identified and anesthetized with local anesthetic. An incision is made, and using a combination of sharp, cautery, and blunt dissection, the pleural cavity carefully entered. The parietal pleura is palpated, a trocar inserted under direct vision, and the thoracoscope advanced into the pleural cavity. Initial visual exploration is performed. The sites for all additional trocar incisions (1 to 2), if necessary, are identified and are anesthetized with local anesthetic. The additional trocar incisions are made in a similar fashion. Access ports as necessary are placed at each incision site for the passage of instruments. Pleural fluid, if present and if appropriate, is sent for cytology and microbiology. The chest and lung are explored, which includes both visual inspection and/or palpation of the parietal pleura, visceral pleura, diaphragm, mediastinum, and each lung lobe. No abnormalities of the visceral and parietal pleura and lung are noted and no biopsies are performed. The anesthetist is asked to inflate the operated lung and it is assessed for both hemostasis and air leakage. The lung is again deflated and the chest cavity is irrigated. A chest tube(s) is inserted through a separate interspace incision(s) to provide evacuation of air and fluid from the chest. All trocar incisions are assessed for hemostasis. A surgical pause is conducted, while an instrument, needle, and sponge count is completed and confirmed by the surgeon. Each incision is closed with multiple layers of suture for the muscle, and the skin reapproximated with a subcuticular stitch.

Clinical Example (32607)

A 56-year-old male presents with worsening dyspnea and progressive bilateral diffuse infiltrates on CT scan. Transbronchialiopsies were nondiagnostic.

Description of Procedure (32607)

The site for the initial trocar site is identified and anesthetized with local anesthetic. An incision is made, and using a combination of sharp, cautery, and blunt dissection the pleural cavity carefully entered. The parietal pleura is palpated, a trocar inserted under direct vision, and the thoracoscope advanced into the pleural cavity. Initial visual exploration is performed. The sites for all additional trocar incisions (1 to 2) are identified and are anesthetized with local anesthetic. The additional trocar incisions are made in a similar fashion. Access ports, as necessary, are placed at each incision site for the passage of instruments. Adhesions between the lung and chest wall are freed. Pleural fluid, if present and if appropriate, is sent for cytology and microbiology. The chest and lung are explored, which includes both visual inspection and/or palpation of the parietal pleura, visceral pleura, diaphragm, mediastinum, and each of the lung lobes. Abnormalities of the lung are noted. A diffuse, infiltrative, non-localized process involving the lung is seen. Both abnormal and normal regions of the lung are identified and their relationship to the pulmonary vasculature and bronchial tree assessed to determine that biopsy is feasible. Using multiple firings of the endoscopic tissue staplers, at least 2 wedge resections of the lung are performed, removing portions of both abnormal and normal lung. Each specimen prior to removal from the chest is placed in a sterile bag to avoid trocar site contamination. As necessary, hemostasis is secured with electrocautery and, if needed, the staple lines reinforced with suture. Sterile portions of the resected lung are prepared and sent for appropriate microbiologic testing. The remaining portions of resected lung are sent for frozen section pathologic evaluation to ensure that adequate biopsy material has been obtained. If not, additional biopsies are taken. The anesthetist is asked to inflate the operated lung and it is assessed for both hemostasis and air leakage. The lung is again deflated and the chest cavity is irrigated. A chest tube(s) is inserted through a separate interspace incision(s) to provide evacuation of air and fluid from the chest. All trocar incisions are assessed for hemostasis. A surgical pause is conducted while an instrument, needle, and sponge count is completed and confirmed by the surgeon. Each incision is closed with multiple layers of suture for the muscle, and the skin reapproximated with a subcuticular stitch.

 Clinical Example (32608)

A 65-year-old male smoker presents with a growing pulmonary nodule, which is suspicious for lung cancer. Multiple other small nodules close to the surface within the same lung are seen on CT.

Description of Procedure (32608)

The site for the initial trocar site is identified and anesthetized with local anesthetic. An incision is made, and using a combination of sharp, cautery, and blunt dissection, the pleural cavity carefully entered. The parietal pleura is palpated, a trocar inserted under direct vision, and the thoracoscope advanced into the pleural cavity. Initial visual exploration is performed. The sites for all additional trocar incisions (1 to 2) are identified and are anesthetized with local anesthetic. The additional trocar incisions are made in a similar fashion. Access ports as necessary are placed at each incision site for the passage of instruments. Adhesions between the lung and chest wall are freed. Pleural fluid, if present and if appropriate, is sent for cytology and microbiology. The chest and lung are explored, which includes both visual inspection and/or palpation of the parietal pleura, visceral pleura, diaphragm, mediastinum, and each of the lung lobes. Abnormalities are noted. Nodularity of the visceral pleura and lung are noted. Biopsy of one of the lung nodules is accomplished by one of several techniques: core cutting needle biopsy, electrocautery excision, ultrasonic scalpel excision, or stapled biopsy. Prior to removal from the chest cavity, the biopsied lung tissue is placed in a sterile bag in order to prevent trocar site contamination. As necessary, hemostasis is secured with electrocautery and, if needed, the biopsy site is reinforced with sutures. If appropriate, sterile portions of the biopsied nodule are prepared and sent for appropriate microbiologic testing. The remaining portions of biopsied nodule are sent for frozen section evaluation to obtain a histopathologic diagnosis. Metastatic lung cancer is confirmed. Because of the extent of metastatic disease, the primary tumor is not resected. After completion of all necessary biopsies(s), the anesthetist is asked to inflate the operated lung and all biopsy sites are assessed for both hemostasis and air leakage. The lung is again deflated and the chest cavity is irrigated. A chest tube(s) is inserted through a separate interspace incision(s) to provide evacuation of air and fluid from the chest. All trocar incisions are assessed for hemostasis. A surgical pause is conducted while an instrument, needle, and sponge count is completed and confirmed by the surgeon. Each incision is closed with multiple layers of suture for the muscle, and the skin reapproximated with a subcuticular stitch.

 Clinical Example (32609)

A 68-year-old male pipefitter presents with progressive dyspnea. A left pleural effusion is found along with generalized parietal pleural thickening. Pleural fluid cytology is nondiagnostic. Pleural biopsy is needed to establish diagnosis.

Description of Procedure (32609)

The site for the initial trocar site is identified and anesthetized with local anesthetic. An incision is made, and using a combination of sharp, cautery, and blunt dissection, the pleural cavity carefully entered. The parietal pleura is palpated, a trocar inserted under direct vision, and the thoracoscope advanced into the pleural cavity. Initial visual exploration is performed. The sites for all additional trocar incisions (1 to 2) are identified and are anesthetized with local anesthetic. The additional trocar incisions are made in a similar fashion. Access ports, as necessary, are placed at each incision site for the passage of instruments. Adhesions between the lung and chest wall are freed. Pleural fluid, if present and if appropriate, is sent for cytology and microbiology. The chest and lung are explored, which includes both visual inspection and/or palpation of the parietal pleura, visceral pleura, diaphragm, mediastinum, and each of the lung lobes. Abnormalities of the visceral and parietal pleura are noted, and the worrisome portions of the pleura are identified and assessed for feasibility of biopsy. Using biopsy forceps or other thoracoscopic instrumentation, pleural biopsies are performed, removing at least 1- to 2-cm portions of pleura. Each specimen prior to removal from the chest is placed in a sterile bag to avoid trocar site contamination. If appropriate, sterile portions of the resected pleura are prepared and sent for appropriate microbiologic testing. The remaining portions of resected pleura are sent for frozen section evaluation to ensure adequate tissue has been obtained, and if possible to obtain histopathologic diagnosis. After completion of all necessary biopsy(s) resection(s), the anesthetist is asked to inflate the operated lung, assessing it for both hemostasis and air leakage. The lung again deflated and the chest cavity is irrigated. A chest tube(s) is inserted through a separate interspace incision(s) to provide evacuation of air and fluid from the chest. All trocar incisions are assessed for hemostasis. A surgical pause is conducted while an instrumentation, needle, and sponge count is completed and confirmed by the surgeon. Each incision is closed with multiple layers of suture for the muscle, and the skin reapproximated with a subcuticular stitch.

 Clinical Example (32663)

A 63-year-old former smoker presents with a 2-cm adenocarcinoma located peripherally in the left lower lobe. The staging workup shows no evidence of metastatic disease. The patient's pulmonary function is such he would tolerate lobectomy.

Description of Procedure (32663)

The site for the initial trocar site is identified and anesthetized with local anesthetic. An incision is made, and using a combination of sharp, cautery, and blunt dissection, the pleural cavity carefully entered. The parietal pleura is palpated, a trocar inserted under direct vision, and the thoracoscope advanced into the pleural cavity. Initial visual exploration is performed. The sites for all additional trocar incisions (3 or 4) are identified and are anesthetized with local anesthetic. The additional trocar incisions are made in a similar fashion, as is the larger accessory incision. Access ports, as necessary, are placed at each incision site for the passage of instruments. Adhesions between the lung and chest wall are freed. Pleural fluid, if present and if appropriate, is sent for cytology and microbiology. The chest and lung are explored, which includes both visual inspection and palpation of the parietal pleura, visceral pleura, diaphragm, mediastinum, and lung. The lung cancer present in the lower lobe is identified. The lung is retracted superiorly to expose the diaphragmatic surface. The inferior pulmonary ligament is divided with electrocautery, and the mediastinal pleura dissected away from the inferior pulmonary vein anteriorly and posteriorly. A right angle clamp is used to carefully dissect around the inferior pulmonary vein away from the superior pulmonary vein to the upper lobe. The endoscopic vascular stapler is passed across the inferior pulmonary vein and fired to divide it. The lower lobe is retracted inferiorly and dissection in the fissure to separate the upper and lower lobes performed. At the base of the fissure, the pulmonary artery is identified and carefully dissected free. The dissection is continued until the branches to the lingual superior segment and the four basilar segments are identified. The arterial branches to the lower lobe are divided using the endoscopic vascular stapler. Underneath the artery the lower lobe bronchus is identified, isolated, and divided using the endoscopic tissue stapler, taking care not to narrow the middle lobe bronchus. Using multiple firings of the endoscopic tissue stapler, the fissures between the lower lobe and upper lobe are completely divided. The resected lower lobe is endoscopically placed in a sterile bag, which is closed and then removed from the chest cavity through the accessory incision. The specimen is sent to pathology for frozen section analysis of the margin, which can require 15 to 20 minutes. For lung cancer, a thoracoscopic mediastinal and regional lymphadenectomy may be performed (separately reported). Once confirmation is obtained indicating that no further surgery is required (eg, benign lesion or margins negative if malignant) the steps for closure are begun. The anesthetist is asked to inflate the operated lung and all staple lines are assessed for both hemostasis and air leakage. The lung is again deflated and the chest cavity is irrigated. A chest tube(s) is inserted through a separate interspace incision(s) to provide evacuation of air and fluid from the chest. All trocar incisions are assessed for hemostasis. The anesthetist is again asked to inflate the operated lung and, with the thoracoscope still in place, observe that the remaining lung completely re-expands. The thoracoscope is then removed. A surgical pause is conducted while an instrument, needle, and sponge count is completed and confirmed by the surgeon. Each incision is closed with multiple layers of suture for the muscle, and the skin reapproximated with a subcuticular stitch.

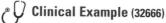

Clinical Example (32666)

A 68-year-old female 2 years status post-right leg resection for osteosarcoma presents with a new solitary pulmonary nodule in the right upper lobe, There is no evidence of local recurrence. Metastatic disease is suspected. The patient is referred for curative resection.

Description of Procedure (32666)

The site for the initial trocar site is identified and anesthetized with local anesthetic. An incision is made, and using a combination of sharp, cautery, and blunt dissection the pleural cavity carefully entered. The parietal pleura is palpated, a trocar inserted under direct vision, and the thoracoscope advanced into the pleural cavity. Initial visual exploration is performed. The sites for all additional trocar incisions (1 or 2) if necessary are identified and are anesthetized with local anesthetic. The additional trocar incisions are made in a similar fashion. Access ports as necessary are placed at each incision site for the passage of instruments. Adhesions between the lung and chest wall are freed. Pleural fluid, if present and if appropriate, is sent for cytology and microbiology. The chest and lung are explored which includes both visual inspection and/or palpation of the parietal pleura, visceral pleura, diaphragm, mediastinum, and lung. The worrisome lung nodule is identified, and its relationship to the pulmonary vasculature and bronchial tree assessed to determine that biopsy is feasible. The lung is mobilized as needed for assistance in exposing the nodule. Using multiple firings of endoscopic tissue staplers a wedge resection of the nodule is performed removing the nodule with at least a 1- to 2 cm free margin of normal lung parenchyma. The specimen prior to removal from the chest is placed in a sterile bag to avoid trocar site contamination. As necessary, hemostasis is secured with electrocautery and if needed, the staple lines reinforced with suture. If necessary, sterile portions of the resected nodule are prepared and sent for appropriate microbiologic testing. The remaining portions of resected lung are sent for frozen section evaluation to obtain a histopathologic diagnosis and ensure that the nodule has been removed with free margins. The anesthetist is asked to inflate the operated lung and all staple lines are assessed for both hemostasis and air leakage. The lung is again deflated and the chest cavity is irrigated. A chest tube(s) is inserted through a separate interspace incision(s) to provide evacuation of air and fluid from the chest. All trocar incisions are assessed for hemostasis. A surgical pause is conducted while an instrumentation, needle, and sponge count is completed and confirmed by the surgeon. Each incision is closed with multiple layers of suture for the muscle, and the skin reapproximated with a subcuticular stitch.

Clinical Example (32667)

A 68-year-old female 2 years status post-right leg resection for osteosarcoma presents with a nodule in the right upper lobe and an additional nodule in the right lower lobe. There is no evidence of local recurrence and patient is referred for curative resections.

The patient has a thoracoscopic wedge resection of the right upper lobe nodule (separately reported). A separate wedge resection of the right lower lobe nodule is performed.

(Please note this is an add-on code.)

Description of Procedure (32667)

If there is more than one lung nodule present, then after the first wedge resection is performed and histopathologic diagnosis confirmed, wedge resection of the additional nodule(s) may be indicated. This entails performing the additional necessary wedge resection(s) in the same fashion as the initial wedge resection utilizing multiple firings of the endoscopic tissue staplers. Some nodules may require electrocautery resection with suture closure of the lung parenchymal defect. All nodules should be removed with ideally 1- to 2-cm free margin. Each specimen prior to removal from the chest is placed in a sterile bag to avoid trocar site contamination. Each of the resected nodules should be sent for histopathologic examination. The anesthetist is asked to inflate the operated lung and all resection sites are assessed for both hemostasis and air leakage.

Clinical Example (32668)

A 62-year-old male smoker is found to have a growing left spiculated pulmonary nodule now measuring 3 cm in size. There is no evidence of metastatic disease. Pulmonary function is normal. Resection is indicated.

The patient undergoes a thoracoscopic diagnostic wedge resection to be followed by an appropriate more extensive resection (reported separately) based upon intraoperative pathology findings. This service represents only the additional services of the thoracoscopic diagnostic wedge resection in a patient who goes on to have a more extensive lung resection procedure based upon the pathology findings.

(Please note this is an add-on code.)

Description of Procedure (32668)

The site for the initial trocar site is identified and anesthetized with local anesthetic. An incision is made, and using a combination of sharp, cautery, and blunt dissection, the pleural cavity carefully entered. The parietal pleura is palpated, a trocar inserted under direct vision, and the thoracoscope advanced into the pleural cavity. Initial visual exploration is performed. The sites for all additional trocar incisions (1 or 2), if necessary, are identified and are anesthetized with local anesthetic. The additional trocar incisions are made in a similar fashion. Access ports as necessary are placed at each incision site for the passage of instruments. Adhesions between the lung and chest wall are freed. Pleural fluid, if present and if appropriate, is sent for cytology and microbiology. The chest and lung are explored, which includes both visual inspection and palpation of the parietal pleura, visceral pleura, diaphragm, mediastinum, and lung. The worrisome lung nodule is located and its relationship to the pulmonary vasculature and bronchial tree assessed to determine that resection is feasible. The lung is mobilized as needed for assistance in exposing the nodule. Using multiple firings of endoscopic tissue staplers a wedge resection of the nodule is performed removing the nodule with at least a 1- to 2-cm margin of normal lung parenchyma. The specimen prior to removal from the chest is placed in a sterile bag to avoid trocar site contamination. As necessary, hemostasis is secured with electrocautery and if needed the staple lines reinforced with suture. If necessary, sterile portions of the resected nodule are prepared and sent for appropriate microbiologic testing. The remaining portions of resected lung are sent for frozen section evaluation to obtain a histopathologic diagnosis. If lung cancer is confirmed, then anatomic resection (eg, VATS or open segmentectomy, lobectomy, pneumonectomy) (separately reported) may be indicated.

Clinical Example (32669)

A 78-year-old male smoker with severe emphysema presents with non-small cell lung cancer limited to the superior segment of the left lower lobe. Patient is felt not to be a candidate for lobectomy and segmental resection is performed.

Description of Procedure (32669)

The site for the initial trocar site is identified and anesthetized with local anesthetic. An incision is made, and using a combination of sharp, cautery, and blunt dissection the pleural cavity carefully entered. The parietal pleura is palpated, a trocar inserted under direct vision, and the thoracoscope advanced into the pleural cavity. Initial visual exploration is performed. The sites for all additional trocar incisions (3 or 4) are identified and are anesthetized with local anesthetic. The additional trocar incisions are made in a similar fashion as is the larger accessory incision. Access ports, as necessary, are placed at each incision site for the passage of instruments. Adhesions between the lung and chest wall are freed. Pleural fluid, if present and if appropriate, is sent for cytology and microbiology. The chest and lung are explored, which includes both visual inspection and/or palpation of the parietal pleura, visceral pleura, diaphragm, mediastinum, and lung. The cancer in the superior segment of the lower lobe is identified. The lung is retracted superiorly to expose the diaphragmatic surface. The inferior pulmonary ligament is divided with electrocautery, and the mediastinal pleura dissected away from the inferior pulmonary vein anteriorly and posteriorly. A right angle clamp is used to carefully dissect around the inferior pulmonary vein avoiding the superior pulmonary vein. The superior segmental vein branch of the inferior pulmonary vein is identified and separately isolated. The endoscopic vascular stapler is passed across the superior segmental vein and fired to divide it. The lower lobe is retracted inferiorly and dissection in the fissure to separate the upper and lower lobes performed. At the base of the fissure the pulmonary artery is identified and carefully dissected free. The dissection is continued until the branches to the superior segment of the lower lobe and the four basilar segments are identified. The arterial branch(s) to the superior segment is divided using the endoscopic vascular stapler. Underneath the artery the superior segmental bronchus to the lower lobe is identified, isolated, and divided using the endoscopic tissue stapler, taking care not to narrow the basilar segmental bronchi. Using multiple firings of the endoscopic tissue stapler, the fissures between the superior segment of the lower lobe and the upper lobe and superior segment and the basilar segments are divided. The resected superior segment is endoscopically placed in a sterile bag which is closed and then removed from the chest cavity through the accessory incision. The specimen is sent to pathology for frozen section analysis of the margin, which can require 15 to 20 minutes. For lung cancer, a thoracoscopic mediastinal and regional lymphadenectomy is performed (separately reported). Once confirmation is obtained indicating that no further surgery is required (eg, benign lesion or margins negative if malignant) the steps for closure are begun. The anesthetist is asked to inflate the operated lung and all staple lines are assessed for both hemostasis and air leakage. The lung is again deflated and the chest cavity is irrigated. A chest tube(s) is inserted through a separate interspace incision(s) to provide evacuation of air and fluid from the chest. All trocar incisions are assessed for hemostasis. The anesthetist is again asked to inflate the operated lung and with the thoracoscope still in place observing that the remaining lung completely re-expands. The thoracoscope is then removed. A surgical pause is conducted while an instrument, needle, and sponge count is completed and confirmed by the surgeon. Each incision is closed with multiple layers of suture for the muscle, and the skin reapproximated with a subcuticular stitch.

 ## Clinical Example (32670)

A 69-year-old male presents with centrally located non-small cell lung cancer which involves both the middle and lower lobe orifices. Bilobar resection (combined resection of middle and lower lobes) is required.

Description of Procedure (32670)

The site for the initial right trocar site is identified and anesthetized with local anesthetic. An incision is made, and using a combination of sharp, cautery, and blunt dissection the pleural cavity carefully entered. The parietal pleura is palpated, a trocar inserted under direct vision, and the thoracoscope advanced into the pleural cavity. Initial visual exploration is performed. The sites for all additional trocar incisions (3 or 4) are identified and are anesthetized with local anesthetic. The additional trocar incisions are made in a similar fashion as is the larger accessory incision. Access ports as necessary are placed at each incision site for the passage of instruments. Adhesions between the lung and chest wall are freed. Pleural fluid, if present and if appropriate, is sent for cytology and microbiology. The chest and lung are explored which includes both visual inspection and/or palpation of the parietal pleura, visceral pleura, diaphragm, mediastinum, and lung. The central lung cancer is identified. The lung is retracted superiorly to expose the diaphragmatic surface. The inferior pulmonary ligament is divided with electrocautery, and the mediastinal pleura dissected away from the inferior pulmonary vein anteriorly and posteriorly. A right angle clamp is used to carefully dissect around the inferior pulmonary vein away from the superior pulmonary vein to the upper lobe. The endoscopic vascular stapler is passed across the inferior pulmonary vein and fired to divide it. In a similar fashion the middle lobe vein is dissected free and isolated from the superior pulmonary vein. It too is divided utilizing the endoscopic vascular stapler. The lower lobe is retracted inferiorly and dissection in the fissure to separate the upper and lower lobes performed. At the base of the fissure the pulmonary artery is identified and carefully dissected free. The dissection is continued until the branches to the middle lobe, superior segment, and the four basilar segments are identified. The arterial branches are divided using the endoscopic vascular stapler. Underneath the artery the bronchus intermedius is identified, isolated, and divided using the endoscopic tissue stapler, taking care not to narrow the upper lobe bronchus. Using multiple firings of the endoscopic tissue stapler, the fissures between the lower lobe and upper lobe, and upper lobe and middle lobe are divided. The resected middle and lower lobes are

⊘=Modifier 51 Exempt   ⊙=Moderate Sedation   ✚=Add-on Code   ⊮=FDA approval pending

endoscopically placed in a sterile bag which is closed and then removed from the chest cavity through the accessory incision. The specimen is sent to pathology for frozen section analysis of the margin, which can require 15 to 20 minutes. For lung cancer, a thoracoscopic mediastinal and regional lymphadenectomy may be performed (separately reported). Once confirmation is obtained indicating that no further surgery is required (eg, benign lesion or margins negative if malignant) the steps for closure are begun. The anesthetist is asked to inflate the operated lung and all staple lines are assessed for both hemostasis and air leakage. The lung is again deflated and the chest cavity is irrigated. A chest tube(s) is inserted through a separate interspace incision(s) to provide evacuation of air and fluid from the chest. All trocar incisions are assessed for hemostasis. The anesthetist is again asked to inflate the operated lung and with the thoracoscope still in place observing that the remaining lung completely re-expands. The thoracoscope is then removed. A surgical pause is conducted while an instrument, needle, and sponge count is completed and confirmed by the surgeon. Each incision is closed with multiple layers of suture for the muscle, and the skin reapproximated with a subcuticular stitch.

Clinical Example (32671)

A 64-year-old female presents with a squamous carcinoma of the left upper lobe involving the left mainstem bronchus requiring pneumonectomy for complete excision.

Description of Procedure (32671)

The site for the initial trocar site is identified and anesthetized with local anesthetic. An incision is made, and using a combination of sharp, cautery, and blunt dissection the pleural cavity carefully entered. The parietal pleura is palpated, a trocar inserted under direct vision, and the thoracoscope advanced into the pleural cavity. Initial visual exploration is performed. The sites for all additional trocar incisions (3 or 4) are identified and are anesthetized with local anesthetic. The additional trocar incisions are made in a similar fashion as is the larger accessory incision. Access ports as necessary are placed at each incision site for the passage of instruments. Adhesions between the lung and chest wall are freed. Pleural fluid, if present and if appropriate, is sent for cytology and microbiology. The chest and lung are explored which includes both visual inspection and/or palpation of the parietal pleura, visceral pleura, diaphragm, mediastinum, and lung. Abnormalities of the visceral and parietal pleura and lung are noted. Retract lung superiorly to expose the diaphragmatic surface. The inferior pulmonary ligament is divided with electrocautery, and the mediastinal pleura dissected away from the inferior pulmonary vein anteriorly and posteriorly. A right angle clamp is used to carefully dissect around the inferior pulmonary vein away from the superior pulmonary vein. The endoscopic vascular stapler is passed across the inferior pulmonary vein and fired to divide it. A right angle clamp is used to carefully dissect around the superior pulmonary vein, and the endoscopic vascular stapler is passed across the superior pulmonary vein and fired to divide it. The lung is retracted inferiorly and posteriorly and the pulmonary artery identified and carefully dissected free. The pulmonary artery is encircled with a vascular loop. The pulmonary artery is divided with the endoscopic vascular stapler. The mainstem bronchus is dissected free. For lung cancer, a thoracoscopic mediastinal and regional lymphadenectomy is performed (separately reported). The mainstem bronchus is then divided with the endoscopic tissue stapler. The resected lung is endoscopically placed in a sterile bag which is closed and then removed from the chest cavity through the accessory incision. The specimen is sent to pathology for frozen section analysis of the margin, which can require 15 to 20 minutes. Once confirmation is obtained indicating that no further surgery is required (eg, benign lesion or margins negative if malignant) the steps for closure are begun. The anesthetist is asked to inflate the operated side and the bronchial staple line is assessed for air leakage. All vascular staple lines are assessed for hemostasis. The chest cavity is irrigated with several liters of saline. A chest tube(s) is inserted through a separate interspace incision(s) to provide for stabilization of the mediastinum. All trocar incisions are assessed for hemostasis. A surgical pause is conducted while an instrumentation, needle, and sponge count is completed and confirmed by the surgeon. Each incision is closed with multiple layers of suture for the muscle, and the skin reapproximated with a subcuticular stitch. With the patient supine and positive pressure from the anesthetist, the chest tube is removed and pursestring skin suture tied.

Clinical Example (32672)

A 45-year-old female with severe COPD and dyspnea presents for LVRS. She has upper lobe predominant emphysema and is an appropriate candidate for LVRS.

Description of Procedure (32672)

The site for the initial trocar site is identified and anesthetized with local anesthetic. An incision is made, and using a combination of sharp, cautery, and blunt dissection the pleural cavity carefully entered. The parietal pleura is palpated, a trocar inserted under direct vision, and the thoracoscope advanced into the pleural cavity. Initial visual exploration is performed. The sites for all additional trocar incisions (2 or 3) are identified and are anesthetized with local anesthetic. The additional trocar incisions are made in a similar fashion as is the larger accessory incision. Access ports as necessary are placed at each incision site for the passage of instruments. Adhesions between the lung and chest wall are carefully freed so as not to injure the severely emphysematous lung. Pleural fluid, if present and if appropriate, is sent for cytology and microbiology. The chest and lung are explored. The target areas of severe emphysematous lung are noted and using many applications of the endoscopic stapling device with specially applied buttressing material a significant portion of emphysematous lung is removed. Typically about two-thirds of the affected lobe is removed. On the ipsilateral side, other areas of destroyed lung may be removed as well from the other lobe(s) (not separately reported). The specimens are removed from the chest in a sterile bag and sent to pathology. The staple lines are reinforced as necessary with additional staple applications, suturing, or by the application of tissue sealants. The anesthetist is asked to inflate the operated lung and all staple lines are assessed for both hemostasis and air leakage. A pleural tent or pleurodesis is done if needed. A chest tube(s) is inserted through a separate interspace incision(s) to provide evacuation of air and fluid from the chest. All trocar incisions are assessed for hemostasis. The anesthetist is again asked to inflate the operated lung and with the thoracoscope still in place observing that the remaining lung completely re-expands. The thoracoscope is then removed. A surgical pause is conducted while an instrumentation, needle, and sponge count is completed and confirmed by the surgeon. Each incision is closed with multiple layers of suture for the muscle, and the skin reapproximated with subcuticular stitch.

Clinical Example (32673)

A 35-year-old male with myasthenia gravis is referred for thymectomy.

Description of Procedure (32673)

The site for the initial trocar site is identified and anesthetized with local anesthetic. An incision is made, and using a combination of sharp, cautery, and blunt dissection the pleural cavity carefully entered. The parietal pleura is palpated, a trocar inserted under direct vision, and the thoracoscope advanced into the pleural cavity. Initial visual exploration is performed. The sites for all additional trocar incisions (1 or 2) if necessary are identified and are anesthetized with local anesthetic. The additional trocar incisions are made in a similar fashion. Access ports as necessary are placed at each incision site for the passage of instruments. Adhesions between the lung and chest wall are freed. Pleural fluid, if present and if appropriate, is sent for cytology and microbiology. The chest and lung are explored, which includes both visual inspection and/or palpation of the parietal pleura, visceral pleura, diaphragm, mediastinum, and lung. The thymus and attached mediastinal fat is carefully dissected off the pericardium from the diaphragm up to the innominate vein. The phrenic nerve is carefully protected. The innominate vein is skeletonized and venous tributaries are ligated or clipped. The two cervical lobes are dissected out above the innominate vein and brought down into the mediastinal space. The pleura on the opposite side is dissected off the thymus and the remainder of the thymus separated from its mediastinal attachments. On occasion it may be necessary to place a trocar in the contralateral pleural space to complete the dissection of the contralateral portion of the thymus gland. The thymus is placed in a sterile bag to avoid trocar site contamination. The operative field is inspected for adequate hemostasis. The chest cavity is irrigated. A chest tube(s) is inserted through a separate interspace incision(s) to provide evacuation of air and fluid from the chest. The anesthetist is asked to inflate the lung. A surgical pause is conducted while an instrumentation, needle, and sponge count is completed and confirmed by the surgeon. Each incision is closed with multiple layers of suture for the muscle, and the skin reapproximated with a subcuticular stitch.

Clinical Example (32674)

A 59-year-old male undergoes a thoracoscopic right upper lobectomy (separately reported) for a clinical stage I adenocarcinoma. Clinical guidelines indicate the need for a complete thoracic regional and mediastinal lymphadenectomy. Mediastinal lymph nodes are not included within the proximity of the lobectomy specimen. Mediastinal lymph nodes include the paratracheal, subcarinal, paraesophageal, and inferior pulmonary ligament. The presence of tumor in any lymph nodes in the mediastinum signifies a significantly worse prognosis and indicates the need for postoperative adjuvant therapy. (Please note this is an add-on code.)

Description of Procedure (32674)

In the ipsilateral chest, thoracoscopically dissect and remove regional and mediastinal lymph nodes. On the right, this includes the separate removal and labeling of lymph nodes from the following locations: paratracheal, subcarinal, inferior pulmonary ligament, paraesophageal, and hilar.

Cardiovascular System

Heart and Pericardium

PERICARDIUM

▶(For thoracoscopic [VATS] pericardial procedures, see 32601, 32604, 32658, 32659, 32661)◀

✍ Rationale

A parenthetical note was placed following the section heading for Pericardium. This parenthetical directs users to the appropriate codes to use to identify thoracoscopic pericardial procedures (Video-Assisted Thoroascopic Surgery, or VATS). For more information regarding VATS procedures, see the rationale listed following the Lungs and Pleura subheading.

⊙**33010** Pericardiocentesis; initial

(For radiological supervision and interpretation, use 76930)

⊙**33011**   subsequent

(For radiological supervision and interpretation, use 76930)

33015 Tube pericardiostomy

33020 Pericardiotomy for removal of clot or foreign body (primary procedure)

33025 Creation of pericardial window or partial resection for drainage

▶(For thoracoscopic [VATS] pericardial window, use 32659)◀

✍ Rationale

A parenthetical note was placed following code 33025. This parenthetical directs users to the appropriate codes to use to identify a thoracoscopic pericardial window procedure (Video-Assisted Thoroascopic Surgery [VATS]). For more information regarding VATS procedures, see the rationale listed following the Lungs and Pleura subheading.

33030 Pericardiectomy, subtotal or complete; without cardiopulmonary bypass

33031   with cardiopulmonary bypass

▲**33050** Resection of pericardial cyst or tumor

▶(For open pericardial biopsy, use 39010)◀

▶(For thoracoscopic [VATS] resection of pericardial cyst, tumor or mass, use 32661)◀

⊘=Modifier 51 Exempt   ⊙=Moderate Sedation   ✚=Add-on Code   ✗=FDA approval pending

✍ Rationale

Parenthetical notes have been placed following code 33050. These parentheticals direct users to the appropriate codes to use to identify an open pericardial biopsy procedure (39010) and thoracoscopic (VATS) resection of pericardial cyst, tumor, or mass (32661). For more information regarding VATS procedures, see the rationale listed following the Lungs and Pleura subheading.

PACEMAKER OR PACING CARDIOVERTER-DEFIBRILLATOR

A pacemaker system includes . . .

A single chamber pacemaker system . . .

▶Like a pacemaker system, a pacing cardioverter-defibrillator (ICD) system includes a pulse generator and electrodes, although pacing cardioverter-defibrillators may require multiple leads, even when only a single chamber is being paced. A pacing cardioverter-defibrillator system may be inserted in a single chamber (pacing in the ventricle) or in dual chambers (pacing in atrium and ventricle). These devices use a combination of antitachycardia pacing, low-energy cardioversion or defibrillating shocks to treat ventricular tachycardia or ventricular fibrillation.◀

Pacing cardioverter-defibrillator pulse generators . . .

The electrodes (leads) of a pacing cardioverter-defibrillator . . .

▶Electrode positioning on the epicardial surface of the heart requires a thoracotomy, or thoracoscopic placement of the leads. Removal of electrode(s) may first be attempted by transvenous extraction (33234, 33235, or 33244). However, if transvenous extraction is unsuccessful, a thoracotomy may be required to remove the electrodes (33238 or 33243). Use 33212, 33213, 33221, 33230, 33231, 33240 as appropriate in addition to the thoracotomy or endoscopic epicardial lead placement codes (33202 or 33203) to report the insertion of the generator if done by the same physician during the same session.

When the "battery" of a pacemaker or pacing cardioverter-defibrillator is changed, it is actually the pulse generator that is changed. Removal of pacemaker or pacing cardioverter-defibrillator pulse generator only is reported with 33233 or 33241. Removal of a pacemaker or pacing cardioverter-defibrillator pulse generator with insertion of a new pulse generator without any replacement or insertion of a lead(s) is reported with 33227-33229 and 33262-33264. Insertion of a new pulse generator, when existing leads are already in place and when no prior pulse generator is removed, is reported with 33212, 33213, 33221, 33230, 33231, 33240. When a pulse generator insertion involves the insertion or replacement of one or more lead(s), use the system codes 33206-33208 for pacemaker or 33249 for pacing cardioverter-defibrillator. Removal of a pulse generator (33233 or 33241) or extraction of transvenous leads (33234, 33235 or 33244) should be reported separately. An exception involves a pacemaker upgrade from single to dual system which includes removal of pulse generator, replacement of new pulse generator, and insertion of new lead, reported with 33214.

Repositioning of a pacemaker electrode, pacing cardioverter-defibrillator electrode(s), or a left ventricular pacing electrode is reported using 33215 or 33226, as appropriate.

The pacemaker and pacing cardioverter-defibrillator device evaluation codes 93279-93299 may not be reported in conjunction with pulse generator and lead insertion or revision codes 33206-33249. Defibrillator threshold testing (DFT) during pacing cardioverter-defibrillator insertion or replacement may be separately reported using 93640, 93641.

Radiological supervision and interpretation related to the pacemaker or pacing cardioverter-defibrillator procedure is included in 33206-33249. To report fluoroscopic guidance for diagnostic lead evaluation without lead insertion, replacement, or revision procedures, use 76000.

The following definitions apply to 33206-33249.

Single lead: a pacemaker or pacing cardioverter-defibrillator with pacing and sensing function in only one chamber of the heart.

Dual lead: a pacemaker or pacing cardioverter-defibrillator with pacing and sensing function in only two chambers of the heart.

Multiple lead: a pacemaker or pacing cardioverter-defibrillator with pacing and sensing function in three or more chambers of the heart.◄

	System	
►Transvenous Procedure	Pacemaker	Implantable Cardioverter-Defibrillator
Insert transvenous single lead only without pulse generator	33216	33216
Insert transvenous dual leads without pulse generator	33217	33217
Insert transvenous multiple leads without pulse generator	33217 + 33224	33217 + 33224
Initial pulse generator insertion only with existing single lead	33212	33240
Initial pulse generator insertion only with existing dual leads	33213	33230
Initial pulse generator insertion only with existing multiple leads	33221	33231
Initial pulse generator insertion or replacement plus insertion of transvenous single lead	33206 (atrial) or 33207 (ventricular)	33249
Initial pulse generator insertion or replacement plus insertion of transvenous dual leads	33208	33249
Initial pulse generator insertion or replacement plus insertion of transvenous multiple leads	33208 + 33225	33249 + 33225
Upgrade single chamber system to dual chamber system	33214 (includes removal of existing pulse generator)	33241 + 33249
Removal pulse generator only (without replacement)	33233	33241
Removal pulse generator with replacement pulse generator only single lead system (transvenous)	33227	33262
Removal pulse generator with replacement pulse generator only dual lead system (transvenous)	33228	33263
Removal pulse generator with replacement pulse generator only multiple lead system (transvenous)	33229	33264
Removal transvenous electrode only single lead system	33234	33244
Removal transvenous electrode only dual lead system	33235	33244
Removal and replacement of pulse generator and transvenous electrodes	33233 + (33234 or 33235) + (33206 or 33207 or 33208) and 33225, when appropriate	33241 + 33244 + 33249 and 33225, when appropriate◄

33202 Insertion of epicardial electrode(s); open incision (eg, thoracotomy, median sternotomy, subxiphoid approach)

33203   endoscopic approach (eg, thoracoscopy, pericardioscopy)

▶(When epicardial lead placement is performed with insertion of the generator, report 33202, 33203 in conjunction with 33212, 33213, 33221, 33230, 33231, 33240)◀

⊙▲**33206** Insertion of new or replacement of permanent pacemaker with transvenous electrode(s); atrial

⊙▲**33207**   ventricular

⊙▲**33208**   atrial and ventricular

(Codes 33206-33208 include subcutaneous insertion of the pulse generator and transvenous placement of electrode[s])

▶(For removal and replacement of pacemaker pulse generator and transvenous electrode(s), use 33233 in conjunction with either 33234 or 33235 and 33206-33208)◀

▶(Do not report 33206-33208 in conjunction with 33227-33229)◀

⊙**33210** Insertion or replacement of temporary transvenous single chamber cardiac electrode or pacemaker catheter (separate procedure)

⊙**33211** Insertion or replacement of temporary transvenous dual chamber pacing electrodes (separate procedure)

⊙▲**33212** Insertion of pacemaker pulse generator only; with existing single lead

⊙▲**33213**   with existing dual leads

#⊙●**33221**   with existing multiple leads

▶(Do not report 33212, 33213, 33221 in conjunction with 33233 for removal and replacement of the pacemaker pulse generator. Use 33227-33229, as appropriate, when pulse generator replacement is indicated)◀

▶(When epicardial lead placement is performed with insertion of generator, report 33202, 33203 in conjunction with 33212, 33213, 33221)◀

⊙**33214** Upgrade of implanted pacemaker system, conversion of single chamber system to dual chamber system (includes removal of previously placed pulse generator, testing of existing lead, insertion of new lead, insertion of new pulse generator)

▶(Do not report 33214 in conjunction with 33227-33229)◀

33215 Repositioning of previously implanted transvenous pacemaker or pacing cardioverter-defibrillator (right atrial or right ventricular) electrode

⊙**33216** Insertion of a single transvenous electrode, permanent pacemaker or cardioverter-defibrillator

⊙**33217** Insertion of 2 transvenous electrodes, permanent pacemaker or cardioverter-defibrillator

(Do not report 33216-33217 in conjunction with 33214)

(For insertion or replacement of a cardiac venous system lead, see 33224, 33225)

⊙▲**33218** Repair of single transvenous electrode, permanent pacemaker or pacing cardioverter-defibrillator

---

►(For repair of single permanent pacemaker or pacing cardioverter-defibrillator electrode with replacement of pulse generator, see 33227-33229 or 33262-33264 and 33218)◄

⊙▲**33220**   Repair of 2 transvenous electrodes for permanent pacemaker or pacing cardioverter-defibrillator

►(For repair of 2 transvenous electrodes for permanent pacemaker or pacing cardioverter-defibrillator with replacement of pulse generator, use 33220 in conjunction with 33228, 33229, 33263, 33264)◄

33221   ►Code is out of numerical sequence. See 33202-33249◄

⊙**33222**   Revision or relocation of skin pocket for pacemaker

⊙**33223**   Revision of skin pocket for cardioverter-defibrillator

▲**33224**   Insertion of pacing electrode, cardiac venous system, for left ventricular pacing, with attachment to previously placed pacemaker or pacing cardioverter-defibrillator pulse generator (including revision of pocket, removal, insertion, and/or replacement of existing generator)

(When epicardial electrode placement is performed, report 33224 in conjunction with 33202, 33203)

✚▲**33225**   Insertion of pacing electrode, cardiac venous system, for left ventricular pacing, at time of insertion of pacing cardioverter-defibrillator or pacemaker pulse generator (including upgrade to dual chamber system and pocket revision) (List separately in addition to code for primary procedure)

►(Use 33225 in conjunction with 33206, 33207, 33208, 33212, 33213, 33214, 33216, 33217, 33221, 33222, 33230, 33231, 33233, 33234, 33235, 33240, 33249)◄

▲**33226**   Repositioning of previously implanted cardiac venous system (left ventricular) electrode (including removal, insertion and/or replacement of existing generator)

33227   ►Code is out of numerical sequence. See 33202-33249◄

33228   ►Code is out of numerical sequence. See 33202-33249◄

33229   ►Code is out of numerical sequence. See 33202-33249◄

33230   ►Code is out of numerical sequence. See 33202-33249◄

33231   ►Code is out of numerical sequence. See 33202-33249◄

⊙▲**33233**   Removal of permanent pacemaker pulse generator only

\#⊙●**33227**   Removal of permanent pacemaker pulse generator with replacement of pacemaker pulse generator; single lead system

\#⊙●**33228**   dual lead system

\#⊙●**33229**   multiple lead system

►(Do not report 33227-33229 in conjunction with 33233)◄

►(For removal and replacement of pacemaker pulse generator and transvenous electrode[s], use 33233 in conjunction with either 33234 or 33235 and 33206-33208)◄

⊙**33234**   Removal of transvenous pacemaker electrode(s); single lead system, atrial or ventricular

⊙**33235**   dual lead system

33236 Removal of permanent epicardial pacemaker and electrodes by thoracotomy; single lead system, atrial or ventricular

33237   dual lead system

33238 Removal of permanent transvenous electrode(s) by thoracotomy

⊙▲**33240** Insertion of pacing cardioverter-defibrillator pulse generator only; with existing single lead

(Use 33240, as appropriate, in addition to the epicardial lead placement codes to report the insertion of the generator when done by the same physician during the same session)

#⊙●**33230**   with existing dual leads

#⊙●**33231**   with existing multiple leads

►(Do not report 33230, 33231, 33240 in conjunction with 33241 for removal and replacement of the pacing cardioverter-defibrillator pulse generator. Use 33262-33264, as appropriate, when pulse generator replacement is indicated)◄

►(When epicardial lead placement is performed with insertion of generator, report 33202, 33203 in conjunction with 33230, 33231, 33240)◄

⊙▲**33241** Removal of pacing cardioverter-defibrillator pulse generator only

►(For removal and replacement of a pacing cardioverter-defibrillator pulse generator and electrode(s), use 33241 in conjunction with either 33243 or 33244 and 33249)◄

#⊙●**33262** Removal of pacing cardioverter-defibrillator pulse generator with replacement of pacing cardioverter-defibrillator pulse generator; single lead system

#⊙●**33263**   dual lead system

#⊙●**33264**   multiple lead system

►(Do not report 33262-33264 in conjunction with 33241)◄

►(For removal of electrode[s] by thoracotomy in conjunction with pulse generator removal or replacement, use 33243 in conjunction with 33241, 33262-33264)◄

►(For removal of electrode[s] by transvenous extraction in conjunction with pulse generator removal or replacement, use 33244 in conjunction with 33241, 33262-33264)◄

(For repair of implantable cardioverter-defibrillator pulse generator and/or leads, see 33218, 33220)

33243 Removal of single or dual chamber pacing cardioverter-defibrillator electrode(s); by thoracotomy

⊙**33244**   by transvenous extraction

⊙▲**33249** Insertion or replacement of permanent pacing cardioverter-defibrillator system with transvenous lead(s), single or dual chamber

►(For removal and replacement of a pacing cardioverter-defibrillator system [pulse generator and electrodes], report 33241 in conjunction with either 33243 or 33244 and 33249)◄

►(For insertion of implantable cardioverter-defibrillator lead(s), without thoracotomy, use 33216 or 33217)◄

✎ Rationale

The AMA/Specialty Society RVS Update Committee (RUC) identified codes 33207, 33208, 33212, 33213, 33233, 33240, 33241, 33249, 71090, and 93641 as being reported together in various combinations more than 75% of the time. In order to accommodate the various combinations of pacemaker or pacing cardioverter-defibrillator services that are reported together, many changes have been made to the codes and guidelines in the Cardiovascular System/Heart and Pericardium/ Pacemaker or Pacing Cardioverter-Defibrillator sections. In addition, radiology code 71090 has been deleted. Please see the discussion of the deletion of code 71090 in the Radiology: Diagnostic Radiology (Diagnostic Imaging)/Chest section of this book.

Codes 33206-33208 have been revised to specify that they describe either the insertion of a new permanent pacemaker or the replacement of a permanent pacemaker. Codes 33212 and 33213 have been revised to describe insertion of a pulse generator. Prior to 2012, these codes described insertion or replacement of the pulse generator. They no longer describe replacement. Code 33212 has been further revised to specify an existing single lead. Code 33213 has also been further revised, and it now specifies existing dual leads. A new code (33221) has been added to this family to identify insertion of a pacemaker pulse generator with multiple existing leads. Code 33221 appears with a number symbol (#) to indicate that the code is out of numerical sequence. A reference note has been added to instruct the user to the appropriate code range of 33202-33249 for placement of code 33221.

Transvenous electrode repair codes 33218 and 33220 have been revised by removing the reference to the number of chambers involved. Code 33224 for insertion of cardiac venous system ventricular pacing electrode with attachment to a previously placed pacemaker or pacing cardioverter-defibrillator pulse generator has been revised to specify that it includes removal, insertion, and/or replacement of an existing generator. Add-on code 33225, which describes the same service when performed at the time of insertion of the pacemaker or pacing cardioverter-defibrillator pulse generator, has been revised to include pocket revision. Code 33226 for repositioning of cardiac venous system electrode has been revised to specify that it includes the removal, insertion and/or replacement of an existing generator.

Code 33233 has been revised to specify that it only describes removal of a permanent pacemaker pulse generator. Codes 33227-33229 have been established to report removal with replacement of a permanent pacemaker pulse generator. Code 33227 specifies a single-lead system, code 33228 specifies a dual-lead system, and code 33229 specifies a multiple-lead system. Codes 33227, 33228, and 33229 appear with a number symbol (#) to indicate that these codes are out of numerical sequence. Three reference notes have been added to instruct the user to the appropriate code range of 33202-33249 for placement of codes 33227, 33228, and 33229.

Code 33240 has been revised by removing reference to chamber and specifying that it only describes insertion of a pacing cardioverter-defibrillator pulse generator with existing single lead. Codes 33230 and 33231 have been established to specify existing dual leads and existing multiple leads, respectively. Codes 33230 and 33231 appear with a number symbol (#) to indicate that these codes are out of numerical sequence. Two reference notes have been added to instruct the user to the appropriate code range of 33202-33249 for placement of codes 33230 and 33231.

Code 33241 has been revised by removing the subcutaneous approach and the reference to chamber and by specifying that it only describes removal of a pacing cardioverter-defibrillator pulse generator. Codes 33262-33264 have been established to report removal and replacement of a pacing cardioverter-defibrillator pulse generator. Code 33262 specifies a single-lead system, code 33263 specifies a dual-lead system, and code 33264 specifies a multiple-lead system. Codes 33262, 33263, and 33264 appear with a number symbol (#) to indicate that these codes are out of numerical sequence. Three reference notes have been added to instruct the user to the appropriate code range of 33202-33249 for placement of codes 33262, 33263, and 33264.

Code 33249 has been revised to describe insertion or replacement of a permanent pacing cardioverter-defibrillator system with transvenous lead(s) for a single or dual chamber. It no longer includes repositioning.

Prior to 2012, radiological supervision and interpretation for pacemaker insertion was reported with radiology code 71090. In 2012, code 71090 has been deleted. Radiological supervision and interpretation are now included in codes 33206-33249.

Several parenthetical notes have been added and revised to provide clear instruction on the appropriate reporting of this revised coding structure. The guidelines have also been updated with instructions on appropriate reporting of the codes and with definitions of some of the terms that are in the code descriptors. A new paragraph has been added to explain that pacemaker and pacing cardioverter-defibrillator device evaluation may not be reported in conjunction with pulse generator and lead insertion or revision, and that defibrillator threshold testing (DFT) during pacing cardioverter-defibrillator insertion or replacement may be separately reported. Another new paragraph has been added to explain the appropriate reporting of radiological services.

A table has been added following the guidelines to assist users in appropriate code selection. There is a column in the table for pacemaker and a column for implantable cardioverter-defibrillator. For example, code 33227 is listed in the Pacemaker-column for removal and replacement of a single-lead (transvenous) system pacemaker pulse generator. Code 33230 is listed in the Implantable Cardioverter-Defibrillator–column for removal and replacement of a single-lead (transvenous) system cardioverter-defibrillator.

 ### Clinical Example (33212)

A 68-year-old patient presents with complete heart block and existing lead placed during a separate surgical procedure. The patient has no signs of systemic infection and needs implantation of a single chamber pacemaker pulse generator and attachment to existing lead.

Description of Procedure (33212)

The appropriate pectoral region is prepared and draped in a sterile manner. An incision is made in the subclavicular region and carried to the pectoralis fascia or the subpectoral region. A pocket for the pacemaker generator is created either in the plane of pectoralis fascia or underneath the pectoral muscles just above the ribcage. The existing lead is dissected free from fibrous tissue. Hemostasis is achieved. The lead is tested for sensing, capture threshold, and impedance. The pocket is irrigated. The pacing lead is connected to the new generator. The generator is inserted into the pocket. The pocket is closed with either suture alone or a combination of suture and staples or suture and tissue adhesive. Programming of the device is performed.

 Clinical Example (33213)

An 8-year-old patient presents with third-degree AV block and existing leads placed during a separate surgical procedure. The patient has no signs of systemic infection and needs implantation of a dual chamber pacemaker pulse generator and attachment to existing leads.

Description of Procedure (33213)

The appropriate pectoral region is prepared and draped in a sterile manner. An incision is made in the subclavicular region and carried to the pectoralis fascia or the subpectoral region. A pocket for the pacemaker generator is created either in the plane of pectoralis fascia or underneath the pectoral muscles just above the ribcage. The existing leads are dissected free from fibrous tissue. Hemostasis is achieved. The leads are tested for sensing, capture threshold, and impedance. The pocket is irrigated. The pacing leads are connected to the new generator. The generator is inserted into the pocket. The pocket is closed with either suture alone or a combination of suture and staples or suture and tissue adhesive. Programming of the device is performed.

 Clinical Example (33221)

A 42-year-old patient with congenital heart disease presents with systolic heart failure and left bundle branch block (LBBB). During a prior surgical procedure, pacemaker leads were placed in the right atrium (RA), right ventricle (RV), and left ventricle (LV) in anticipation of need for pacing and tunneled subcutaneously. The patient now meets indications for biventricular pacing.

Description of Procedure (33221)

The appropriate pectoral region is prepared and draped in a sterile manner. An incision is made in the subclavicular region and carried to the pectoralis fascia or the subpectoral region. A pocket for the pacemaker generator is created either in the plane of pectoralis fascia or underneath the pectoral muscles just above the ribcage. The existing leads are dissected free from fibrous tissue. Hemostasis is achieved. The leads are tested for sensing, capture threshold, and impedance. The pocket is irrigated. The pacing leads are connected to the new generator. The generator is inserted into the pocket. The pocket is closed with either suture alone or a combination of suture and staples or suture and tissue adhesive. Programming of the device is performed.

○=Modifier 51 Exempt   ⊙=Moderate Sedation   ✚=Add-on Code   ✗=FDA approval pending

Clinical Example (33227)

An 85-year-old patient presents with a history of complete heart block whose pacemaker generator is at elective replacement indicator. The patient has no evidence of systemic infection or decompensated congestive heart failure (CHF).

Description of Procedure (33227)

The appropriate pectoral region is prepared and draped in a sterile manner. An incision is made of the existing generator and carried down to the level of the capsule surrounding the generator. The existing generator is dissected free and the lead is freed from fibrous scar tissue. This must be performed in a manner preventing damage to the lead. Often extensive removal of scar tissue/capsule is required. During the procedure adequate hemostasis and sterility are maintained. The existing lead is tested to assess the adequacy, including capture threshold, sensing, and impedance. The pocket may need to be modified to accommodate the shape and size of the new generator. The pocket is copiously irrigated. The new generator is inserted in the pocket and attached to the existing lead. The pocket is closed with either suture alone or a combination of suture and staples or suture and tissue adhesive. Programming of the device is performed.

Clinical Example (33228)

An 82-year-old patient presents with a history of sick sinus syndrome and intermittent paroxysmal atrial fibrillation. The pacemaker is at elective replacement indicator. The patient has no evidence of systemic infection. The patient is complaining of dyspnea felt to be related to a rate or mode change due to the device reaching elective replacement indicator.

Description of Procedure (33228)

The appropriate pectoral region is prepared and draped in a sterile manner. An incision is made of the existing generator and carried down to the level of the capsule surrounding the generator. The existing generator is dissected free and the leads are freed from fibrous scar tissue. Often extensive removal of scar tissue/capsule is required. This must be performed in a manner preventing damage to the leads. During the procedure adequate hemostasis and sterility are maintained. The existing leads are tested to assess the adequacy, including capture threshold, sensing, and impedance. The pocket may need to be modified to accommodate the shape and size of the new generator. The pocket is copiously irrigated. The new generator is inserted in the pocket and attached to the existing leads. The pocket is closed with either suture alone or a combination of suture and staples or suture and tissue adhesive. Programming of the device is performed.

Clinical Example (33229)

An 84-year-old patient presents with moderate to severe congestive heart failure (CHF) and left bundle branch block (LBBB) and does not wish to have implantable cardioverter-defibrillator (ICD) therapy. The biventricular pacemaker is at elective replacement indicator. There is no evidence of systemic infection.

Description of Procedure (33229)

The appropriate pectoral region is prepared and draped in a sterile manner. An incision is made of the existing generator and carried down to the level of the capsule surrounding the generator. The existing generator is dissected free and the leads are freed from fibrous scar tissue. Often extensive removal of scar tissue/capsule is required. This must be performed in a manner preventing damage to the leads. During the procedure adequate hemostasis and sterility are maintained. The existing leads are tested to assess the adequacy, including capture threshold, sensing, and impedance. The pocket may need to be modified to accommodate the shape and size of the new generator. The pocket is copiously irrigated. The new generator is inserted in the pocket and attached to the existing leads. The pocket is closed with either suture alone or a combination of suture and staples or suture and tissue adhesive. Programming of the device is performed.

 Clinical Example (33240)

A 64-year-old patient presents with history of coronary artery disease, old myocardial infarction approximately 3 to 4 years ago with depressed left ventricular function with ejection fraction of 34% and existing lead placed during a separate surgical procedure. The patient has no signs of systemic infection and needs implantation of a single chamber ICD generator and attachment to existing lead to complete a functional system.

Description of Procedure (33240)

The appropriate pectoral region is prepared and draped in a sterile manner. An incision is made in the subclavicular region and carried to the pectoralis fascia or the subpectoral region. A pocket for the pacemaker generator is created either in the plane of pectoralis fascia or underneath the pectoral muscles just above the ribcage. The existing lead is dissected free from fibrous tissue. Hemostasis is achieved. The lead is tested for sensing, capture threshold, and impedance. The pocket is irrigated. The pacing lead is connected to the new generator. The generator is inserted into the pocket. The pocket is closed with either suture alone or a combination of suture and staples or suture and tissue adhesive. Programming of the device is performed.

Clinical Example (33230)

A 67-year-old patient presents with systolic heart failure and existing leads placed during a separate surgical procedure. The patient has no signs of systemic infection and needs implantation of a dual chamber ICD generator and attachment to existing leads to complete a functional system.

Description of Procedure (33230)

The appropriate pectoral region is prepared and draped in a sterile manner. An incision is made in the subclavicular region and carried to the pectoralis fascia or the subpectoral region. A pocket for the pacemaker generator is created either in the plane of pectoralis fascia or underneath the pectoral muscles just above the ribcage. The existing leads are dissected free from fibrous tissue. Hemostasis is achieved. The leads are tested for sensing, capture threshold, and impedance. The pocket is irrigated. The pacing leads are connected to the new generator. The generator is inserted into the pocket. The pocket is closed with either suture alone or a combination of suture and staples or suture and tissue adhesive. Programming of the device is performed.

⃠=Modifier 51 Exempt   ⊙=Moderate Sedation   ✚=Add-on Code   𝑵=FDA approval pending

Clinical Example (33231)

A 62-year-patient presents with systolic heart failure and LBBB block. During a separate surgical procedure, right atrial (RA), right ventricular (RV), and left ventricular (LV) leads were placed. The patient requires implantation of a biventricular ICD generator with attachment with existing leads to complete the ICD system.

Description of Procedure (33231)

The appropriate pectoral region is prepared and draped in a sterile manner. An incision is made in the subclavicular region and carried to the pectoralis fascia or the subpectoral region. A pocket for the pacemaker generator is created either in the plane of pectoralis fascia or underneath the pectoral muscles just above the ribcage. The existing leads are dissected free from fibrous tissue. Hemostasis is achieved. The leads are tested for sensing, capture threshold, and impedance. The pocket is irrigated. The pacing leads are connected to the new generator. The generator is inserted into the pocket. The pocket is closed with either suture alone or a combination of suture and staples or suture and tissue adhesive. Programming of the device is performed.

Clinical Example (33262)

A 60-year-old patient presents with systolic congestive heart failure (CHF) from prior myocardial infarction whose implantable cardioverter-defibrillator (ICD) is at elective replacement indicator. The patient has no signs of systemic infection or unstable coronary syndrome.

Description of Procedure (33262)

The appropriate pectoral region is prepared and draped in a sterile manner. An incision is made of the existing generator and carried down to the level of the capsule surrounding the generator. The existing generator is dissected free and the lead is freed from fibrous scar tissue. This must be performed in a manner preventing damage to the lead. Often extensive removal of scar tissue/capsule is required. During the procedure adequate hemostasis and sterility are maintained. The existing lead is tested to assess the adequacy, including capture threshold, sensing, and impedance. The pocket may need to be modified to accommodate the shape and size of the new generator. The pocket is copiously irrigated. The new generator is inserted in the pocket and attached to the existing lead. The pocket is closed with either suture alone or a combination of suture and staples or suture and tissue adhesive. Programming of the device is performed.

Clinical Example (33263)

A 70-year-old patient with systolic congestive heart failure (CHF) from prior myocardial infarction (MI), who also has bradycardia, presents with an implantable cardioverter-defibrillator (ICD) at elective replacement indicator. The patient has no signs of systemic infection or unstable coronary syndrome.

Description of Procedure (33263)

The appropriate pectoral region is prepared and draped in a sterile manner. An incision is made of the existing generator and carried down to the level of the capsule surrounding the generator. The existing generator is dissected free and the leads are freed from fibrous scar tissue. Often extensive removal of scar tissue/capsule is required. This must be performed in a manner preventing damage to the leads. During the procedure adequate hemostasis and sterility are maintained. The existing leads are tested to assess the adequacy, including capture threshold, sensing, and impedance. The pocket may need to be modified to accommodate the shape and size of the new generator. The pocket is copiously irrigated. The new generator is inserted in the pocket and attached to the existing leads. The pocket is closed with either suture alone or a combination of suture and staples or suture and tissue adhesive. Programming of the device is performed.

Clinical Example (33264)

A 73-year-old patient with systolic congestive heart failure (CHF), Class III symptoms, and left bundle branch block (LBBB) presents with an implantable cardioverter-defibrillator (ICD) at elective replacement indicator. The patient has no signs of systemic infection.

Description of Procedure (33264)

The appropriate pectoral region is prepared and draped in a sterile manner. An incision is made of the existing generator and carried down to the level of the capsule surrounding the generator. The existing generator is dissected free and the leads are freed from fibrous scar tissue. Often extensive removal of scar tissue/capsule is required. This must be performed in a manner preventing damage to the leads. During the procedure adequate hemostasis and sterility are maintained. The existing leads are tested to assess the adequacy, including capture threshold, sensing, and impedance. The pocket may need to be modified to accommodate the shape and size of the new generator. The pocket is copiously irrigated. The new generator is inserted in the pocket and attached to the existing leads. The pocket is closed with either suture alone or a combination of suture and staples or suture and tissue adhesive. Programming of the device is performed.

CARDIAC ASSIST

The insertion of a ventricular assist device (VAD) can be performed via percutaneous (0048T) or transthoracic (33975, 33976, 33979) approach. The location of the ventricular assist device may be intracorporeal or extracorporeal.

Removal of a ventricular assist device (33977, 33978, 33980, 0050T) includes removal of the entire device, including the cannulas.

▶Replacement of a ventricular assist device pump (ie, 33981-33983) includes the removal of the pump and insertion of a new pump, connection, de-airing, and initiation of the new pump.◀

▶Replacement of the entire ventricular assist device system, ie, pump(s) and cannulas, is reported using the insertion codes (ie, 33975, 33976, 33979). Removal (ie, 33977, 33978, 33980) of the ventricular assist device system being replaced is not separately reported.◀

Rationale

The Cardiac Assist guidelines have been revised to delineate applicable code ranges. The specific codes for replacement, insertion, and removal were added as

⊘=Modifier 51 Exempt ⊙=Moderate Sedation ✚=Add-on Code 𝑵=FDA approval pending

follows: (1) codes 33981, 33982, and 33983 were added in parentheses with an "ie" to delineate the codes describing the replacement of a ventricular-assist device pump; (2) codes 33975, 33976, and 33979 were added in parentheses with an "ie" to delineate the codes describing insertion of a ventricular assist device; and (3) codes 33977, 33978, and 33980 were added in parentheses with an "ie" to delineate the codes describing the removal of the ventricular assist device.

▲33960   Prolonged extracorporeal circulation for cardiopulmonary insufficiency; initial day

▲33961   each subsequent day

✎ Rationale

Codes 33960 and 33961 have been revised by changing the unit of service from hours to days and by changing the status of code 33961 from add-on to stand alone. Hence, code 33960 now describes the initial day of prolonged extracorporeal circulation for cardiopulmonary insufficiency, and code 33961 describes each subsequent day of service. This change clarifies that these codes are intended to identify physician services provided each day and prevents any misinterpretation that a full 24 hours of monitoring is required in order to report these codes.

The parenthetical note following code 33961 instructing users to report code 33961 in conjunction with code 33960 has been deleted.

Arteries and Veins

ENDOVASCULAR REPAIR OF ABDOMINAL AORTIC ANEURYSM

34800   Endovascular repair of infrarenal abdominal aortic aneurysm or dissection; using aorto-aortic tube prosthesis

34802   using modular bifurcated prosthesis (1 docking limb)

34803   using modular bifurcated prosthesis (2 docking limbs)

(For endovascular repair of abdominal aortic aneurysm or dissection involving visceral vessels using a fenestrated modular bifurcated prosthesis (2 docking limbs), use Category III codes 0078T, 0079T)

34804   using unibody bifurcated prosthesis

34805   using aorto-uniiliac or aorto-unifemoral prosthesis

►(For radiological supervision and interpretation, use 75952 in conjunction with 34800-34805)◄

+34813   Placement of femoral-femoral prosthetic graft during endovascular aortic aneurysm repair (List separately in addition to code for primary procedure)

(Use 34813 in conjunction with 34812)

►(For femoral artery grafting, see 35521, 35533, 35539, 35540, 35556, 35558, 35566, 35621, 35646, 35654-35661, 35666, 35700)◄

34825   Placement of proximal or distal extension prosthesis for endovascular repair of infrarenal abdominal aortic or iliac aneurysm, false aneurysm, or dissection; initial vessel

+34826   each additional vessel (List separately in addition to code for primary procedure)

(Use 34826 in conjunction with 34825)

▶(Use 34825, 34826 in addition to 34800-34805, 34900 as appropriate)◀

(For radiological supervision and interpretation, use 75953)

✍ Rationale

A number of revisions have been made to codes used to identify vascular surgery procedures. The changes provide improved instructions and better identify the intended use for many of the codes included within the sections for report of these types of services.

In conjunction with these revisions, a parenthetical note used to direct users to the correct code to report radiological supervision and interpretation (S&I) has been moved from a location following code 34808 to a more appropriate location following code 34805 because 34805 is a main body endovascular abdominal aortic aneurysm repair (EVAR) code. This parenthetical is more appropriately placed following codes 34800-34805 because it is intended for use for guidance imaging that is necessary for main body endovascular abdominal aortic aneurysm repair, and not for the report of guidance imaging for implantation of an iliac artery occlusion device (34808). The parenthetical listed following code 75952 has also been revised to reflect this.

Coinciding with the deletion of bypass graft codes 35548, 35549, 35551, and 35651, the parenthetical note following code 34813 has been revised with the removal of these deleted codes.

The parenthetical note that notifies users regarding appropriate use of staged procedure modifier 58 (listed following code 34826) has been deleted. The procedure identified by code 34826 is more often provided as a "related" procedure than a "staged" procedure. As a result, the removal of this parenthetical note more accurately reflects the intent for report of this service.

In addition, the code range referenced in the second parenthetical note following code 34826 has been revised to direct users to the more appropriate code range (34800-34805) for procedures that are to be additionally reported, as appropriate.

ENDOVASCULAR REPAIR OF ILIAC ANEURYSM

▶Code 34900 represents a procedure to report introduction, positioning, and deployment of an endovascular graft for treatment of aneurysm, pseudoaneurysm, or arteriovenous malformation or trauma of the iliac artery (common, hypogastric, external). All balloon angioplasty and/or stent deployments within the target treatment zone for the endoprosthesis, either before or after endograft deployment, are included in the work of 34900 and are not separately reportable. Open femoral or iliac artery exposure (eg, 34812, 34820), introduction of guidewires and catheters (eg, 36200, 36245-36248), and extensive repair or replacement of an artery (eg, 35206-35286) should be additionally reported. ◀

For fluoroscopic guidance in conjunction . . .

Other interventional procedures performed . . .

34900   Endovascular repair of iliac artery (eg, aneurysm, pseudoaneurysm, arteriovenous malformation, trauma) using ilio-iliac tube endoprosthesis

✍️ Rationale

The guidelines for Endovascular Repair of Iliac Aneurysm have been revised. The code range examples included for introduction of guidewires and catheters have been revised to cite a more appropriate code range for the procedures performed (eg, 36200, 36245-36248).

BYPASS GRAFT

Vein

+35500   Harvest of upper extremity vein, 1 segment, for lower extremity or coronary artery bypass procedure (List separately in addition to code for primary procedure)

▶(Use 35500 in conjunction with 33510-33536, 35556, 35566, 35570, 35571, 35583-35587)◀

(For harvest of more than one vein segment, see 35682, 35683) (For endoscopic procedure, use 33508)

35501   Bypass graft, with vein; common carotid-ipsilateral internal carotid

▶(35548 has been deleted. To report, see 35537, 35539, 35565)◀

▶(35549 has been deleted. To report, see 35537, 35538, 35539, 35540, 35565)◀

▶(35551 has been deleted. To report, see 35539, 35540, 35556, 35583)◀

Other Than Vein

35601   Bypass graft, with other than vein; common carotid-ipsilateral internal carotid

▶(35651 has been deleted. To report, see 35646, 35647, 35656)◀

ADJUVANT TECHNIQUES

+35686   Creation of distal arteriovenous fistula during lower extremity bypass surgery (non-hemodialysis) (List separately in addition to code for primary procedure)

▶(Use 35686 in conjunction with 35556, 35566, 35570, 35571, 35583-35587, 35623, 35656, 35666, 35671)◀

EXCISION, EXPLORATION, REPAIR, REVISION

+35700   Reoperation, femoral-popliteal or femoral (popliteal)-anterior tibial, posterior tibial, peroneal artery, or other distal vessels, more than 1 month after original operation (List separately in addition to code for primary procedure)

▶(Use 35700 in conjunction with 35556, 35566, 35570, 35571, 35583, 35585, 35587, 35656, 35666, 35671)◄

Rationale

A number of revisions have been made to codes used to identify vascular surgery procedures. The changes provide improved instructions and better identify the intended use for many of the codes included within the sections for report of these types of services.

Bypass graft codes 35548, 35549, 35551, and 35651 have been deleted, as these procedures are now represented by more granular codes. Cross-reference notes have been added for these deleted codes to direct users to the appropriate codes.

The parentheticals following codes 35500, 35686, and 35700 have all been revised to include reference to code 35570. Because this code was created to describe bypass using vein conduit from a tibial artery to a tibial artery and may correctly be reported with the aforementioned codes, the revision has been made to reflect the intended use.

VASCULAR INJECTION PROCEDURES

Listed services for injection procedures include necessary local anesthesia, introduction of needles or catheter, injection of contrast media with or without automatic power injection, and/or necessary pre- and postinjection care specifically related to the injection procedure.

Selective vascular catheterization should be coded to include introduction and all lesser order selective catheterization used in the approach (eg, the description for a selective right middle cerebral artery catheterization includes the introduction and placement catheterization of the right common and internal carotid arteries).

Additional second and/or third order arterial catheterization within the same family of arteries or veins supplied by a single first order vessel should be expressed by 36012, 36218, or 36248.

Additional first order or higher catheterization in vascular families supplied by a first order vessel different from a previously selected and coded family should be separately coded using the conventions described above.

(For radiological supervision and interpretation, see Radiology)

(For injection procedures in conjunction with cardiac catheterization, see 93452-93461, 93563-93568)

(For chemotherapy of malignant disease, see 96401-96549)

Rationale

The Vascular Injection Procedures guidelines have been revised to remove reference to "Catheters, drugs, and contrast media are not included in the listed service for the injection procedures" because several of the procedures listed in this section include catheters.

⊘ =Modifier 51 Exempt   ⊙=Moderate Sedation   ✚=Add-on Code   ☏=FDA approval pending

Intra-Arterial—Intra-Aortic

36120   Introduction of needle or intracatheter; retrograde brachial artery

36140   extremity artery

(For insertion of arteriovenous cannula, see 36810-36821)

(36145 has been deleted. To report see 36147, 36148)

▶***Diagnostic Studies of Arteriovenous (AV) Shunts for Dialysis:*** For diagnostic studies, the arteriovenous (AV) dialysis shunt (AV shunt) is defined as beginning with the arterial anastomosis and extending to the right atrium. This definition includes all upper and lower extremity AV shunts (arteriovenous fistulae [AVF] and arteriovenous grafts [AVG]). Code 36147 includes the work of directly accessing and imaging the entire AV shunt. Antegrade and/or retrograde punctures of the AV shunt are typically used for imaging, and contrast may be injected directly through a needle or through a catheter placed into the AV shunt. Occasionally the catheter needs to be advanced further into the shunt to adequately visualize the arterial anastomosis or the central veins, and all manipulation of the catheter for diagnostic imaging of the AV shunt is included in 36147. Advancement of the catheter to the vena cava to adequately image that segment of the AV shunt is included in 36147 and is not separately reported. Advancement of the catheter tip through the arterial anastomosis to adequately visualize the anastomosis is also considered integral to the work of 36147 and is not separately reported.

Ultrasound guidance for puncture of the AV shunt is not included in 36147. Particularly in the case of new or failing AVF, ultrasound may be necessary to safely and effectively puncture the AV access for evaluation, and this may be reported separately with 76937 if all the appropriate elements for reporting 76937 are performed.

Evaluation of the peri-anastomotic portion of the inflow is considered an integral part of the dialysis fistulagram and is included in the work of 36147. The peri-anastomotic portion of the vessel at the arterial anastomosis includes the short segment of the artery immediately adjacent to the anastomosis, the anastomosis itself, and the portion of the vessel or graft immediately distal to the anastomosis.

The arterial inflow to the AV access is considered a separate vessel. If a more proximal inflow problem separate from the peri-anastomotic segment is suspected and additional catheter work and imaging must be done for adequate evaluation, this work is not included in 36147. If a catheter is selectively advanced from the AV shunt puncture into the inflow artery, an additional catheterization code may be reported. In the typical case of an upper extremity AV shunt, 36215 is used to report this work, and includes placement of the catheter retrograde into the inflow artery and into the aorta if necessary (ie, 36200 may not be also reported since that work is included in the work defined by 36215).◀

▶***Interventions for Arteriovenous (AV) Shunts Created for Dialysis (AV Grafts and AV Fistulae):*** For the purposes of coding interventional procedures in arteriovenous (AV) shunts created for dialysis (both arteriovenous fistulae [AVF] and arteriovenous grafts [AVG]), the AV shunt is artificially divided into two vessel segments. The first segment is peripheral and extends from the peri-arterial anastomosis through the axillary vein (or entire cephalic vein in the case of cephalic venous outflow). The second segment includes the veins central to the axillary and cephalic veins, including the subclavian and innominate veins through the vena cava. Interventions performed in a single segment, regardless of the number of lesions treated, are coded as a single intervention.

The AV shunt is considered to be venous and most interventions are coded with the venous intervention codes (ie, angioplasty is reported with venous angioplasty codes 35476, 75978). Codes 35476 and 75978 would be reported once to describe all angioplasty work performed in one segment of the AV dialysis shunt, regardless of the number of distinct lesions treated within that segment, the number of times the balloon is inflated, or the number of balloon catheters required to open all lesions.

There is an exception to the use of venous interventional codes. When there is a stenosis at the arterial anastomosis, it typically extends across the anastomosis and involves the artery just proximal to and at the anastomosis as well as the outflow vessel or graft. This segment is called the peri-anastomotic (or juxta-anastomotic) region, and even though the stenosis can involve multiple vessels, it is typically a single lesion with a single etiology crossing the anastomosis, and treatment to open this lesion crosses from the artery into the vein or venous graft. An intervention treated in this peri-anastomotic segment is coded as an arterial intervention (35475, 75962). Since the entire segment of the AV shunt from the peri-arterial anastomosis through the axillary vein is considered a single vessel for coding of interventions, the arterial angioplasty codes include the work of opening the peri-anastomotic stenosis, as well as all other stenoses treated within this segment of the vessel. Codes 35475 and 75962 are reported once to describe all work done to angioplasty any lesion from the peri-arterial anastomosis through the axillary vein in procedures that involve angioplasty of the peri-arterial anastomosis of the AV shunt. In these special instances, venous angioplasty codes would not be reported additionally for this first or most peripheral shunt segment, even if balloon angioplasty is performed on segments of the AV dialysis shunt that are purely venous anatomy within this specific vessel segment.

It is never appropriate to report removal of the arterial plug during a declot/thrombectomy procedure as an arterial or venous angioplasty (35475, 35476). Removal of the arterial plug is included in the work of a fistula thrombectomy (36870), even if a balloon catheter is used to mechanically dislodge the resistant thrombus.

The central veins (eg, subclavian, innominate, and cava) are considered an additional, separate venous vessel segment for purposes of interventional coding for AV dialysis shunt interventions. If one or more central venous stenoses are treated with angioplasty, this is reported as a single venous angioplasty (35476, 75978), regardless of the number of discrete lesions treated within this segment, and also independent of the number of balloon inflations or number of balloon catheters or sizes required. This additional work should be clearly documented in the patient record and in the recorded images.

The codes for stents placed in AV dialysis accesses are generic for intravascular work and not specific for arterial or venous anatomy. However, the same rules used for angioplasty apply to stent placements for AV dialysis shunts with respect to the number of interventions reported for each patient. Stent codes (37205, 75960) are reported once to describe all work of stenting lesions within the defined AV dialysis shunt segment from the peri-arterial anastomosis through the axillary and cephalic veins, regardless of the number of stents placed or the number of discrete lesions treated within that vessel segment. If additional stenting is required for central venous stenosis, this may be reported as an additional stent placement (37206, 75960), describing all the work of stent placement within the central venous segment.

The work of catheterizing all the veins in the dialysis AV shunt is included in 36147 (and, if appropriate, 36148). Selective catheterization of the inferior/superior vena cava and central veins cannot be separately reported when performed from a direct puncture of the AVF/AVG.

However, if additional venous side branches off of the conduit, known as accessory veins, are separately catheterized for intervention such as embolization of a large competing accessory vein, this additional work may be separately reported using the appropriate selective venous catheterization codes (36011 and 36012). The embolization may be reported using 37204, 75894.◀

Rationale

New guidelines for Diagnostic Studies of Arteriovenous (AV) Shunts for Dialysis have been added to the Surgery, Cardiovascular System, Arteries and Veins, Vascular Injection Procedures subsection for CPT 2012. The new guidelines have been added to clarify appropriate reporting for codes 36147 and 36215.

New guidelines for Interventions for Arteriovenous (AV) Shunts Created for Dialysis (AV Grafts and AV Fistulae) have been added to the Surgery, Cardiovascular System, Arteries and Veins, Vascular Injection Procedures subsection. The new guidelines clarify appropriate reporting for codes 35475, 35476, 36011, 36012, 36147, 36148, 36870, 37204, 37205, 37206, 75894, 75960, 75962, and 75978.

⊙▲36200 Introduction of catheter, aorta

⊙▲36245 Selective catheter placement, arterial system; each first order abdominal, pelvic, or lower extremity artery branch, within a vascular family

⊙▲36246 initial second order abdominal, pelvic, or lower extremity artery branch, within a vascular family

⊙▲36247 initial third order or more selective abdominal, pelvic, or lower extremity artery branch, within a vascular family

⊙+▲36248 additional second order, third order, and beyond, abdominal, pelvic, or lower extremity artery branch, within a vascular family (List in addition to code for initial second or third order vessel as appropriate)

Rationale

Codes 36200, 36245, 36246, 36247, 36248 have been revised, adding the conscious sedation symbol, to note that moderate sedation is inherently included as part of this procedure.

Clinical Example (36200)

A 75-year-old female with peripheral arterial disease and history of aortobifemoral bypass presents with acute left buttock claudication and absent left femoral pulse. After review of the medical history, physical, labs, and imaging studies, she is brought to the angiography suite. Via right femoral approach, a catheter is introduced into her abdominal aorta for angiography.

Description of Procedure (36200)

Administer or supervise administration of conscious sedation. The access vessel is palpated and local anesthesia is administered. Using Seldinger technique, the vessel is punctured, a guidewire is passed, and a vascular sheath is introduced into the artery. This is then flushed with sterile saline. Over guidewire, catheter and guidewire are manipulated into the diseased iliac vessels, and then ultimately into the diseased aorta. Sterile saline flush and test injection of contrast are performed to ensure intraluminal and safe position of catheter. Depending on imaging portion of procedure, the catheter may be repositioned or exchanged over appropriate guidewire for different caliber or shaped catheter to facilitate imaging and pressure measurement. Following the imaging portion of the procedure (performed and reported separately), manual compression or closure device are utilized for closure of the arteriotomy to achieve hemostasis.

Clinical Example (36246)

A 74-year-old female with hypertension and a 2.5-cm splenic artery aneurysm presents for diagnostic angiogram for surgical or endovascular planning. After review of the medical history, physical, labs, and imaging studies, she is brought to the angiography suite. Via right femoral approach, a catheter is introduced into the aorta with selective catheterization of the celiac and splenic artery to define neck size and number of feeding vessels.

Description of Procedure (36246)

Administer or supervise administration of conscious sedation. Access vessel is palpated and local anesthesia is administered. Using Seldinger technique, the vessel is punctured, a guidewire is passed, and a catheter and guidewire are manipulated into the diseased aorta. After the nonselective imaging portion of the procedure is performed (separately), the catheter is exchanged over guidewire for appropriate selective catheter, which is manipulated under fluoroscopic guidance into the origin of the chosen branch vessel. Sterile saline flush and test injection of contrast are performed to ensure intraluminal and safe position of catheter. Using guidewire and catheter techniques, the catheter is advanced beyond the first-branch point into the second-order portion of the vessel (eg, splenic, common hepatic, left gastric). Flush and test injection are repeated throughout the procedure to ensure safe position and patency of catheter system. The catheter may be repositioned or exchanged over appropriate guidewire to be seated safely in the vessel. Following the imaging portion of the procedure (performed and reported separately), manual compression or closure device are utilized for closure of the arteriotomy to achieve hemostasis.

Clinical Example (36247)

A 67-year-old female with history of pancreatitis presents with hematemesis, hypotension, and tachycardia. Endoscopy localizes the bleeding to the upper GI tract. After review of the medical history, physical, labs, and imaging studies, she is brought to the angiography suite. Via right femoral approach, a catheter is introduced into the aorta, celiac and common hepatic artery. Through the base catheter, a microcatheter is introduced into the gastroduodenal artery (GDA). Angiography is performed.

Description of Procedure (36247)

Administer or supervise administration of conscious sedation. The access vessel is palpated and local anesthesia is administered. Using Seldinger technique, the vessel is punctured, a guidewire is passed, and a catheter and guidewire are manipulated into the aorta. After the nonselective imaging portion of the procedure

⊘=Modifier 51 Exempt   ⊙=Moderate Sedation   ✚=Add-on Code   ⊮=FDA approval pending

is performed (separately reported), the catheter is exchanged over guidewire for appropriate selective catheter, which is manipulated under fluoroscopic guidance into the origin of the chosen branch vessel. Sterile saline flush and test injection of contrast are performed to ensure intraluminal and safe position of catheter. Using guidewire and catheter techniques, the catheter is advanced beyond the first-branch point into the second-order portion of the vessel (eg, splenic, common hepatic, left gastric). Flush and test injection are repeated throughout the procedure to ensure safe position and patency of catheter systems. Through the base catheter (typically 4-5 French), a second microcatheter (typically 3 French) is prepared on the back sterile table with assistant. This microcatheter and wire are introduced into the base catheter with sterile pressurized heparin flush connected and infused. Microcatheter is advanced under guidance into the third-order branch vessel (GDA, proper hepatic). Following the imaging portion of the procedure (performed and reported separately), manual compression or closure device are utilized for closure of the arteriotomy to achieve hemostasis.

▶Interventions for Arteriovenous (AV) Shunts Created for Dialysis (AV Grafts and AV Fistulae)◀

⊙●**36251**   Selective catheter placement (first-order), main renal artery and any accessory renal artery(s) for renal angiography, including arterial puncture and catheter placement(s), fluoroscopy, contrast injection(s), image postprocessing, permanent recording of images, and radiological supervision and interpretation, including pressure gradient measurements when performed, and flush aortogram when performed; unilateral

⊙●**36252**   bilateral

⊙●**36253**   Superselective catheter placement (one or more second order or higher renal artery branches) renal artery and any accessory renal artery(s) for renal angiography, including arterial puncture, catheterization, fluoroscopy, contrast injection(s), image postprocessing, permanent recording of images, and radiological supervision and interpretation, including pressure gradient measurements when performed, and flush aortogram when performed; unilateral

    ▶(Do not report 36253 in conjunction with 36251 when performed for the same kidney)◀

⊙●**36254**   bilateral

    ▶(Do not report 36254 in conjunction with 36252)◀

    ▶(Placement of closure device at the vascular access site is not separately reported with 36251-36254)◀

✍ Rationale

The AMA/Specialty Society RVS Update Committee (RUC) identified renal catheterization and angiography procedure codes in the "Codes Reported Together 75% or More" screen. As a result, the services described by these codes have been combined as appropriate by establishing codes 36251-36254 and deleting renal angiography codes 75722 and 75724. See the Radiology/Diagnostic Radiology (Diagnostic Imaging)/Vascular Procedures/Aorta and Arteries section of this book for an explanation of the deletion of codes 75722 and 75724.

Codes 36251-36254 include arterial puncture and catheter placement(s), fluoroscopy, contrast injection(s), image postprocessing, permanent recording of images, and radiological supervision and interpretation. Pressure gradient measurements and flush aortogram are also included when performed. Moderate sedation is an inclusive component of the procedures, which is indicated with the Moderate Sedation (⊙) symbol.

Codes 36251 and 36252 describe first-order selective catheter placement in the main renal artery and any accessory renal artery(s) for renal angiography. Code 36251 describes a unilateral procedure, and code 36252 describes a bilateral procedure. Codes 36253 and 36254 describe superselective catheter placement. Code 36253 describes a unilateral procedure, and code 36254 describes a bilateral procedure.

A parenthetical note has been added following code 36253 instructing users not to report code 36253 with code 36251 when performed for the same kidney. Two instructional parenthetical notes were added following code 36254. The first note directs users not to report code 36254 with code 36252. The second note instructs users not to report placement of closure device at the vascular access site separately with codes 36251-36254.

Clinical Example (36251)

A 63-year-old diabetic male with Stage II chronic kidney disease is being evaluated for uncontrolled hypertension. A renal duplex scan has shown an atrophic right kidney with no flow identified in the right renal artery. The left kidney is normal-sized, but the left renal artery is partially obscured by overlying bowel gas and could not be adequately seen. To limit exposure to contrast material, it was elected to perform a diagnostic catheter angiogram to further evaluate the renal arteries.

Description of Procedure (36251)

Administer or supervise administration of conscious sedation. The access vessel is palpated and local anesthesia is administered. Using Seldinger technique, the vessel is punctured, a guidewire is passed, and a flush catheter and guidewire are manipulated into the aorta. After forming the catheter, a small amount of contrast is injected to confirm appropriate and safe position. DSA imaging of the aorta and renal ostia is performed. After the nonselective imaging portion of the procedure is performed, the catheter is exchanged over guidewire for appropriate selective catheter, which is manipulated under fluoroscopic guidance and formed in the aorta. The origin of the renal artery is probed for and ultimately engaged with the catheter advanced into the main renal. Sterile saline flush and test injection of contrast are performed to ensure intraluminal and safe position of catheter. Selective DSA imaging with injection of contrast or CO_2 is performed in multiple projections. If appropriate, pressure measurements are performed with withdrawal of catheter across the vessel origin. Several minutes of time may be dedicated to monitoring of pressure measurements, and wave forms with subsequent interpretation. The selective catheter is unformed under fluoroscopic observation in the thoracic aorta and subsequently removed. Manual compression or closure device are utilized for closure of the arteriotomy to achieve hemostasis.

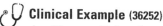

Clinical Example (36252)

An 80-year-old female with Stage III chronic kidney disease and hypertension, which requires three medications to control, is being evaluated for renal artery stenosis. A magnetic resonance angiography was done which suggested there may be ostial stenosis of the right main renal artery and possible stenosis of the origin of the left renal artery. Diagnostic bilateral renal catheter arteriogram is performed.

Description of Procedure (36252)

Administer or supervise administration of conscious sedation. The access vessel is palpated and local anesthesia is administered. Using Seldinger technique, the vessel is punctured, a guidewire is passed, and a flush catheter and guidewire are manipulated into the aorta. After forming the catheter, a small amount of contrast is injected to confirm appropriate and safe position. DSA imaging of the aorta and renal ostia is performed. After the nonselective imaging portion of the procedure is performed, the catheter is exchanged over guidewire for appropriate selective catheter which is manipulated under fluoroscopic guidance and formed in the aorta. The origin of the renal artery is probed for and ultimately engaged. Sterile saline flush and test injection of contrast are performed to ensure intraluminal and safe position of catheter. Selective DSA imaging with injection of contrast or CO_2 is performed in multiple projections. If appropriate, pressure measurements are performed with withdrawal of catheter across the vessel origin. Several minutes of time may be dedicated to monitoring of pressure measurements, and wave forms with subsequent interpretation. The selective catheter is advanced out of the renal artery and the contralateral renal artery is probed for and ultimately selected. Repeat test injection, DSA imaging, and pressure measurements are performed as described on the initial side. The selective catheter is unformed under fluoroscopic observation in the thoracic aorta and subsequently removed. Manual compression or closure device are utilized for closure of the arteriotomy to achieve hemostasis.

Clinical Example (36253)

A 60-year-old female presents with acute onset of hematuria. She recently had a left renal biopsy performed for chronic kidney disease evaluation.

Description of Procedure (36253)

Administer or supervise administration of conscious sedation. The access vessel is palpated and local anesthesia is administered. Using Seldinger technique, the vessel is punctured, a guidewire is passed, and a flush catheter and guidewire are manipulated into the aorta. After forming the catheter, a small amount of contrast is injected to confirm appropriate and safe position. DSA imaging of the aorta and renal ostia is performed. After the nonselective imaging portion of the procedure is performed, the catheter is exchanged over guidewire for appropriate selective catheter which is manipulated under fluoroscopic guidance and formed in the aorta. The origin of the renal artery is probed for and ultimately engaged. Sterile saline flush and test injection of contrast are performed to ensure intraluminal and safe position of catheter. Selective DSA imaging with injection of contrast or CO_2 is performed in multiple projections. A second microcatheter is prepared on the back sterile table with assistant. Through the base catheter, this microcatheter and wire are introduced into the base catheter with sterile pressurized heparin flush connected and infused. Using careful fluoroscopic guidance, alternating wire and catheter maneuvers are performed, and the microcatheter is advanced into the second or third order branch vessel of the renal artery. Magnification DSA imaging using contrast or CO_2 is performed in multiple projections. The microcatheter is withdrawn and the base catheter is unformed under fluoroscopic observation in the thoracic aorta and subsequently removed. Manual compression or closure device are utilized for closure of the arteriotomy to achieve hemostasis.

Clinical Example (36254)

A 48-year-old male is undergoing evaluation for hypertension. Renal duplex scanning and computed tomographic angiography have identified branch renal artery aneurysms bilaterally. Renal arteriography is ordered to get more detailed anatomy of the aneurysms to plan repair.

Description of Procedure (36254)

Administer or supervise administration of conscious sedation. The access vessel is palpated and local anesthesia is administered. Using Seldinger technique, the vessel is punctured, a guidewire is passed, and a flush catheter and guidewire are manipulated into the aorta. After forming the catheter, a small amount of contrast is injected to confirm appropriate and safe position. DSA imaging of the aorta and renal ostia is performed. After the nonselective imaging portion of the procedure is performed, the catheter is exchanged over guidewire for appropriate selective catheter which is manipulated under fluoroscopic guidance and formed in the aorta. The origin of the renal artery is probed for and ultimately engaged. Sterile saline flush and test injection of contrast are performed to ensure intraluminal and safe position of catheter. Selective DSA imaging with injection of contrast or CO_2 is performed in multiple projections. If appropriate, pressure measurements are performed with withdrawal of catheter across the vessel origin. Several minutes of time may be dedicated to monitoring of pressure measurements, and wave forms with subsequent interpretation. A second microcatheter is prepared on the back sterile table with assistant. Through the base catheter, this microcatheter and wire are introduced into the base catheter with sterile pressurized heparin flush connected and infused. Using careful fluoroscopic guidance, alternating wire and catheter maneuvers are performed, and the microcatheter is advance into the second or third order branch vessel of the renal artery. Magnification DSA imaging using contrast or CO_2 is performed in multiple projections. The microcatheter is withdrawn and the selective catheter is advanced out of the renal artery and the contralateral renal artery is probed for and ultimately selected. Repeat test injection, DSA imaging, and pressure measurements are performed as described on the initial side. The microcatheter is prepped and re-advanced through the base catheter, and using guidance, the contralateral second or third order branches are selected with repeat magnification imaging performed as indicated. The base catheter is unformed under fluoroscopic observation in the thoracic aorta and subsequently removed. Manual compression or closure device are utilized for closure of the arteriotomy to achieve hemostasis.

⊘=Modifier 51 Exempt   ⊙=Moderate Sedation   ✚=Add-on Code   ✗=FDA approval pending

Venous

36475 Endovenous ablation therapy of incompetent vein, extremity, inclusive of all imaging guidance and monitoring, percutaneous, radiofrequency; first vein treated

+36476   second and subsequent veins treated in a single extremity, each through separate access sites (List separately in addition to code for primary procedure)

(Use 36476 in conjunction with 36475)

▶(Do not report 29581, 29582, 36475, 36476 in conjunction with 36000-36005, 36410, 36425, 36478, 36479, 37204, 75894, 76000, 76001, 76937, 76942, 76998, 77022, 93970, 93971)◀

36478 Endovenous ablation therapy of incompetent vein, extremity, inclusive of all imaging guidance and monitoring, percutaneous, laser; first vein treated

+36479   second and subsequent veins treated in a single extremity, each through separate access sites (List separately in addition to code for primary procedure)

(Use 36479 in conjunction with 36478)

▶(Do not report 36478, 36479 in conjunction with 29581, 29582, 36000-36005, 36410, 36425, 36475, 36476, 37204, 75894, 76000, 76001, 76937, 76942, 76998, 77022, 93970, 93971)◀

✐ Rationale

In support of the establishment of codes 29582-29584, the exclusionary parenthetical notes following codes 36476 and 36479 have been revised to preclude the reporting of the application of multilayer compressions system codes 29581 and 29582 in conjunction with these services.

TRANSCATHETER PROCEDURES

Other Procedures

⊙●**37191** Insertion of intravascular vena cava filter, endovascular approach including vascular access, vessel selection, and radiological supervision and interpretation, intraprocedural roadmapping, and imaging guidance (ultrasound and fluoroscopy), when performed

▶(For open surgical interruption of the inferior vena cava through a laparotomy or retroperitoneal exposure, use 37619)◀

⊙●**37192** Repositioning of intravascular vena cava filter, endovascular approach including vascular access, vessel selection, and radiological supervision and interpretation, intraprocedural roadmapping, and imaging guidance (ultrasound and fluoroscopy), when performed

▶(Do not report 37192 in conjunction with 37191)◀

⊙●**37193** Retrieval (removal) of intravascular vena cava filter, endovascular approach including vascular access, vessel selection, and radiological supervision and interpretation, intraprocedural roadmapping, and imaging guidance (ultrasound and fluoroscopy), when performed

▶(Do not report 37193 in conjunction with 37203, 75961)◀

⊙**37203** Transcatheter retrieval, percutaneous, of intravascular foreign body (eg, fractured venous or arterial catheter)

(For radiological supervision and interpretation, use 75961)

▶(For removal of a vena cava filter, use 37193)◀

Rationale

In response to the AMA/Specialty Society RVS Update Committee (RUC) analyses and in support of deletion of codes 37620 and 75940, three new codes for reporting intravascular vena cava filter procedures via endovascular approach (37191-37193) have been added to CPT 2012.

Code 37191 is intended to report insertion of intravascular vena cava filter; 37192 is intended to report repositioning of an intravascular vena cava filter; and 37193 is intended to be used to report retrieval (removal) of an intravascular vena cava filter. Each of these codes include vascular access, vessel selection, and radiological supervision and interpretation, intraprocedural roadmapping, and image guidance (ultrasound and fluoroscopy), when performed.

A cross-reference has been added following code 37191 to direct users to report code 37619 for open surgical interruption of the inferior vena cava through a laparotomy or retroperitoneal exposure.

An exclusionary parenthetical note has been added following code 37192 to indicate that 37192 should not be reported in conjunction with 37191.

An exclusionary parenthetical note has been added following 37193 to indicate that 37193 should not be reported in conjunction with codes 37203 and 75961.

In concert with these revisions, a cross-reference was added following code 37203 to direct users to report removal of a vena cava filter with code 37193.

Clinical Example (37191)

A 56-year-old female has deep venous thrombosis of the leg and pulmonary embolus. Anticoagulation is contraindicated because of gastrointestinal bleeding. An inferior vena cava filter is placed.

Description of Procedure (37191)

Conscious sedation is administered and adequate conscious sedation monitoring is verified. A suitable access vein is cannulated using micropuncture technique and ultrasound guidance. A 5 French vascular sheath is placed. A standard access 0.035 wire and catheter are manipulated into the IVC with fluoroscopic guidance either via the femoral vein or in a transatrial fashion via the internal jugular vein. Breath-hold DSA imaging is obtained with calibrated pigtail catheter for sizing, documentation of anatomy, and assessment for central thromboembolism or stenosis. The position and number of renal veins is documented and marked to plan for optimal filter placement. A second stiff guidewire is advanced and the pigtail catheter is removed. Sequential dilation of the venotomy site is performed and using fluoroscopic guidance the filter delivery sheath is advanced. The filter is slowly deployed under fluoroscopic guidance subjacent to the lowest renal vein. Proper filter deployment is confirmed under magnified fluoroscopy and/or spot imaging in at least two projections. Final venography is performed to ensure proper alignment of the filter with the cava and appropriate position relative to

⊘=Modifier 51 Exempt ⊙=Moderate Sedation ✚=Add-on Code ✕=FDA approval pending

the most inferior renal vein. The filter delivery sheath is removed and hemostasis is obtained with manual compression (with or without hemostasis assist device) or surgical closure of the venotomy.

Clinical Example (37192)

A 56-year-old female with pulmonary embolus had placement of a temporary IVC filter. Follow-up CT scan has identified migration and angulation of the IVC filter. The patient has an ongoing contraindication to anticoagulation (gastrointestinal bleeding). Filter repositioning is performed.

Description of Procedure (37192)

Conscious sedation is administered and adequate conscious sedation monitoring is verified. A suitable access vein is cannulated using micropuncture technique and ultrasound guidance. A 5 French vascular sheath is placed. A standard access 0.035 wire and catheter are manipulated into the IVC with fluoroscopic guidance typically in a transatrial fashion via the internal jugular vein. Initial fluoroscopy and or spot imaging is obtained to assess for position of the existing filter. Breath-hold DSA imaging is obtained in at least two obliquities with calibrated pigtail catheter for sizing, documentation of anatomy, and assessment for central thromboembolism or stenosis. Based on preliminary venography the existing filter is extensively evaluated for trapped thromboembolism, fibrin sheath, and filter cone positioning relative to the caval wall. Presence or absence of filter fixation leg penetration is inspected and additionally imaging is obtained as necessary to satisfactorily inspect these variables. A stiff 0.035 guidewire is advanced and the pigtail catheter is removed. Sequential dilation of the venotomy site is performed and using fluoroscopic guidance the telescoping filter retrieval sheaths are advanced adjacent to the filter. The snare device is advanced and initial attempts are made to snare the filter cone. Once the filter cone is grasped with either the initial snare device, subsequent snare device, or blunt dissection tool, attempts are made to slowly collapse the filter into the telescoping sheath system while paying close fluoroscopic and clinical attention to limit the potential for caval laceration. Once the filter is collapsed the filter is repositioned under fluoroscopic guidance to a more suitable location based on anatomic landmarks and venocavagram. The filter is then redeployed in an appropriate position based on prior and intraprocedural imaging. Proper filter deployment is confirmed under magnified fluoroscopy and/or spot imaging in at least two projections. Final venography is performed to ensure proper alignment of the filter with the cava and appropriate position relative to the renal veins. The filter delivery sheath is removed and hemostasis is obtained with manual compression (with or without hemostasis assist device) or surgical closure of the venotomy.

Clinical Example (37193)

A 56-year-old male had placement of an inferior vena cava filter for deep venous thrombosis and gastrointestinal bleeding. The filter is no longer needed and is retrieved using an endovascular approach.

Description of Procedure (37193)

Conscious sedation is administered and adequate conscious sedation monitoring is verified. A suitable access vein is cannulated using micropuncture technique and ultrasound guidance. A 0.018 wire is advanced centrally and the access needle is removed. The micropuncture dilator is placed and the 0.018 guidewire is exchanged for a standard access 0.035 wire. The micropuncture dilator is removed and a 5 French vascular sheath is placed. The 0.035 wire and 4 or 5 French catheter are manipulated into the IVC with fluoroscopic guidance typically in a trans-atrial fashion via the internal jugular vein. Initial fluoroscopy and/or spot imaging is obtained to assess for position of the existing filter. Breath-hold DSA imaging is obtained in at least two obliquities with calibrated pigtail catheter for sizing, documentation of anatomy, and assessment for central thromboembolism or stenosis. Based on preliminary venography the existing filter is extensively evaluated for trapped thromboembolism, fibrin sheath, and filter cone positioning relative to the caval wall. Presence or absence of filter fixation leg penetration is determined and additional imaging is obtained as necessary to satisfactorily inspect these variables. A stiff 0.035 guidewire is advanced and the pigtail catheter is removed. Sequential dilation of the venotomy site is performed and using fluoroscopic guidance, the telescoping filter retrieval sheaths are advanced adjacent to the filter. The snare device is advanced and initial attempts are made to snare the filter cone. Once the filter cone is grasped with either the initial snare device, subsequent snare device, or blunt dissection tool, attempts are made to slowly collapse the filter into the telescoping sheath system while paying close fluoroscopic and clinical attention to limit the potential for caval laceration. Once the filter is collapsed it is removed under fluoroscopic guidance along with the inner telescoping sheath. The filter is inspected and venography is repeated to ensure caval integrity and to assess for residual clot and/or fibrin sheath at the filter site. The filter delivery sheath is removed and hemostasis is obtained with manual compression (with or without hemostasis assist device) or surgical closure of the venotomy.

ENDOVASCULAR REVASCULARIZATION (OPEN OR PERCUTANEOUS, TRANSCATHETER)

Codes 37220-37235 are to be used . . .

▶These lower extremity endovascular revascularization codes all include the work of accessing and selectively catheterizing the vessel, traversing the lesion, radiological supervision and interpretation directly related to the intervention(s) performed, embolic protection if used, closure of the arteriotomy by pressure and application of an arterial closure device or standard closure of the puncture by suture, and imaging performed to document completion of the intervention in addition to the intervention(s) performed. Extensive repair or replacement of an artery may be additionally reported (eg, 35226 or 35286). These codes describe endovascular procedures performed percutaneously and/or through an open surgical exposure. These codes include balloon angioplasty (eg, low-profile, cutting balloon, cryoplasty), atherectomy (eg, directional, rotational, laser), and stenting (eg, balloon-expandable, self-expanding, bare metal, covered, drug-eluting). Each code in this family (37220-37235) includes balloon angioplasty, when performed.◀

These codes describe revascularization therapies . . .

✍️ Rationale

Changes have been made to this guideline language to clarify the specific type of closure proceduress that are included for these lower extremity endovascular procedures. Language has been added to inform users that pressure application of the arterial closure device or standard closure of the puncture site by suture is inherently included as part of the procedure. Language was also included to specify services that should be separately reported (including extensive repair or replacement of an artery, such as code 35226 or 35286).

+⊙**37222**   Revascularization, endovascular, open or percutaneous, iliac artery, each additional ipsilateral iliac vessel; with transluminal angioplasty (List separately in addition to code for primary procedure)

+⊙**37223**   with transluminal stent placement(s), includes angioplasty within the same vessel, when performed (List separately in addition to code for primary procedure)

        ▶(Use 37223 in conjunction with 37221, 37229, 37231)◀

+⊙**37232**   Revascularization, endovascular, open or percutaneous, tibial/peroneal artery, unilateral, each additional vessel; with transluminal angioplasty (List separately in addition to code for primary procedure)

+⊙**37233**   with atherectomy, includes angioplasty within the same vessel, when performed (List separately in addition to code for primary procedure)

        ▶(Use 37233 in conjunction with 37229, 37231)◀

+⊙**37234**   with transluminal stent placement(s), includes angioplasty within the same vessel, when performed (List separately in addition to code for primary procedure)

        ▶(Use 37234 in conjunction with 37229, 37230, 37231)◀

✍️ Rationale

The parenthetical notes following endovascular codes 37223, 37233, and 37234 were revised and updated to instruct the user to the appropriate code ranges to report.

LIGATION

●**37619**   Ligation of inferior vena cava

        ▶(For endovascular delivery of an inferior vena cava filter, use 37191)◀

        ▶(37620 has been deleted. To report, see 37191 for endovascular placement of intravascular filter or 37619 for open surgical ligation of the inferior vena cava)◀

✍️ Rationale

In response to the AMA/Specialty Society RVS Update Committee (RUC) analyses, ligation code 37620 and radiology code 75940 have been deleted. Code 37619 has been established for reporting ligation of the inferior vena cava. A cross-reference note has been added following code 37619 to instruct users to report code 37191 for endovascular delivery of an inferior vena cava filter. A second parenthetical indicates that code 37620 has been deleted and directs users to code 37191, for endovascular placement of an intravascular filter or code 37619 for open surgical ligation of the inferior vena cava.

Clinical Example (37619)

A 56-year-old male sustains penetrating trauma to the flank. He is emergently taken for exploratory laparotomy and a retroperitoneal hematoma is identified. Exploration reveals a complex injury to the inferior vena cava below the level of the renal veins. His tenuous condition requires that the inferior vena cava be ligated.

Description of Procedure (37619)

Rapidly perform laparotomy incision and explore abdomen to identify site of hemorrhage. Assess location and status of renal vein and hepatic veins as well as adjacent organs including liver, spleen, and bowel mesentery. Communicate with anesthesiologist as to overall status of the patient, collaborating regarding fluid and transfusion therapy to ensure adequate volume replacement. Rapidly configure ring forceps with sponges to occlude the flow of blood through the inferior vena cava to stop bleeding, and manually compress vena cava and or clamp aorta if patient has exsanguinating hemorrhage, avoiding injury to adjacent viscera. Perform Kocher maneuver to expose the vena cava by rotating the colon, duodenum, and pancreas medially. Rapidly dissect soft tissue from surface of bleeding inferior vena cava taking care to avoid injury to the right renal vessels. Use digital pressure to control hemorrhage, employing vascular clamps as required. Assess the injury to the vena cava to determine if any form of repair can be performed. Since repair is always preferred over ligation, the typical patient will undergo significant efforts at repair prior to decision to ligate (and in this situation there would be no way to report the failed work of attempted repair). Once determined that the vena cava is not able to be repaired, rapidly expose the vessel ends sufficiently to allow ligation. Suture ligate the superior and inferior ends of the IVC. Apply additional sutures as needed to control hemorrhage. Listen with Doppler to the renal vessels to assure adequate flow pattern and determine there is no injury to the renal artery or vein during the ligation. Correct coagulopathy with fresh frozen plasma, platelets, and cryoprecipitate. Re-explore abdomen to ensure there are no other injuries. Irrigate wound to wash out hematoma. Confirm final sponge and instrument count. Check again for hemostasis and close laparotomy fascia. Evaluate lower legs for impaired venous return and the potential need for prophylactic lower extremity four compartment fasciotomies.

Hemic and Lymphatic Systems

General

BONE MARROW OR STEM CELL SERVICES/PROCEDURES

38207   Transplant preparation of hematopoietic progenitor cells; cryopreservation and storage

⊘ =Modifier 51 Exempt   ⊙=Moderate Sedation   ✚ =Add-on Code   ✗ =FDA approval pending

(For diagnostic cryopreservation and storage, use 88240)

▲38208   thawing of previously frozen harvest, without washing, per donor

(For diagnostic thawing and expansion of frozen cells, use 88241)

▲38209   thawing of previously frozen harvest, with washing, per donor

Rationale

The Bone Marrow or Stem Cell services codes 38208 and 38209 were revised to state "per donor" to allow for multiple units to be reported, as the use of multiple cord blood units has become relatively common.

38220   Bone marrow; aspiration only

38221   biopsy, needle or trocar

(For bone marrow biopsy interpretation, use 88305)

▲38230   Bone marrow harvesting for transplantation; allogeneic

●38232   autologous

(For autologous and allogeneic blood-derived peripheral stem cell harvesting for transplantation, see 38205-38206)

Rationale

Code 38232 has been added to describe autologous bone marrow harvesting for transplantation. Code 38230 has been revised to state allogeneic to differentiate it from the addition of code 38232 for autologous harvest. These changes provide consistency with the other stem cell collection codes, which differentiate the work of allogeneic and autologous harvesting.

Clinical Example (38230)

Patient is a 65-year-old female with aplastic anemia who has failed antithymocyte immunoglobulin therapy with cyclosporine. The patient has a sibling donor who is fully HLA matched.

Description of Procedure (38230)

The donor is brought to the operating room and general anesthesia is administered. Approximately 400 needle sticks are administered to collect bone marrow from the posterior iliac crest. Blood is given to the donor for red blood cell support, and as needed, irradiated packed RBCs are provided. The donor is moved to supine position, is extubated and transferred to the recovery room.

Clinical Example (38232)

Patient is a 66-year-old male with multiple myeloma, who is unable to have a peripheral blood stem cell collection because of the use of pretransplant Revlimid. The patient's marrow cellularity is approximately 20%.

Description of Procedure (38232)

The patient is brought to the operating room and general anesthesia is administered. Approximately 400 needle sticks are administered to collect bone marrow from the posterior iliac crest. Blood is given to the patient for red blood cell support as needed. The patient is moved to supine position, is extubated and transferred to the recovery room.

Lymph Nodes and Lymphatic Channels

RADICAL LYMPHADENECTOMY (RADICAL RESECTION OF LYMPH NODES)

+▲38746   Thoracic lymphadenectomy by thoracotomy, mediastinal and regional lymphadenectomy (List separately in addition to code for primary procedure)

▶(On the right, mediastinal lymph nodes include the paratracheal, subcarinal, paraesophageal, and inferior pulmonary ligament)◀

▶(On the left, mediastinal lymph nodes include the aortopulmonary window, subcarinal, paraesophageal, and inferior pulmonary ligament)◀

▶(Report 38746 in conjunction with 32440, 32442, 32445, 32480, 32482, 32484, 32486, 32488, 32503, 32504, 32505)◀

▶(To report mediastinal and regional lymphadenectomy via thoracoscopy [VATS], see 32674)◀

 Rationale

Code 38746 has been editorially revised to more specifically identify the intended use for this code. This has been accomplished by revision of descriptor language that identifies the location of the node resections (ie, regional nodes of the mediastinum) and approach for the resection (ie, by thoracotomy). Other clarifications have been provided for users via citation of parenthetical notes that identify: (1) the nodes that are included as mediastinal lymph nodes on both the left and the right; (2) the codes with which add-on code 38746 is intended to be reported; and (3) the appropriate code to report mediastinal and regional lymphadenectomy via thoracoscopy (VATS).

For more information regarding VATS procedures, see the rationale listed following the Lungs and Pleura subheading.

 Clinical Example (38746)

A 60-year-old female has a right lower lobectomy by thoracotomy (separately reported) for a clinical stage I adenocarcinoma. Clinical guidelines indicate the need for a complete thoracic regional and mediastinal lymphadenectomy. Mediastinal lymph nodes include the paratracheal, subcarinal, paraesophageal, and inferior pulmonary ligament. The presence of tumor in any lymph nodes in the mediastinum signifies a significantly worse prognosis and indicates the need for postoperative adjuvant therapy.

(Please note this is an add-on code.)

Description of Procedure (38746)

In the ipsilateral open chest, dissect, and remove regional and mediastinal lymph nodes. On the right this includes the separate removal and labeling of lymph nodes from the following locations: paratracheal, subcarinal, inferior pulmonary ligament, paraesophageal, and hilar.

INTRODUCTION

38790   Injection procedure; lymphangiography

▲38792   radioactive tracer for identification of sentinel node

(For excision of sentinel node, see 38500-38542)

(For nuclear medicine lymphatics and lymph gland imaging, use 78195)

▶(For intraoperative identification (eg, mapping) of sentinel lymph node(s) including injection of non-radioactive dye, see 38900)◀

✎ Rationale

The term "radioactive tracer" has been added to code 38792 to clarify that this code should be reported only for injection of a radioactive tracer for sentinel node identification. A parenthetical note has been added following code 38792 to direct users to code 38900, when the injection for sentinel node identification is of nonradioactive dye.

Mediastinum and Diaphragm

Mediastinum

INCISION

39000   Mediastinotomy with exploration, drainage, removal of foreign body, or biopsy; cervical approach

39010   transthoracic approach, including either transthoracic or median sternotomy

▶(For VATS pericardial biopsy, use 32604)◀

✎ Rationale

A parenthetical note has been placed following code 39010 to direct users to the appropriate code for VATS pericardial biopsy (32604). For more information regarding VATS procedures, see the rationale listed following the Lungs and Pleura subheading.

▶Excision/Resection◀

▲**39200**   Resection of mediastinal cyst

▲**39220**   Resection of mediastinal tumor

(For substernal thyroidectomy, use 60270)

(For thymectomy, use 60520)

▶(For thoracoscopic [VATS] resection of mediastinal cyst, tumor, or mass, use 32662)◀

🖎 Rationale

In conjunction with other editorial revisions for services listed for lung-related procedures, codes 39200 and 39220 have been editorially revised to include the term "resection" to more specifically identify the intended use for these codes. In compliance with this, the section heading has also been revised to reflect inclusion of services that use either term.

ENDOSCOPY

▲**39400**   Mediastinoscopy, includes biopsy(ies), when performed

🖎 Rationale

Code 39400 has been editorially revised to reflect conventional CPT coding language. This is reflected by the replacement of the terms " . . . with or without biopsy" with the terms ". . . includes biopsy(ies) when performed."

Digestive System

Stomach

LAPAROSCOPY

43647   Laparoscopy, surgical; implantation or replacement of gastric neurostimulator electrodes, antrum

43648   revision or removal of gastric neurostimulator electrodes, antrum

(For open approach, see 43881, 43882)

(For insertion of gastric neurostimulator pulse generator, use 64590)

(For revision or removal of gastric neurostimulator pulse generator, use 64595)

(For electronic analysis and programming of gastric neurostimulator pulse generator, see 95980-95982)

▶(For laparoscopic implantation, revision, or removal of gastric neurostimulator electrodes, lesser curvature [morbid obesity], use 43659)◀

⊘=Modifier 51 Exempt   ⊙=Moderate Sedation   ✚=Add-on Code   ✗=FDA approval pending

Rationale

In support of the deletion of Category III codes 0155T and 0156T, the cross-reference note following code 43648 has been updated.

OTHER PROCEDURES

43882 Revision or removal of gastric neurostimulator electrodes, antrum, open

(For laparoscopic approach, see 43647, 43648)

(For insertion of gastric neurostimulator pulse generator, use 64590)

(For revision or removal of gastric neurostimulator pulse generator, use 64595)

(For electronic analysis and programming of gastric neurostimulator pulse generator, see 95980-95982)

▶(For open implantation, revision, or removal of gastric neurostimulator electrodes, lesser curvature [morbid obesity], use 43999)◀

(For electronic analysis and programming of gastric neurostimulator, lesser curvature, use Category III code 0162T)

Rationale

In support of the deletion of Category III codes 0157T and 0158T, the cross-reference note following code 43882 has been updated.

Anus

ENDOSCOPY

46600 Anoscopy; diagnostic, with or without collection of specimen(s) by brushing or washing (separate procedure)

46615 with ablation of tumor(s), polyp(s), or other lesion(s) not amenable to removal by hot biopsy forceps, bipolar cautery or snare technique

▶(For delivery of thermal energy to the muscle of the anal canal, use 0288T)◀

Rationale

A parenthetical note was added below code 46615 to direct the use of Category III code 0288T for anoscopy with delivery of thermal energy to the muscle of the anal canal (eg, for fecal incontinence).

Liver

INCISION

⊙▲**47000** Biopsy of liver, needle; percutaneous

Rationale

Code 47000 has been revised, adding the conscious sedation symbol, to note that moderate sedation is inherently included as part of this procedure.

Abdomen, Peritoneum, and Omentum

INCISION

▶(49080, 49081 have been deleted. To report, see 49082-49084)◀

● **49082**   Abdominal paracentesis (diagnostic or therapeutic); without imaging guidance

● **49083**   with imaging guidance

▶(Do not report 49083 in conjunction with 76942, 77002, 77012, 77021)◀

● **49084**   Peritoneal lavage, including imaging guidance, when performed

▶(Do not report 49084 in conjunction with 76942, 77002, 77012, 77021)◀

Rationale

As a result of the AMA/Specialty Society RVS Update Committee (RUC) analyses, codes 49080 and 49081 have been identified as codes for which the dominant providers have changed from when these codes were originally surveyed. For this reason, codes 49080 and 49081 and related cross-references have been deleted from the CPT 2012 code set. Instead, abdominal paracentesis codes 49082 and 49083 and peritoneal lavage code 49084 have been established. Code 49082 is intended to report abdominal paracentesis without imaging. Code 49083 is intended to report abdominal paracentesis with imaging. Code 49084 is intended to report peritoneal lavage including imaging guidance when performed.

A parenthetical note has been added to instruct users to see codes 49082, 49083, 49084 for reporting the services previously described by deleted codes 49080 and 49081. A parenthetical note has been added following code 49083 to preclude reporting code 49083 in conjunction with codes 76942, 77002, 77012, and 77021. A second parenthetical note has been added following code 49084 to preclude reporting code 49084 in conjunction with codes 76942, 77002, 77012, and 77021.

Clinical Example (49082)

A 45-year-old male with cirrhosis and symptomatic ascites that has not responded to medical and dietary management

Description of Procedure (49082)

The patient is examined, the presence of ascites confirmed with physical examination, and an appropriate location for paracentesis is identified using palpation and percussion. The patient's abdomen is sterilely prepared with skin antiseptic (eg, iodine, providine, chlorhexidine, etc) and draped with sterile sheets. The skin and deeper tissues down to the peritoneum are infiltrated with a local anesthetic. A small incision is made. A needle or catheter is advanced into the peritoneal space and fluid aspirated. A sample of fluid is sent for laboratory analysis. The needle or

⊘ =Modifier 51 Exempt   ⊙=Moderate Sedation   ✚ =Add-on Code   ✗ =FDA approval pending

catheter is then attached to a vacuum bottle and ascites fluid is drained. The catheter position is adjusted periodically as needed during ascites drainage to mitigate adherent bowel due to suction thus ensuring maximum drainage The needle or catheter is removed. If necessary, a suture is placed.

Clinical Example (49083)

A 59-year-old female with metastatic ovarian cancer and previously demonstrated loculated ascitic for removal for reaccumulating symptomatic ascitic fluid.

Description of Procedure (49083)

The patient is examined and the presence of ascites confirmed with physical examination. Ultrasound is used to interrogate the abdomen for extent and appropriate pockets of ascites, presence of echogenic complex fluid, or loculations, and identification of subjacent organs and abdominal wall vasculature. Images are recorded. The skin and deeper tissues down to the peritoneum are infiltrated with a local anesthetic under ultrasound guidance taking care to avoid vessels. A small incision is made. Using real-time ultrasound guidance a needle is advanced into the peritoneal space and fluid aspirated. A sample of fluid is sent for laboratory analysis. Using Seldinger technique, a centesis catheter is advanced into the ascites and secured in place temporarily. The catheter is then attached to a vacuum bottle and a variable amount of fluid (~3-5 liters) is drained. The catheter position is adjusted to avoid adhering to bowel due to suction, thus ensuring maximum drainage. Ultrasound is used to help in repositioning.

Clinical Example (49084)

A 55-year-old male is seen in the emergency room, hemodynamically unstable with multiple trauma following a motor vehicle collision. Peritoneal lavage is performed to assess for blood, the presence of enteric contents, and for further laboratory analysis.

Description of Procedure (49084)

A vertical skin incision is made one-third of the distance from the umbilicus to the symphysis pubis (above the umbilicus if pelvic fracture is suspected). The linea alba is divided and the peritoneum entered after it has been picked up to prevent bowel perforation. A catheter is inserted towards the pelvis and aspiration of material attempted using a syringe. If no blood is aspirated, 1 liter of warm 0.9% saline is infused. Five minutes are allowed for equilibration. The IV bag is then lowered to allow for retrieval of intraperitoneal fluid via siphoning effect. Altering position of patient/catheter is performed to maximize retrieval of effluent. Effluent is sent for analysis.

INTRODUCTION, REVISION, REMOVAL

⊙49418 Insertion of tunneled intraperitoneal catheter (eg, dialysis, intraperitoneal chemotherapy instillation, management of ascites), complete procedure, including imaging guidance, catheter placement, contrast injection when performed, and radiological supervision and interpretation, percutaneous

⊙49419 Insertion of tunneled intraperitoneal catheter, with subcutaneous port (ie, totally implantable)

(For removal, use 49422)

▶(49420 has been deleted. To report open placement of a tunneled intraperitoneal catheter for dialysis, use 49421. To report open or percutaneous peritoneal drainage or lavage, see 49020, 49021, 49040, 49041, 49082-49084, as appropriate. To report percutaneous insertion of a tunneled intraperitoneal catheter without subcutaneous port, use 49418)◀]

✍ Rationale

The parenthetical note following code 49419 has been revised to note that code 49421 is for open placement of an "intraperitoneal" tunneled catheter, and that 49418 is the code for percutaneous insertion of an "intraperitoneal" tunneled catheter "without subcutaneous port." In addition, the reference for reporting open or percutaneous peritoneal drainage has been revised to specify the intent of these codes to report lavage and the listed codes were revised to direct users to codes 49020, 49021, 49040, 49041, 49080, 49081, 49082, 49083, and 49084.

Female Genital System

(For pelvic laparotomy, use 49000)

(For excision or destruction of endometriomas, open method, see 49203-49205, 58957, 58958)

▶(For paracentesis, see 49082, 49083, 49084)◀

(For secondary closure of abdominal wall evisceration or disruption, use 49900)

(For fulguration or excision of lesions, laparoscopic approach, use 58662)

(For chemotherapy, see 96401-96549)

✍ Rationale

In support of the establishment of codes 49082, 49083, and 49084 the above parenthetical note has been added to direct users to these new codes.

Vagina

REPAIR

57282 Colpopexy, vaginal; extra-peritoneal approach (sacrospinous, iliococcygeus)

57283 intra-peritoneal approach (uterosacral, levator myorrhaphy)

▶(Do not report 57283 in conjunction with 57556, 58263, 58270, 58280, 58292, 58294)◀

✍ Rationale

A parenthetical note has been added following intraperitoneal colpopexy code 57283 instructing users not to report code 57283 with codes 57556, 58263, 58270, 58280, 58292, and 58294. All these codes describe procedures with enterocele repair, which is performed via intraperitoneal colpopexy. Colpopexy is an inclusive component of these codes and should not be reported separately.

⊘=Modifier 51 Exempt   ⊙=Moderate Sedation   ✚ =Add-on Code   ✗ =FDA approval pending

Corpus Uteri

EXCISION

Hysterectomy Procedures

58260   Vaginal hysterectomy, for uterus 250 g or less;

58263   with removal of tube(s), and/or ovary(s), with repair of enterocele

 Rationale

In support of the clarifying parenthetical note that has been added following code 57283, the parenthetical note following code 58263 instructing users not to report code 58263 with code 57283 has been deleted. Please see the discussion of the new parenthetical note following code 57283 in the Surgery/Female Genital System/Vagina/Repair section of this book.

INTRODUCTION

▶(To report insertion of non-biodegradable drug delivery implant for contraception, use 11981. To report removal of implantable contraceptive capsules with subsequent insertion of non-biodegradable drug delivery implant, use 11976 and 11981)◀

58300   Insertion of intrauterine device (IUD)

 Rationale

In support of the deletion of codes 11975 and 11977, the parenthetical note above code 58300 has been revised by adding instructions for reporting insertion of a nonbiodegradable drug delivery implant for contraception and reporting removal of implantable contraceptive capsules with subsequent insertion of a nonbiodegradable drug delivery implant. Please see the discussion of the deletion of codes 11975 and 11977 in the Surgery/Integumentary System/Introduction section of this book.

Endocrine System

Parathyroid, Thymus, Adrenal Glands, Pancreas, and Carotid Body

EXCISION

60520   Thymectomy, partial or total; transcervical approach (separate procedure)

60521   sternal split or transthoracic approach, without radical mediastinal dissection (separate procedure)

60522   sternal split or transthoracic approach, with radical mediastinal dissection (separate procedure)

▶(For thoracoscopic [VATS] thymectomy, see 32673)◀

Rationale

A parenthetical note has been added following code 60522 to direct users to the appropriate code for reporting thoracoscopic thymectomy.

Nervous System

Skull, Meninges, and Brain

NEUROSTIMULATORS (INTRACRANIAL)

61885 Insertion or replacement of cranial neurostimulator pulse generator or receiver, direct or inductive coupling; with connection to a single electrode array

61886   with connection to 2 or more electrode arrays

(For percutaneous placement of cranial nerve (eg, vagal, trigeminal) neurostimulator electrode(s), use 64553)

▶(For revision or removal of cranial nerve (eg, vagal, trigeminal) neurostimulator electrode array, use 64569)◀

 Rationale

The cross-reference following code 61886 was revised by replacing code 64585 with 64569, which appropriately references the revision or removal of a cranial nerve neurostimulator electrode array.

Spine and Spinal Cord

INJECTION, DRAINAGE, OR ASPIRATION

Injection of contrast during fluoroscopic . . .

For radiologic supervision and interpretation . . .

Code 62263 describes a catheter-based . . .

Code 62264 describes multiple adhesiolysis . . .

Codes 62263 and 62264 include the procedure . . .

▶Fluoroscopy (for localization) may be used in the placement of injections reported with 62310-62319, but is not required. If used, fluoroscopy should be reported with 77003. For epidurography, use 72275.

The placement and use of a catheter to administer one or more epidural or subarachnoid injections on a single calendar day should be reported in the same manner as if a needle had been used, ie, as a single injection using either 62310 or 62311. Such injections should not be reported with 62318 or 62319.

Threading a catheter into the epidural space, injecting substances at one or more levels and then removing the catheter should be treated as a single injection (62310, 62311). If the catheter is left in place to deliver substance(s) over a prolonged period (ie, more than a single calendar day) either continuously or via intermittent bolus, use 62318, 62319 as appropriate.

⊘=Modifier 51 Exempt   ⊙=Moderate Sedation   ✚=Add-on Code   ✔=FDA approval pending

When reporting 62310-62319, code choice is based on the region at which the needle or catheter entered the body (eg, lumbar). Codes 62310-62319 should be reported only once, when the substance injected spreads or catheter tip insertion moves into another spinal region (eg, 62311 is reported only once for injection or catheter insertion at L3-4 with spread of the substance or placement of the catheter tip to the thoracic region).

Percutaneous spinal procedures are done with indirect visualization (eg, image guidance or endoscopic approaches) and without direct visualization (including through a microscope). Endoscopic assistance during an open procedure with direct visualization is reported using excision codes (eg, 63020-63035).◀

(Report 01996 for daily hospital management of continuous epidural or subarachnoid drug administration performed in conjunction with 62318-62319)

▲**62287** Decompression procedure, percutaneous, of nucleus pulposus of intervertebral disc, any method utilizing needle based technique to remove disc material under fluoroscopic imaging or other form of indirect visualization, with the use of an endoscope, with discography and/or epidural injection(s) at the treated level(s), when performed, single or multiple levels, lumbar

▶(This includes endoscopic approach)◀

▶(Do not report 62287 in conjunction with 62267, 62290, 62311, 77003, 77012, 72295, when performed at same level)◀

▶(For non-needle based technique for percutaneous decompression of nucleus pulposus of intervertebral disc, see codes 0276T, 0277T)◀

🖎 Rationale

A number of changes have been implemented within this section to identify the correct intent for identifying open versus percutaneous procedures for decompression procedures for the spine. The changes include additions, deletions, and revisions to guidelines, parenthetical notes, and code descriptors. The changes have been provided to differentiate percutaneous spinous procedures from their open counterparts and to instruct users regarding the intended use of these codes.

New guideline language has been included in the Injection, Drainage, or Aspiration subsection for Spine and Spinal Cord procedures. The language has been added to: (1) provide a definition for services that should be identified as "percutaneous spinal procedures"; (2) to instruct users that percutaneous spinal procedures do not include services done via use of a microscope; and (3) to direct users to the appropriate codes to use for endoscopically-assisted open spinal procedures (eg, use of code 63020-63035).

Changes were also made to code 62287 through the addition of descriptor language that specifies that this code is intended to identify indirect decompressive spinal procedures. The language ". . . utilizing needle-based technique to remove disc material **under fluoroscopic imaging or other form of indirect visualization,** with the use of an endoscope, with discography and/or epidural injection(s) at the treated level(s) . . ." provides users with specific directions noting that this code is intended to identify *percutaneous needle removal of disc material **via use of indirect visualization.***

A number of parenthetical notes have also been placed following code 62287, which note: (1) that this procedure ". . . includes endoscopic approach"; (2) services that are precluded from use with code 62287; and (3) appropriate codes to use to report non-needle based techniques for percutaneous decompression procedures of the nucleus pulposus of the disc.

▲**62310**   Injection(s), of diagnostic or therapeutic substance(s) (including anesthetic, antispasmodic, opioid, steroid, other solution), not including neurolytic substances, including needle or catheter placement, includes contrast for localization when performed, epidural or subarachnoid; cervical or thoracic

▲**62311**   lumbar or sacral (caudal)

▲**62318**   Injection(s), including indwelling catheter placement, continuous infusion or intermittent bolus, of diagnostic or therapeutic substance(s) (including anesthetic, antispasmodic, opioid, steroid, other solution), not including neurolytic substances, includes contrast for localization when performed, epidural or subarachnoid; cervical or thoracic

▲**62319**   lumbar or sacral (caudal)

Rationale

For CPT 2012, the codes that describe epidural or subarachnoid injection(s) of diagnostic or therapeutic substance(s), codes 62310, 62311, 62318, and 62319, were editorially revised.

Codes 62310-62311 are intended to report epidural or subarachnoid injection(s) of the cervical, thoracic, lumbar, or sacral regions. These codes are reported when a catheter is placed to administer one or more epidural or subarachnoid injections on a single calendar day, as a single injection. Additionally, threading a catheter into the epidural space and injecting substances at one or more levels and then removing the catheter should be treated as a single injection and reported with 62310 or 62311, as appropriate. Code selection is based upon the region at which the needle or catheter entered the body. Code 62310 is reported for the cervical or thoracic region, and code 62311 for the lumbar or sacral region.

Codes 62318 and 62319 are intended to be reported if the catheter is left in place to deliver substance(s) over a prolonged period (ie, more than a single calendar day) either continuously or via intermittent bolus. Again, code selection is based on the region at which the needle or catheter entered the body (eg, lumbar): code 62318 for the cervical or thoracic region and code 62319 for the lumbar or sacral region. Codes 62310-62319 should be reported only once, when the substance injected spreads or catheter tip insertion moves into another spinal region.

Fluoroscopy (for localization) may be used in the placement of injections reported with codes 62310-62319 but is not required. If used, fluoroscopy should be reported separately with code 77003.

RESERVOIR/PUMP IMPLANTATION

▲ **62367**   Electronic analysis of programmable, implanted pump for intrathecal or epidural drug infusion (includes evaluation of reservoir status, alarm status, drug prescription status); without reprogramming or refill

62368   with reprogramming

(For refilling and maintenance of an implantable infusion pump for spinal or brain drug therapy, see 95990-95991)

● **62369**   with reprogramming and refill

● **62370**   with reprogramming and refill (requiring physician's skill)

▶(Do not report 62367-62370 in conjunction with 95990, 95991. For refilling and maintenance of a reservoir or an implantable infusion pump for spinal or brain drug delivery without reprogramming, see 95990, 95991)◀

 Rationale

The AMA/Specialty Society RVS Update Committee (RUC) identified codes 62367, 62368, 95990, and 95991 in the "Codes Reported Together 75% or More" screen. As a result, the services described by these codes have been combined as appropriate by revising code 62367, adding two new codes to this code family, and revising codes 95990 and 95991. See the Medicine/Neurology and Neuromuscular Procedures/Other Procedures section of this book for an explanation of the revisions to codes 95990 and 95991.

Code 62367 has been revised to specify that it does not include refilling of a programmable, implanted pump that is used for intrathecal or epidural drug infusion. Codes 62369 and 62370 were added to this code family to report electronic analysis of a programmable, implanted pump for intrathecal or epidural drug infusion, including reprogramming and refilling of the pump. Code 62369 is reported when a physician's skill is not required to perform the service. Code 62370 should be reported when the service does require a physician's skill.

Codes 62367-62370 should not be reported with codes 95990 and 95991. Codes 95990 and 95991 should be reported for refilling and maintenance without reprogramming (when performed) on a reservoir or an implantable infusion pump for spinal or brain drug delivery.

 Clinical Example (62367)

A 65-year-old male presents for an electronic analysis of an implanted infusion pump that delivers opiates and has successfully controlled his pain due to prostate cancer and metastases to multiple bone sites in the lower body and resultant bilateral leg and pelvic bone pain (rated 8/10). Because of the multiple sites of bone involvement and lack of response to chemotherapy, no radiation therapy or further chemotherapy is planned. His expected survival time from his cancer is 9 months. The electronic analysis of the implanted pump device, which determines the rate of infusion and the amount of morphine solution remaining in the pump reservoir, indicates a satisfactory infusion rate and residual volume; so no reprogramming or refill is needed.

Description of Procedure (62367)

Electronic analysis is performed to determine reservoir status, alarm status, and the drug prescription status. Because the electronic analysis of the implanted pump device indicates a satisfactory infusion rate and residual volume; no reprogramming or refill is needed.

 Clinical Example (62369)

A 65-year-old male has prostate cancer and metastases to multiple bone sites in the lowerbody and resultant bilateral leg and pelvic bone pain. A permanent implantable subcutaneous programmable infusion pump and an intrathecal infusion catheter were implanted for a long-term intrathecal infusion of narcotic. Because of inadequate pain control, the patient now presents for refill and reprogramming of his pump, not requiring physician's skill.

Description of Procedure (62369)

The nurse fills the pump under physician supervision and then electronic analysis is performed to determine reservoir status, alarm status, and the drug prescription status. Electronic analysis of the pump function verifies the infusion rate. Based on the patient's evaluation, the pump is then reprogrammed to adjust the rate of infusion and control the increased level of pain. The pump alarm settings and reservoir levels are programmed as well as any changes made to the drug infusion concentration or mixture. Refill date estimates are also made.

 Clinical Example (62370)

A 65-year-old male has prostate cancer and metastases to multiple bone sites in the lower body and resultant bilateral leg and pelvic bone pain. A permanent implantable subcutaneous programmable infusion pump and an intrathecal infusion catheter were implanted for a long-term intrathecal infusion of narcotic. Because of inadequate pain control the patient now presents for refill (requiring physician's skill because of difficult access or other medical issues or complex reprogramming of his pump).

Description of Procedure (62370)

Electronic analysis is performed to determine reservoir status, alarm status, drug prescription status. The subcutaneous pump is palpated and identified. The entire area over the pump is prepped and draped. Throughout all this procedure, sterile technique is meticulous to prevent infection. A pump refill kit is then opened and extra required supplies added to the kit. The solution's container is checked to be sure that the drug, the drug volume, and the drug's concentration are all correct according to what was ordered. Using sterile technique, the drug to be injected into the pump is then drawn from its transport vial into a sterile syringe using a filter needle. The syringe is then connected to a Huber needle with an extension tube in the kit. The needle is advanced and probed to find the actual center of the pump reservoir and advanced through the injection septum of the pump into the reservoir to the proper depth. The residual volume of the solution is aspirated from the pump/reservoir and is measured and checked against the medical records and/or pump status printout to make sure the entire volume of the pump/reservoir has been removed. The syringe containing the new solution attached to the tubing and then very slowly injected into the pump/reservoir. The patient is examined and pump/reservoir are then checked for any possible error in administration. The pump is then reprogrammed to adjust the rate of infusion and control the increased level of pain. The pump alarm settings and reservoir levels are programmed as well as any changes made to the drug infusion concentration or mixture. Refill date estimates are also made.

POSTERIOR EXTRADURAL LAMINOTOMY OR LAMINECTOMY FOR EXPLORATION/ DECOMPRESSION OF NEURAL ELEMENTS OR EXCISION OF HERNIATED INTERVERTEBRAL DISCS

▶Endoscopically assisted laminotomy (hemilaminectomy) requires open and direct visualization. When visualization is only endoscopic and/or image guidance, the procedure is percutaneous and reported using 0274T, 0275T.◀

(When 63001-63048 are followed by arthrodesis, see 22590-22614)

▲63020   Laminotomy (hemilaminectomy), with decompression of nerve root(s), including partial facetectomy, foraminotomy and/or excision of herniated intervertebral disc; 1 interspace, cervical

(For bilateral procedure, report 63020 with modifier 50)

▲63030   1 interspace, lumbar

(For bilateral procedure, report 63030 with modifier 50)

+▲63035   each additional interspace, cervical or lumbar (List separately in addition to code for primary procedure)

(Use 63035 in conjunction with 63020-63030)

(For bilateral procedure, report 63035 with modifier 50)

▶(For percutaneous endoscopic approach, see 0274T, 0275T)◀

✍ Rationale

Introductory guidelines have been added to the spinal procedures section to note that endoscopically assisted laminotomy (hemilaminectomy) procedures require open and direct visualization. If the visualization is performed via endoscope and/or image guidance, then the procedure is considered to be percutaneous. In these circumstances, codes 0274T and/or 0275T should be used to identify the laminotomy procedure performed. To further clarify this, the common descriptor of the parent code 63020 has been revised by deleting the phrase ". . . including open and endoscopically assisted approaches . . .," further clarifying that codes 63020-63035 are intended to be used for open laminotomies done with direct visualization. A cross-reference has also been inserted following code 63035 directing users to codes 0274T and 0275T for reporting percutaneous endoscopic approaches for lamoninotomies.

Extracranial Nerves, Peripheral Nerves, and Autonomic Nervous System

NEUROSTIMULATORS (PERIPHERAL NERVE)

▶Codes 64553-64595 apply to both simple and complex neurostimulators. For initial or subsequent electronic analysis and programming of neurostimulator pulse generators, see codes 95970-95975. An electrode array is a catheter or other device with more than one contact. The function of each contact may be capable of being adjusted during programming services.◀

▶(For implantation of trial or permanent electrode arrays or pulse generators for peripheral subcutaneous field stimulation, see 0282T-0284T)◀

64550   Application of surface (transcutaneous) neurostimulator

▲**64553**   Percutaneous implantation of neurostimulator electrode array; cranial nerve

(For open placement of cranial nerve (eg, vagal, trigeminal) neurostimulator pulse generator or receiver, see 61885, 61886, as appropriate)

▲**64555**   peripheral nerve (excludes sacral nerve)

(Do not report 64555 in conjunction with 64566)

▶(64560 has been deleted)◀

▲**64561**   sacral nerve (transforaminal placement)

▲**64565**   neuromuscular

64566   Posterior tibial neurostimulation, percutaneous needle electrode, single treatment, includes programming

(Do not report 64566 in conjunction with 64555, 95970-95972)

64568   Incision for implantation of cranial nerve (eg, vagus nerve) neurostimulator electrode array and pulse generator

(Do not report 64568 in conjunction with 61885, 61886, 64570)

64569   Revision or replacement of cranial nerve (eg, vagus nerve) neurostimulator electrode array, including connection to existing pulse generator

(Do not report 64569 in conjunction with 64570 or 61888)

(For replacement of pulse generator, use 61885)

64570   Removal of cranial nerve (eg, vagus nerve) neurostimulator electrode array and pulse generator

(Do not report 64570 in conjunction with 61888)

(64573 has been deleted)

▲**64575**   Incision for implantation of neurostimulator electrode array; peripheral nerve (excludes sacral nerve)

▶(64577 has been deleted)◀

▲**64580**   neuromuscular

▲ **64581** sacral nerve (transforaminal placement)

▲ **64585** Revision or removal of peripheral neurostimulator electrode array

 Rationale

Changes have been made to the neurostimulation codes throughout the CPT codebook to provide language that is the same for these procedures as well as to more clearly portray the intended use for these procedures. This includes revision to the guidelines following the neurostimulator heading, which has been revised to provide a definition for the term "electrode array" identifying that an array includes more than a single contact capable of being adjusted. This change accommodates the addition of the term "array" to codes 64553, 64555, 64561, 64565, 64575, 64580, 64581, and 64585, which have been revised to reflect the more appropriate term "electrode array."

In addition, codes 64560 and 64577 have been deleted, as these codes included obsolete language.

In support of the new peripheral field stimulation codes 0282T-0285T, a parenthetical note has been added in the Neurostimulators (Peripheral Nerve) section directing users to codes 0282T-0284T for peripheral field stimulation electrode array or pulse generator implantation procedures. Please see the discussion of codes 0282T-0285T in the Category III section of this book.

DESTRUCTION BY NEUROLYTIC AGENT (EG, CHEMICAL, THERMAL, ELECTRICAL OR RADIOFREQUENCY)

▶Codes 64600-64681 include the injection of other therapeutic agents (eg, corticosteroids). Do not report diagnostic/therapeutic injections separately. (For therapies that are not destructive of the target nerve [eg, pulsed radiofrequency], use 64999)◀

Somatic Nerves

64620 Destruction by neurolytic agent, intercostal nerve

▶(64622-64627 have been deleted. For image guided neurolysis of facet joint nerve(s), see 64633-64636)◀

▶(Imaging guidance [fluoroscopy, CT] are inclusive components of 64633-64636)◀

▶(Image guidance [fluoroscopy or CT] and any injection of contrast are inclusive components of 64633-64636. Image guidance and localization are required for the performance of paravertebral facet joint nerve destruction by neurolytic agent described by 64633-64636. If CT or fluoroscopic imaging is not used, report 64999)◀

▶(For paravertebral facet destruction by neurolysis of the T12-L1 joint, or nerves innervating that joint, use 64633)◀

#●**64633** Destruction by neurolytic agent, paravertebral facet joint nerve(s) with imaging guidance (fluoroscopy or CT); cervical or thoracic, single facet joint

▶(For bilateral procedure, report 64633 with modifier 50)◀

#+●64634   cervical or thoracic, each additional facet joint (List separately in addition to code for primary procedure)

▶(Use 64634 in conjunction with 64633)◀

▶(For bilateral procedure, report 64634 with modifier 50)◀

#●64635   lumbar or sacral, single facet joint

▶(For bilateral procedure, report 64635 with modifier 50)◀

#+●64636   lumbar or sacral, each additional facet joint (List separately in addition to code for primary procedure)

▶(Use 64636 in conjunction with 64635)◀

▶(For bilateral procedure, report 64636 with modifier 50)◀

▶(Do not report 64633-64636 in conjunction with 77003, 77012)◀

64630   Destruction by neurolytic agent; pudendal nerve

64632   plantar common digital nerve

(Do not report 64632 in conjunction with 64455)

64633   ▶Code is out of numerical sequence. See 64600-64640◀

64634   ▶Code is out of numerical sequence. See 64600-64640◀

64635   ▶Code is out of numerical sequence. See 64600-64640◀

64636   ▶Code is out of numerical sequence. See 64600-64640◀

🖎 Rationale

The paravertebral facet joint nerve codes 64622, 64623, 64626, and 64627 have been deleted. Four new codes have been established to more accurately reflect the work and anatomical site involved in these procedures. Prior to 2012, the unit of service used to report these procedures was a single nerve at a single vertebral level. However, two nerves innervate each facet joint, and there are two facet joints at each vertebral level. One or two facet joints at the same level potentially could be treated. As such, the vertebral level is of less significance than the number of facet joints treated, so using vertebral level as the unit of service did not adequately reflect the work performed. To address this issue, the unit of service is a single facet joint in new codes 64633, 64634, 64635, and 64636, rather than a vertebral level. If both facet joints at the same vertebral level are treated, then the parent code (64633 or 64635) should be reported with modifier 50 appended. It is important to note that the number of nerves injected for a single facet joint does not affect code selection. Therefore, the new codes indicate "nerve(s)" in the descriptors.

To be consistent with other procedures involving vertebra in the CPT code set, these codes are structured based on spinal region. Codes 64633 and 64634 specify the cervical or thoracic region. Codes 64635 and 64636 specify the lumbar or sacral region. Note that codes 64634 and 64636 are add-on codes. These codes should be reported for each additional facet joint at a different vertebral level in the same spinal region for which this procedure is performed.

The guidelines for the Extracranial Nerves, Peripheral Nerves, and Autonomic Nervous System/Destruction by Neurolytic Agent section have been updated to instruct users not to report diagnostic/therapeutic injections separately.

Several parenthetical notes have been deleted, revised, and added to provide guidance on the reporting of these services.

The guidelines regarding imaging guidance for destruction of facet joint nerves by neurolytic agent have changed for 2012. Previously, imaging guidance was separately reported using code 77003. Effective 2012, imaging guidance using fluoroscopy or CT is no longer separately reported and is considered an inclusive component of codes 64633-64636. To reflect these changes, code 77003 has been revised by removing the reference to neurolytic agent destruction. See the Radiology/Diagnostic Radiology (Diagnostic Imaging)/Radiologic Guidance/Fluoroscopic Guidance section of this book for an explanation of the revision of code 77003. Image guidance and localization are required for the performance of paravertebral facet joint nerve destruction by neurolytic agent as described by codes 64633-64636. If CT or fluoroscopic imaging is not used, then the Nervous System unlisted procedure code, 64999, should be reported.

The parenthetical note following code 64622 that instructed users to report code 77003 for fluoroscopic guidance and localization has been deleted. A parenthetical note has been added following code 64636 instructing users not to report codes 64633-64636 with imaging guidance codes 77003 and 77012.

Codes 64633, 64634, 64635, and 64636 appear with a number symbol (#) to indicate that these codes are out of numerical sequence. Four reference notes have been added to instruct the user to the appropriate code range of 64600-64640 for the placement of codes 64633, 64634, 64635, and 64636.

Clinical Example (64633)

A 65-year-old female involved in a flexion extension injury from an automobile accident presents with constant neck pain. The patient's history includes imaging studies with findings of minimal degenerative disc disease and cervical spondylosis. The patient had no relief with conservative treatments such as physical therapy, NSAIDs, or trigger point injections. Previous trials of cervical medial branch blocks provided significant short-term relief. She undergoes radiofrequency neurotomy of the two medial branch nerves innervating the symptomatic facet joint.

Description of Procedure (64633)

The patient is monitored with continuous pulse oximetry, blood pressure, and ECG. A C-arm fluoroscopy machine is rotated and adjusted until the targeted facet joint and the bony landmarks are optimally visualized. The skin and subcutaneous tissues are anesthetized with local anesthetic. A needle is directed towards the lateral facet pillar and groove under intermittent fluoroscopic guidance. Care must be taken to avoid vital neural structures or blood vessels. The patient is stimulated with appropriate frequencies for sensory and motor stimulation to verify that the needle is in the correct position. Appropriate positioning of the needle tip is confirmed with multiple fluoroscopic views, including A-P and lateral projections. Anesthetic is injected. Radiofrequency ablation of the nerve is performed. The probe is repositioned, to complete additional lesion(s) along the nerve. The entire procedure is repeated for the second medial branch nerve. After both nerves are lesioned, a dressing is applied.

Clinical Example (64634)

A 65-year-old female involved in a flexion extension injury from an automobile accident presents with constant neck pain. The patient's history includes imaging studies with findings of minimal degenerative disease and cervical spondylosis. The patient received no relief with conservative treatments such as physical therapy, NSAIDs, or trigger point injections. Previous trials of cervical medial branch blocks provided significant short-term relief. She undergoes radiofrequency neurotomy two medial branch nerves innervating the additional symptomatic facet joint.

Description of Procedure (64634)

The patient is monitored with continuous pulse oximetry, blood pressure, and ECG. A C-arm fluoroscopy machine is rotated and adjusted until the targeted facet joint and the bony landmarks are optimally visualized. The skin and subcutaneous tissues are anesthetized with local anesthetic. A needle is directed towards the lateral facet pillar and groove under intermittent fluoroscopic guidance. Care must be taken to avoid vital neural structures or blood vessels. The patient is stimulated with appropriate frequencies for sensory and motor stimulation to verify that the needle is in the correct position. Appropriate positioning of the needle tip is confirmed with multiple fluoroscopic views, including A-P and lateral projections. Anesthetic is injected. Radiofrequency ablation of the nerve is performed. The probe is repositioned, to complete additional lesion(s) along the nerve. The entire procedure is repeated for the second medial branch nerve. After both nerves are lesioned, a dressing is applied.

Clinical Example (64635)

A 65-year-old female involved in a flexion-extension injury from an automobile accident presents with constant low back pain. The patient's history includes imaging studies with findings of minimal degenerative disc disease and no facet arthropathy. The patient had no relief with conservative treatments such as physical therapy, NSAIDs, or trigger point injections. Previous trials of lumbar medial branch blocks provided significant short-term relief of her low back pain. She undergoes radiofrequency neurotomy of the two medial branch nerves innervating the symptomatic facet joint.

Description of Procedure (64635)

The patient is monitored with continuous pulse oximetry, blood pressure and ECG. A C-arm fluoroscopy machine is rotated and adjusted until the targeted facet joint and the bony landmarks are optimally visualized. The skin and subcutaneous tissues are anesthetized with local anesthetic. A needle is directed towards the lateral facet pillar and groove under intermittent fluoroscopic guidance. Care must be taken to avoid vital neural structures or blood vessels. The patient is stimulated with appropriate frequencies for sensory and motor stimulation to verify that the needle is in the correct position. Appropriate positioning of the needle tip is confirmed with multiple fluoroscopic views, including A-P and lateral projections. Anesthetic is injected. Radiofrequency ablation of the nerve is performed. The probe is repositioned, to complete additional lesion(s) along the nerve. The entire procedure is repeated for the second medial branch nerve. After both nerves are lesioned, a dressing is applied.

Clinical Example (64636)

A 65-year-old female involved in a flexion extension injury from an automobile accident presents with constant low back pain. The patient's history includes imaging studies with findings of minimal degenerative disc disease and no facet arthropathy. The patient had no relief with conservative treatments such as physical therapy, NSAIDs, or trigger point injections. Previous trials of lumbar medial branch blocks provided significant short-term relief. She undergoes radiofrequency neurotomy of the two medial branch nerves innervating the additional symptomatic facet joint.

Description of Procedure (64636)

The patient is monitored with continuous pulse oximetry, blood pressure, and ECG. A C-arm fluoroscopy machine is rotated and adjusted until the targeted facet joint and the bony landmarks are optimally visualized. The skin and subcutaneous tissues are anesthetized with local anesthetic. A needle is directed towards the lateral facet pillar and groove under intermittent fluoroscopic guidance. Care must be taken to avoid vital neural structures or blood vessels. The patient is stimulated with appropriate frequencies for sensory and motor stimulation to verify that the needle is in the correct position. Appropriate positioning of the needle tip is confirmed with multiple fluoroscopic views, including A-P and lateral projections. Anesthetic is injected. Radiofrequency ablation of the nerve is performed. The probe is repositioned, to complete additional lesion(s) along the nerve. The entire procedure is repeated for the second medial branch nerve. After both nerves are lesioned, a dressing is applied.

Eye and Ocular Adnexa

Eyeball

REPAIR OF LACERATION

65270   Repair of laceration; conjunctiva, with or without nonperforating laceration sclera, direct closure

65280   cornea and/or sclera, perforating, not involving uveal tissue

65285   cornea and/or sclera, perforating, with reposition or resection of uveal tissue

▶(65280 and 65285 are not used for repair of a surgical wound)◀

Rationale

A parenthetical note has been added following codes 65280 and 65285 to note that these codes are not used for surgical wound repair, as they are intended to be reported for trauma to the globe.

Anterior Segment

CORNEA

Other Procedures

65775 Corneal wedge resection for correction of surgically induced astigmatism

▶(For fitting of contact lens for treatment of disease, see 92071, 92072)◀

(For unlisted procedures on cornea, use 66999)

 Rationale

The parenthetical note following code 65775 has been revised to reference the new codes that have replaced code 92070 for the fitting of contact lenses, listed as 92071 for fitting of contact lens for the treatment of ocular surface disease and 92072 for fitting of contact lens for the management of keratoconus.

Auditory System

Inner Ear

INCISION AND/OR DESTRUCTION

69801 Labyrinthotomy, with perfusion of vestibuloactive drug(s); transcanal

▶(69802 has been deleted)◀

Rationale

Code 69802 has been deleted, as labyrinthotomy with mastoidectomy has become an obsolete procedure. It was determined that this service is considered obsolete and did not warrant referencing an unlisted code.

⊘=Modifier 51 Exempt   ⊙=Moderate Sedation   ✚=Add-on Code   ✔=FDA approval pending

Radiology

Ten new codes have been added to the Radiology section. Revisions have been made to eight codes and eighteen codes have been deleted. Significant changes have been made to the codes included in the Nuclear Medicine Respiratory System section to simplify the use for these testing procedures. In addition, new guidelines have been added in the Radiation Treatment Management subsection and revisions have been made to the Diagnostic Ultrasound guidelines.

Radiology

Diagnostic Radiology (Diagnostic Imaging)

Head and Neck

▲70355   Orthopantogram (eg, panoramic x-ray)

 Rationale

Code 70355 was editorially revised. The parenthetical example listed within the descriptor of code 70355 has been changed, citing "panoramic X ray" as an example of the type of service that is included when reporting the "orthopantogram" code. This example was included to verify the intended use for code 70355 as the correct code to use for panoramic X rays. To further exemplify this, a parenthetical note has been included following codes 76101 and 76102 directing users to code 70355 for reporting a panoramic X ray. An additional note has been included following codes 76101 and 76102 to limit reporting of these codes to once per day.

Chest

71060   Bronchography, bilateral, radiological supervision and interpretation

▶(71090 has been deleted. To report pacemaker or pacing cardioverter-defibrillator lead insertion, replacement, or revision procedures with fluoroscopic guidance, see 33206-33249. To report fluoroscopic guidance for diagnostic lead evaluation without lead insertion, replacement, or revision procedures, use 76000)◀

 Rationale

As a part of the changes to reporting of pacemaker and pacing cardioverter-defibrillator services, code 71090 has been deleted. Imaging guidance is now included in codes 33206-33249. A cross-reference has been added to the Radiology section instructing users to report codes 33206-33249 for pacemaker or pacing cardioverter-defibrillator lead insertion, replacement, or revision procedures with fluoroscopic guidance and to report code 76000 for fluoroscopic guidance for diagnostic lead evaluation without lead insertion, replacement, or revision. Please see the discussion of the changes to the pacemaker and pacing cardioverter-defibrillator services in the Surgery/Cardiovascular System/Heart and Pericardium/Pacemaker or Pacing Cardioverter-Defibrillator section of this book.

Spine and Pelvis

72100   Radiologic examination, spine, lumbosacral; 2 or 3 views

72110   minimum of 4 views

▲72114   complete, including bending views, minimum of 6 views

▲**72120**   bending views only, 2 or 3 views

(Contrast material in CT of spine is either by intrathecal or intravenous injection. For intrathecal injection, use also 61055 or 62284. IV injection of contrast material is part of the CT procedure.

🖎 Rationale

In response to the AMA/Specialty RVS Update Committee (RUC) deliberations and analyses, Radiology spine X-ray codes 72114 and 72120 were revised to clearly define the number of views for each code and to accurately reflect the work performed.

Code 72114 is intended to report spine, lumbosacral radiologic examination, complete, including bending views, minimum of 6 views.

Code 72120 is intended to report spine, lumbosacral radiological examination, bending views only, 2 or 3 views.

72170   Radiologic examination, pelvis; 1 or 2 views

72190   complete, minimum of 3 views

(For pelvimetry, use 74710)

▶(For a combined computed tomography (CT) or computed tomographic angiography abdomen and pelvis study, see 74174, 74176-74178)◀

72191   Computed tomographic angiography, pelvis, with contrast material(s), including noncontrast images, if performed, and image postprocessing

▶(Do not report 72191 in conjunction with 73706 or 75635. For CTA aorto-iliofemoral runoff, use 75635)◀

▶(Do not report 72191 in conjunction with 74175. For a combined computed tomographic angiography abdomen and pelvis study, use 74174)◀

🖎 Rationale

In support of the establishment of CT angiography code 74174, a cross-reference note was added following 72190 instructing users to report 74174 or 74176-74178 for a combined computed tomography (CT) or computed tomographic angiography abdomen and pelvis study.

Following 72191, two exclusionary parenthetical notes were added. The first note limits the use of 72191 in conjunction with 73706 or 75635. The note also indicates that 75635 should be reported for CTA aorto-iliofemoral runoff. The second note limits the use of 72191 in conjunction with 74175. The second note also indicates that code 74174 should be reported for combined computed tomographic angiography abdomen and pelvis study.

⚕ Clinical Example (72114)

A 32-year-old female presents with trauma to the lumbosacral spine from an auto accident. There is clinical concern for instability.

⊘=Modifier 51 Exempt   ⊙=Moderate Sedation   ✚=Add-on Code   ⊿=FDA approval pending

Description of Procedure (72114)

Supervise technologist performing the examination. Interpret radiographs of the lumbosacral spine. Compare with prior studies, if applicable. Dictate report.

 Clinical Example (72120)

A 45-year-old male presents with known Grade I spondylolisthesis from prior exams. There is clinical concern for instability. Bending views are ordered to evaluate for abnormal movement.

Description of Procedure (72120)

Supervise technologist performing the examination. Interpret radiographs of the lumbosacral spine. Compare with prior studies, if applicable. Dictate report.

Lower Extremities

73540   Radiologic examination, pelvis and hips, infant or child, minimum of 2 views

▶(73542 has been deleted, for arthrography use 27096)◀

 Rationale

Radiology arthrography code 73542 has been deleted. Code 27096 has been updated and now includes arthrography, when performed. An instructional note has been added following 73540 to indicate this change and direct the user to the appropriate code.

Abdomen

●74174   Computed tomographic angiography, abdomen and pelvis, with contrast material(s), including noncontrast images, if performed, and image postprocessing

▶(Do not report 74174 in conjunction with 72191, 73706, 74175, 75635, 76376, 76377)◀

▶(For CTA aorto-iliofemoral runoff, use 75635)◀

74175   Computed tomographic angiography, abdomen, with contrast material(s), including noncontrast images, if performed, and image postprocessing

▶(Do not report 74175 in conjunction with 73706 or 75635. For CTA aorto-iliofemoral runoff, use 75635)◀

▶(Do not report 74175 in conjunction with 72191. For a combined computed tomographic angiography abdomen and pelvis study, use 74174)◀

 Rationale

As part of the AMA/Specialty Society RVS Update Committee (RUC) analysis and as a result of the identification of high frequency of reporting CTA of the pelvis with contrast material (72191) and CTA of the pelvis with contrast material (74175) for the same patient, a combination code 74174 has been established to report computed tomography angiography (CTA) of the abdomen and pelvis study.

The stand-alone codes 72191 and 74175 have not been deleted and will remain the same for reporting those services in which a CTA of only the abdomen or pelvis is performed.

To aid users, cross-references and exclusionary notes have been added following codes 72191, 74174, 74175, and 75635 to report these services. Interchangeable exclusionary notes following codes 72191, 74174, and 74175 have been added restricting its use with CTA of the lower extremity 73706 and CTA of the abdominal aorta 75635 and notes that for a combined CTA of the abdomen and pelvis study report 74174. It also instructs to report code 75635 for CTA of the aorto-iliofemoral runoff study.

Clinical Example (74174)

A 67-year-old male has a 6 cm abdominal aortic aneurysm detected on routine screening ultrasound. He is undergoing computed tomographic angiography of the abdomen and pelvis for pre-operative evaluation prior to aortic endograft placement.

Description of Procedure (74174)

Supervise insertion of IV catheter, selection of contrast media, and set-up of mechanical injector. Supervise acquisition of scout views, prescribe area to be scanned, and supervise acquisition of unenhanced axial CT image data. Review the initial unenhanced series of CT image data to assure adequacy of anatomic coverage and assess need for additional sections, additional delayed images, or reconstruction of thin sections in specific locations. Supervise use of mechanical power injector for administration of a rapid (4-7 mL/sec) bolus of intravenous contrast during test-bolus or computer-assisted bolus tracking, and select optimal contrast delay that will result in peak contrast enhancement of major vessels. Supervise scanning for acquisition of axial source image sections in multiple phases of contrast enhancement. Supervise monitoring for contrast reaction or contrast extravasation during injection. Review the arterial and delayed phases of CT image data to assure adequacy of anatomic coverage and assess need for additional sections, additional delayed images, or reconstruction of thin sections in specific locations. Supervise reconstruction of coronal and/or sagittal 2D multiplanar reformatted (MPR) and 3D (such as volume rendering, maximum intensity projection [MIP]) images in multiple projections/views on scanner console or freestanding work-station, and assess need for oblique or other 2D or 3D images. Review and interpret scout radiographs, all source images, additional sections, multiplanar reformations, and 3D images—typically 800 images are acquired which increases to 1800 images when reviewed with the various requisite window/level settings. Axial and multiplanar reformatted images are interpreted in arterial phase and delayed phases using "soft-tissue windows" to provide detailed evaluation of each of the following organs: lower mediastinum, liver, spleen, gallbladder, adrenal glands, kidneys, ureters, bladder, retroperitoneal soft-tissues, stomach, duodenum, small bowel, appendix, colon, pelvic genito-urinary/reproductive organs, all lymph node chains, major abdominal arterial and venous vasculature, and supporting musculature. Axial and 2D reformatted images are interpreted using "vascular" windows to assess vessel contour and detect thrombus, "bone windows"

⊘=Modifier 51 Exempt   ⊙=Moderate Sedation   ✦=Add-on Code   ✗=FDA approval pending to assess the skeletal structures, "liver windows" to assess the liver and "lung windows" to assess the lung base visualized on the scan, 3D volume rendered and/or MIP images are interpreted. Perform measurements for selection of appropriate endovascular graft. Compare current findings to previous studies. Dictate report for the medical record.

Vascular Procedures

AORTA AND ARTERIES

75635   Computed tomographic angiography, abdominal aorta and bilateral iliofemoral lower extremity runoff, with contrast material(s), including noncontrast images, if performed, and image postprocessing

▶(Do not report 75635 in conjunction with 72191, 73706, 74175 or 74174)◀

75716   Angiography, extremity, bilateral, radiological supervision and interpretation

▶(75722 has been deleted. To report, see 36251, 36253)◀

▶(75724 has been deleted. To report, see 36252, 36254)◀

Rationale

In support of the establishment of code 74174, an exclusionary parenthetical note has been added following code 75635 precluding the reporting of code 75635 in conjunction with 72191, 73706, 74175 or 74174.

The Joint CPT/RUC Workgroup identified renal catheterization and angiography procedure codes in the "Codes Reported Together 75% or More" screen. As a result, the services described by these codes have been appropriately combined by deleting renal angiography codes 75722 and 75724, and establishing codes 36251-36254. See the Surgery/Cardiovascular System/Arteries and Veins/Vascular Injection/Procedures/Intra-Arterial—Intra-Aortic section of this book for an explanation of codes 36251-36254.

TRANSCATHETER PROCEDURES

75902   Mechanical removal of intraluminal (intracatheter) obstructive material from central venous device through device lumen, radiologic supervision and interpretation

(For procedure, use 36596)

(For venous catheterization, see 36010-36012)

▶(75940 has been deleted. To report, use 37191)◀

Rationale

In support of the deletion of ligation code 37620, code 75940 has also been deleted. A cross-reference has been added in the Radiology Transcatheter subsection to direct users to code 37191 to report endovascular insertion of intravascular vena cava filter.

75952 Endovascular repair of infrarenal abdominal aortic aneurysm or dissection, radiological supervision and interpretation

▶(For implantation of endovascular grafts, see 34800-34805)◀

▶(For radiologic supervision and interpretation of endovascular repair of abdominal aortic aneurysm involving visceral vessels, see Category III codes 0080T, 0081T)◀

75961 Transcatheter retrieval, percutaneous, of intravascular foreign body (eg, fractured venous or arterial catheter), radiological supervision and interpretation

(For procedure, use 37203)

🖎 Rationale

A number of revisions have been made to codes used to identify vascular surgery procedures. The changes were provided as an editorial enhancement that will provide improved instructions and better identify the intended use for many of the codes.

A parenthetical note directing users to the correct code to report radiological supervision and interpretation (S&I) that was located after code 34808 has been moved to a more appropriate location, ie, to follow code 34805 because 34805 is a main body endovascular abdominal aortic aneurysm repair (EVAR) code. This parenthetical is more appropriately placed following codes 34800-34805 because it is intended for use for guidance imaging that is necessary for main body endovascular abdominal aortic aneurysm repair and not for the report of guidance imaging for implantation of an iliac artery occlusion device (34808). The parenthetical following code 75952 has also been revised to reflect this.

An additional parenthetical listed after code 75952 has been revised to note that the code 0080T is the appropriate code to use to identify radiologic S&I for the Category III surgical procedures.

▶(For removal of a vena cava filter, use 37193)◀

▲**75962** Transluminal balloon angioplasty, peripheral artery other than renal, or other visceral artery, iliac or lower extremity, radiological supervision and interpretation

(For radiological supervision and interpretation for transluminal balloon angioplasty in iliac, femoral, popliteal, and tibial/peroneal arteries, see 37220-37235)

▶(For procedure, see 35458, 35475)◀

✚▲**75964** Transluminal balloon angioplasty, each additional peripheral artery other than renal, or other visceral artery, iliac or lower extremity, radiological supervision and interpretation (List separately in addition to code for primary procedure)

(Use 75964 in conjunction with 75962)

🖎 Rationale

In conjunction with the addition of code 37193, a cross-reference has been added following code 75961 (above code 75962) directing user to the appropriate code for reporting the removal of the vena cava filter.

⃠=Modifier 51 Exempt   ⊙=Moderate Sedation   ✚=Add-on Code   𝒩=FDA approval pending

Radiology codes 75962 and add-on code 75964 were editorially revised to remove the term "cervical carotid" from the code descriptor. Code 75964 was further revised by replacing the word "and" with "or."

A cross-reference was added to direct users to the appropriate codes for transluminal angioplasty services, 35458 (open) and 35475 (percutaneous).

Other Procedures

76101   Radiologic examination, complex motion (ie, hypercycloidal) body section (eg, mastoid polytomography), other than with urography; unilateral

76102   bilateral

►(Do not report 76101, 76102 more than once per day)◄

►(For panoramic X-ray, use 70355)◄

(For nephrotomography, use 74415)

 Rationale

Two parenthetical notes have been included following codes 76101 and 76102. These notes have been placed: (1) to verify that they are intended to be reported only once per day; and (2) to direct users to the correct code to report panoramic X rays.

76376   3D rendering with interpretation and reporting of computed tomography, magnetic resonance imaging, ultrasound, or other tomographic modality; not requiring image postprocessing on an independent workstation

(Use 76376 in conjunction with code[s] for base imaging procedure[s])

►(Do not report 76376 in conjunction with 31627, 70496, 70498, 70544-70549, 71275, 71555, 72159, 72191, 72198, 73206, 73225, 73706, 73725, 74174, 74175, 74185, 74261-74263, 75557, 75559, 75561, 75563, 75565, 75571-75574, 75635, 76377, 78000-78999, 0159T)◄

76377   requiring image postprocessing on an independent workstation

(Use 76377 in conjunction with code[s] for base imaging procedure[s])

►(Do not report 76377 in conjunction with 70496, 70498, 70544-70549, 71275, 71555, 72159, 72191, 72198, 73206, 73225, 73706, 73725, 74174, 74175, 74185, 74261-74263, 75557, 75559, 75561, 75563, 75565, 75571-75574, 75635, 76376, 78000-78999, 0159T)◄

 Rationale

In support of the establishment of code 74174, the exclusionary parenthetical note following codes 76376 and 76377 has been revised precluding the reporting of the combined CTA of the abdomen and pelvis study 74174 in conjunction with these services.

Diagnostic Ultrasound

All diagnostic ultrasound examinations require permanently recorded images with measurements, when such measurements are clinically indicated. For those codes whose sole diagnostic goal is a biometric measure (ie, 76514, 76516, and 76519), permanently recorded images are not required. A final, written report should be issued for inclusion in the patient's medical record. The prescription form for the intraocular lens satisfies the written report requirement for 76519. For those anatomic regions that have "complete" and "limited" ultrasound codes, note the elements that comprise a "complete" exam. The report should contain a description of these elements or the reason that an element could not be visualized (eg, obscured by bowel gas, surgically absent).

If less than the required elements for a "complete" exam are reported (eg, limited number of organs or limited portion of region evaluated), the "limited" code for that anatomic region should be used once per patient exam session. A "limited" exam of an anatomic region should not be reported for the same exam session as a "complete" exam of that same region.

▶Evaluation of vascular structures using both color and spectral Doppler is separately reportable. To report, see **Noninvasive Vascular Diagnostic Studies** (93880-93990). However, color Doppler alone, when performed for anatomic structure identification in conjunction with a real-time ultrasound examination, is not reported separately.◀

Ultrasound guidance procedures also require permanently recorded images of the site to be localized, as well as a documented description of the localization process, either separately or within the report of the procedure for which the guidance is utilized.

Use of ultrasound, without thorough evaluation of organ(s) or anatomic region, image documentation, and final, written report, is not separately reportable.

Definitions

A-mode implies a one-dimensional ultrasonic measurement procedure.

M-mode implies a one-dimensional ultrasonic measurement procedure with movement of the trace to record amplitude and velocity of moving echo-producing structures.

B-scan implies a two-dimensional ultrasonic scanning procedure with a two-dimensional display.

Real-time scan implies a two-dimensional ultrasonic scanning procedure with display of both two-dimensional structure and motion with time.

▶(To report diagnostic vascular ultrasound studies, see 93880-93990)◀

(For focused ultrasound ablation treatment of uterine leiomyomata, see Category III codes 0071T, 0072T)

✍ Rationale

Because of the deletion of code 93875, the Diagnostic Ultrasound guidelines have been revised to remove the reference to deleted code 93875 and added a reference to new code 93880.

⃠=Modifier 51 Exempt   ⊙=Moderate Sedation   ✚=Add-on Code   𝓝=FDA approval pending

Abdomen and Retroperitoneum

76776   Ultrasound, transplanted kidney, real time and duplex Doppler with image documentation

(For ultrasound of transplanted kidney without duplex Doppler, use 76775)

►(For ultrasound and duplex Doppler of a transplanted kidney, do not report 76776 in conjunction with 93975, 93976)◄

✍ Rationale

The parenthetical note following code 76776 was editorially revised to clarify its intent of applying only to procedures in which both ultrasound (76776) and duplex Doppler studies (93975 or 93976) are performed on the same transplanted kidney on the same day of service. The revision clarifies that when grey scale ultrasound and duplex Doppler studies of a transplanted kidney are performed the same day as Doppler studies of a different anatomical area or organ, it is appropriate to report code 76776 and also one of the duplex Doppler codes (93975 or 93976) for a different anatomic area or organ. Coinciding with this change is the deletion of the parenthetical note directing not to report code 76776 with 93975 and 93976, as these codes may be reported together when a different area or organ is studied.

Ultrasonic Guidance Procedures

+ 76937   Ultrasound guidance for vascular access requiring ultrasound evaluation of potential access sites, documentation of selected vessel patency, concurrent realtime ultrasound visualization of vascular needle entry, with permanent recording and reporting (List separately in addition to code for primary procedure)

►(Do not report 76937 in conjunction with 37191, 37192, 37193, 37760, 37761, 76942)◄

(If extremity venous non-invasive vascular diagnostic study is performed separate from venous access guidance, use 93965, 93970 or 93971)

✍ Rationale

In support of the addition of the intravascular vena cava (IVC) transcatheter procedures (37191-37193), the exclusionary parenthetical note following 76937 has been updated to include these procedures.

76942   Ultrasonic guidance for needle placement (eg, biopsy, aspiration, injection, localization device), imaging supervision and interpretation

►(Do not report 76942 in conjunction with 27096, 37760, 37761, 43232, 43237, 43242, 45341, 45342, 64479-64484, 64490-64495, 76975, 0228T-0231T, 0232T, 0249T)◄

(For injection(s) of platelet rich plasma, use 0232T)

✍ Rationale

The exclusionary parenthetical note following code 76942 has been updated to indicate the services that should not be reported in conjunction with 76942.

Fluoroscopic Guidance

▲**77003** Fluoroscopic guidance and localization of needle or catheter tip for spine or paraspinous diagnostic or therapeutic injection procedures (epidural or subarachnoid)

▶(Injection of contrast during fluoroscopic guidance and localization [77003] is included in 22526, 22527, 27096, 62263, 62264, 62267, 62270-62282, 62310-62319)◀

(Fluoroscopic guidance for subarachnoid puncture for diagnostic radiographic myelography is included in supervision and interpretation codes 72240-72270)

(For epidural or subarachnoid needle or catheter placement and injection, see 62270-62282, 62310-62319)

▶(For sacroiliac joint arthrography, see 27096)◀

▶(For paravertebral facet joint injection, see 64490-64495. For paravertebral facet joint nerve destruction by neurolysis, see 64633-64636. For transforaminal epidural needle placement and injection, see 64479-64484)◀

▶(Do not report 77003 in conjunction with 27096, 64479–64484, 64490-64495, 64633-64636)◀

(For percutaneous or endoscopic lysis of epidural adhesions, 62263, 62264 include fluoroscopic guidance and localization)

✒ Rationale

The guidelines regarding imaging guidance for destruction of facet joint nerves by neurolytic agent have changed for 2012. Previously, imaging guidance was separately reported using code 77003. Effective 2012, imaging guidance using fluoroscopy or CT is no longer separately reported and is considered an inclusive component of codes 27096 and 64633-64636. See the Musculoskeletal System/Pelvis and Hip Joint/Introduction or Removal section of this book for an explanation of code 27096. See the Nervous System/Extracranial Nerves, Peripheral Nerves, and Autonomic Nervous System/Destruction by Neurolytic Agent (eg, Chemical, Thermal, Electrical, or Radiofrequency) section of this book for an explanation of codes 64633-64636.

To reflect these changes, code 77003 has been revised by removing the reference to sacroiliac joint and neurolytic agent destruction. The parenthetical notes following code 77003 have been updated to reflect this change in reporting imaging guidance with destruction of facet joint nerves by neurolytic agent or for sacroiliac joint arthrography.

Computed Tomography Guidance

77012 Computed tomography guidance for needle placement (eg, biopsy, aspiration, injection, localization device), radiological supervision and interpretation

▶(Do not report 77012 in conjunction with 27096, 64479-64484, 64490-64495, 64633-64636, 0232T)◀

(For injection(s) of platelet rich plasma, use 0232T)

✏️ Rationale

In support of the changes to the destruction of facet joint nerves by neurolytic agent codes, the parenthetical note following code 77012 has been revised by adding codes 64633-64636 to the list of codes that should not be reported with code 77012. See the Nervous System/Extracranial Nerves, Peripheral Nerves, and Autonomic Nervous System/Destruction by Neurolytic Agent (eg, Chemical, Thermal, Electrical, or Radiofrequency) section of this book for an explanation of codes 64633-64636.

Bone/Joint Studies

77078 Computed tomography, bone mineral density study, 1 or more sites; axial skeleton (eg, hips, pelvis, spine)

►(77079 has been deleted)◄

77080 Dual-energy X-ray absorptiometry (DXA), bone density study, 1 or more sites; axial skeleton (eg, hips, pelvis, spine)

77081 appendicular skeleton (peripheral) (eg, radius, wrist, heel)

77082 vertebral fracture assessment

(For dual energy x-ray absorptiometry [DXA] body composition study, use 76499)

►(77083 has been deleted)◄

✏️ Rationale

As part of the AMA/Specialty Society RVS Update Committee (RUC) analysis, the bone studies described in codes 77079 and 77083 are no longer being performed and so the codes have been deleted and replaced by ones describing other technology. It was determined that these services are considered obsolete and did not warrant referencing an unlisted code.

Radiation Oncology

Radiation Treatment Delivery

77421 Stereoscopic X-ray guidance for localization of target volume for the delivery of radiation therapy

(Do not report 77421 in conjunction with 77432, 77435)

►(Do not report 77421 more than once per treatment delivery session)◄

(For placement of interstitial device[s] for radiation therapy guidance, see 31627, 32553, 49411, 55876)

Rationale

A parenthetical note has been added following code 77421 to instruct reporting of 77421 no more than once per treatment session.

#●77424   Intraoperative radiation treatment delivery, x-ray, single treatment session

#●77425   Intraoperative radiation treatment delivery, electrons, single treatment session

Neutron Beam Treatment Delivery

77422   High energy neutron radiation treatment delivery; single treatment area using a single port or parallel-opposed ports with no blocks or simple blocking

77423   1 or more isocenter(s) with coplanar or non-coplanar geometry with blocking and/or wedge, and/or compensator(s)

77424   ▶Code is out of numerical sequence. See 77401-77425◀

77425   ▶Code is out of numerical sequence. See 77401-77425◀

Radiation Treatment Management

▶Radiation treatment management is reported in units of five fractions or treatment sessions, regardless of the actual time period in which the services are furnished. The services need not be furnished on consecutive days. Multiple fractions representing two or more treatment sessions furnished on the same day may be counted separately as long as there has been a distinct break in therapy sessions, and the fractions are of the character usually furnished on different days. Code 77427 is also reported if there are three or four fractions beyond a multiple of five at the end of a course of treatment; one or two fractions beyond a multiple of five at the end of a course of treatment are not reported separately.

Radiation treatment management requires **and includes** a minimum of one examination of the patient by the physician for medical evaluation and management (eg, assessment of the patient's response to treatment, coordination of care and treatment, review of imaging and/or lab test results with documentation) for each reporting of the radiation treatment management service. Code 77469 represents only the intraoperative session management and does not include medical evaluation and management outside of that session.

The professional services furnished during treatment management typically include:

■ Review of port films;

■ Review of dosimetry, dose delivery, and treatment parameters;

■ Review of patient treatment set-up.◀

●77469   Intraoperative radiation treatment management

▲77470   Special treatment procedure (eg, total body irradiation, hemibody radiation, per oral or endocavitary irradiation)

○=Modifier 51 Exempt   ⊙=Moderate Sedation   ✛=Add-on Code   𝒩=FDA approval pending

(77470 assumes that the procedure is performed 1 or more times during the course of therapy, in addition to daily or weekly patient management)

▶(For intraoperative radiation treatment delivery and management, see 77424, 77425, 77469)◀

✍ Rationale

The development of codes 77424-77469 and the revisions to code 77470 and the guidelines for this section were provided to allow separate identification of intraoperative radiation treatment (IORT) delivery and management.

Historically, treating a patient during surgery involved transport of the anesthetized patient with the open surgical site into the radiation oncology department of the hospital where the treatment machine resides. Recent improvements have allowed for treatment machines that are either mobile or have the ability to be installed in a surgical environment.

Codes 77424 and 77425 are both used to identify intraoperative radiation treatment delivery (single sessions) whether performed using X rays or photons (as identified by code 77424) or by electrons (77425). Separate codes are necessary for these modalities as there are significant differences in the type of radiation protection that is necessary for delivery of photons vs electrons. Additionally, code 77469 has been added to identify treatment management for either of these services. To accommodate the addition of specific codes to identify IORT, existing code 77470, used to identify special treatment procedures, has been revised removing the phrase ". . . or intraoperative cone . . ." from the language. Prior to the development of the new codes, 77470 was the only code that identified intraoperative radiation treatment procedures. The new codes specify different types of IORT treatment. As a result, code 77470 should no longer be used to identify this type of radiation treatment. In congruity with this descriptor language change, a parenthetical note has been included following code 77470 to direct users to the appropriate codes to use for IORT.

IORT services are intended to include simulations necessary for radiation treatment delivery but are not intended to include evaluation and management services (E/M) provided outside of the treatment management session (77469). As a result, a guideline has been included to note that 77469 ". . . *represents only the intraoperative session management and does not include medical evaluation and management outside of that session.*"

Codes 77424 and 77425 appear with a number symbol (#) to indicate that these codes are out of numerical sequence. Two reference notes have been added to instruct the user to the appropriate code range of 77401-77425 for placement of codes 77424 and 77425.

🩺 Clinical Example (77424)

A 48-year-old female presents with a 2-cm mass in the upper outer quadrant of the left breast. A lumpectomy is performed. Before closure of the wound, intraoperative radiation therapy is delivered to the tumor bed.

Clinical Example (77425)

A 52-year-old male with a 4-cm mass in the pancreas presents for surgical resection. Frozen sections reveal adenocarcinoma with positive deep margins. Intraoperative radiation is delivered to the tumor bed.

Clinical Example (77469)

A 60-year-old male with a history of alcohol and tobacco abuse presents with a squamous cell cancer of the tongue with involved cervical lymph nodes. He receives combined modality chemotherapy and radiation with complete regression of tumor. Sixteen months later recurrent neck node is detected. PET/CT shows no other disease. Following resection of the recurrence via radical neck dissection, intraoperative radiation is delivered to the tumor bed.

Description of Procedure (77469)

Review operative specimen with surgeon. Review margins with pathologist to determine target areas, depth of penetration required, energy, etc. Review surgical field with surgeon for tumor areas and normal structures. Applicator selected for appropriate size and shape. The cone is manipulated into position. Position of the cone over the target must be assured and all normal structures in the field or deep to the field must be identified. With applicator in position, the angle of incidence is measured with radiation device specific level (to ensure that the angle does not exceed the design specifications of the radiation machine) and adjusted as indicated. At the discretion of the RO, a surface bolus may be attached to the applicator to maximize surface dose. In-field lead shielding is selected, cut, or fashioned to meet needs and shielding is placed. Applicator is positioned and held in place with a modified Bookwalter retractor system. RO makes certain all important structures have been retracted out from the radiation field. Suction is used to keep the target area as dry as possible (fluid will alter the depth of the penetration of the radiation beam). Wet gauze is placed over exposed tissues that are not in field. Accelerator is set up for treatment. Operative table is unlocked and the team collaborates to move the table and patient into position under the accelerator. Final position placement achieved. Table is relocked. Geometric alignment of the applicator with the gantry head of the accelerator is achieved with a laser alignment system. This soft docking alignment is verified through respiratory cycle. Once this is completed the team moves to the sub sterile room. Radiation oncologist remains in gown and gloves to be able to adjust device as needed. The prescribed radiation dose is administered. Treatment dose is interrupted instantaneously if the patient experiences a problem and the physicians must re-enter the room. (This is common from either machine faults, respiratory movements causing misalignment, etc.) The docking of the radiation device is reversed and the machine backed away from the patient without trauma to the area. Team returns operative table under the surgical lights. After the proper positioning of the applicator is reconfirmed, the applicator is removed. All bolus and shielding is removed.

Nuclear Medicine

Diagnostic

GASTROINTESTINAL SYSTEM

78215   Liver and spleen imaging; static only

78216   with vascular flow

    ▶(78220 has been deleted)◀

    ▶(78223 has been deleted. To report hepatobiliary system imaging, see 78226, 78227)◀

●**78226**   Hepatobiliary system imaging, including gallbladder when present;

●**78227**   with pharmacologic intervention, including quantitative measurement(s) when performed

Rationale

As part of the AMA/Specialty Society RVS Update Committee (RUC) analysis of codes, it became clear that codes 78220 and 78223 no longer reflected current technology and practice and needed to be redefined. As a result, code 78220 for liver function study was deleted, as the radiopharmaceutical associated with this procedure is no longer used and the procedure is outmoded. Code 78226 was established as one of the two replacement codes that more accurately describe the current technology and medical practice formerly described in code 78220. Code 78223 for hepatobiliary ductal system imaging was replaced with establishment of code 78227 to distinguish the differences in physician and technical work required to perform a study that includes pharmacological stimulation of gallbladder and contraction during the study, whether there is quantification of gallbladder or hepatic function (78227), from the work of imaging alone (78226). Unlike the previous codes 78220 and 78233, the image and pharmacologic study of the gallbladder is not required, but is included, if done, as noted in the code language for 78226 and 78227.

Clinical Example (78226)

A 58-year-old female presents with acute onset of right upper quadrant abdominal pain associated with nausea and vomiting. Ultrasonography of the gallbladder was unremarkable except for some right upper quadrant tenderness in the region of the gallbladder. A hepatobiliary study is ordered for suspected acute cholecystitis.

Description of Procedure (78226)

Hepatobiliary scintigraphy is a diagnostic radionuclide imaging study that evaluates hepatocellular function and patency of the biliary system by tracing the production and flow of bile from the liver, and its passage through the biliary system into the gallbladder (when present) and into the small intestine. Sequential digital imaging data of the liver, biliary tree, and gut are obtained.

Under the supervision of the physician, the technologist administers the radio-pharmaceutical. The study consists of planar imaging typically for 60 minutes postintravenous injection of the radiopharmaceutical, with additional views, eg, right lateral, left or right anterior oblique(s), as needed to clarify anatomy. The physician verifies the adequacy of the imaging data before completion of the study, and directs the technologist to obtain additional views or reprocess data when necessary. The data are formatted for film and/or digital display. The physician reviews the study for artifacts and abnormal distribution. The processed and raw images that are acquired are compared to relevant prior studies and formally interpreted, ie, a report is dictated for the medical record.

Clinical Example (78227)

A 47-year-old female presents with a history of intermittent right upper quadrant abdominal pain often associated with ingestion of a fatty meal. Work up, including gallbladder ultrasonography and upper endoscopy, is unremarkable. A hepatobiliary study is ordered for evaluation, including gallbladder function.

Description of Procedure (78227)

Hepatobiliary scintigraphy with pharmacological intervention is a diagnostic radionuclide imaging study that evaluates hepatocellular function and patency of the biliary system by tracing the production and flow of bile from the liver, and its passage through the biliary system into the gallbladder (when present) and into the small intestine. Pharmacological interventions during imaging are employed according to varying indications and individual patient needs. Under the supervision of the physician, the technologist administers the radiopharmaceutical(s) and drug(s). The study consists of sequential digital imaging of the liver, biliary tree, and gut for up to 60 minutes postintravenous injection of the radiopharmaceutical, with additional views, eg, right lateral, left or right anterior oblique as needed to clarify anatomy. To measure gallbladder function (ejection fraction), sequential imaging data of the visualized gallbladder is acquired during a prolonged (45-60 minutes) intravenous infusion of sincalide. The physician determines the timing and quantity of an intravenous administration of sincalide and the time of the administration is noted for calculations of gallbladder ejection fraction (GBEF). The physician verifies the completeness and adequacy of the images before completion of the study and directs the technologist to obtain additional views or reprocess data when necessary. The digital data are formatted for film and/or digital display and analysis. Cinematic display of images may be done to assist the physician, review measurements of gallbladder or hepatic function, if performed. The physician reviews the study for artifacts, correct regions-of-interest placement, and abnormal distribution. The processed and raw images are compared to relevant prior studies and formally interpreted, ie, a report is dictated for the medical record.

RESPIRATORY SYSTEM

●78579   Pulmonary ventilation imaging (eg, aerosol or gas)

▲78580   Pulmonary perfusion imaging (eg, particulate)

⊘=Modifier 51 Exempt   ⊙=Moderate Sedation   ✛=Add-on Code   ✐=FDA approval pending

● **78582**   Pulmonary ventilation (eg, aerosol or gas) and perfusion imaging

● **78597**   Quantitative differential pulmonary perfusion, including imaging when performed

● **78598**   Quantitative differential pulmonary perfusion and ventilation (eg, aerosol or gas), including imaging when performed

▶(Report 78579, 78580, 78582-78598 only once per imaging session)◀

▶(Do not report 78580, 78582-78598 in conjunction with 78451-78454)◀

▶(78584-78596 have been deleted. To report, see 78579, 78582-78598)◀

78599   Unlisted respiratory procedure, diagnostic nuclear medicine

Rationale

Changes have been made to the codes included in the **Nuclear Medicine Respiratory System** section of the CPT code set. These changes have been made to simplify the reporting for these testing procedures. The changes that have been made in this section have therefore been made to more accurately reflect the true intent for use of these codes.

Codes 78579 and 78582-78598 have all been added, and code 78580 has been revised to: (1) clarify that these codes may be used when imaging is performed for aerosols or gases (because testing for aerosols or gases are performed using the same methods); and (2) eliminate confusion regarding pulmonary function quantification by differentiating between ventilation procedures and perfusion procedures. As a result, each of the codes that have been added or revised within this section identify services that should be distinctly identified according to the type of testing procedure that is done and not according to the type of product being tested (ie, ventilation testing vs perfusion imaging and not gas vs aerosol). This includes development of codes that identify multiple services (eg, ventilation and perfusion identified by code 78582).

In addition, codes 78584-78596 have been deleted because these procedures included separate codes for aerosol imaging and gaseous product imaging. Because these are procedures that require no differentiation of work or materials to complete the procedures, these codes have been deleted and replaced by the new codes for these services.

Clinical Example (78579)

A 52-year-old male has recent onset of obstructive pulmonary disease. A pulmonary ventilation study is ordered to determine the extent of disease.

Description of Procedure (78579)

Lung ventilation scintigraphy is a radionuclide diagnostic imaging study that records the bronchopulmonary distribution of an inhaled radioactive aerosol or gas within the lungs. Multiple images of the lungs are acquired. Under the supervision of the physician, the technologist gives specific breathing instructions to the patient while administering the radiopharmaceutical. The study consists of multiple images (eg, anterior, posterior, right and left anterior and posterior obliques, right and left laterals) and documentation of patient position. The physician verifies the adequacy of the imaging data before completion of the study, and directs the technologist to obtain additional views, when necessary. The data are formatted for film and/or digital display and analysis. The physician reviews the study for artifacts and abnormal distribution. The processed and raw images (eg, upright or supine, posterior, left anterior oblique, etc) are compared to a current chest X ray and relevant prior studies, and formally interpreted, ie, a report is dictated for the medical record.

Clinical Example (78580)

Two days post-minor surgical procedure, a 60-year-old female presents with chest pain. There is clinical concern for pulmonary embolism. A perfusion lung study, without a ventilation study, is ordered.

Description of Procedure (78580)

Lung perfusion scintigraphy is a radionuclide diagnostic imaging study that records the distribution of pulmonary arterial blood flow within the lungs. Multiple images of the lungs are acquired. Under the supervision of the physician, the technologist administers the radiopharmaceutical. The study consists of multiple images, in multiple projections (eg, anterior, posterior, right and left anterior and posterior obliques, right and left laterals), and documentation regarding patient position. The physician verifies the adequacy of the imaging data before completion of the study, and directs the technologist to obtain additional views, when necessary. The data are formatted for film and/or digital display and analysis. The physician reviews the study for artifacts and abnormal distribution. The processed and raw images (eg, upright or supine, posterior, anterior, obliques and laterals, etc) are compared to a current chest X ray.

Clinical Example (78582)

Shortly after an overseas airplane trip, a 53-year-old male has chest pain. There is a concern for a pulmonary embolus. A ventilation and perfusion study is ordered.

Description of Procedure (78582)

Lung ventilation and perfusion scintigraphy is a combination of two radionuclide diagnostic imaging procedures that record both the bronchopulmonary distribution of an inhaled radioactive aerosol or gas and the distribution of pulmonary arterial blood flow within the lungs. Multiple images of pulmonary ventilation and perfusion are acquired and compared. Under the supervision of the physician, the technologist gives specific breathing instructions to the patient while administering the radiopharmaceuticals. The complete study consists of administration of two different radiopharmaceuticals, one by inhalation and the other by intravenous injection, acquisition of two (2) sets of multiple images in a variety of projections, (eg, anterior, posterior, right and left anterior and posterior obliques, right and left laterals) and documentation of patient position. The physician verifies the adequacy of the imaging data before completion of the study, and directs the technologist to obtain additional views, when necessary. The data are formatted for film and/or digital display and analysis. The physician reviews the study for artifacts and abnormal distribution. The processed and raw images (eg, upright or supine, posterior, anterior, obliques and laterals, etc) of both ventilation and perfusion imaging sets are compared to a current chest X ray and any additional relevant prior studies, and formally interpreted, ie, a report is dictated for the medical record.

 Clinical Example (78597)

A 61-year-old male with pulmonary fibrosis has a non-small cell lung cancer for which a lobectomy is planned. There is concern for post-operative residual lung function. A quantitative perfusion lung study is ordered.

Description of Procedure (78597)

Quantitative lung perfusion scintigraphy is a radionuclide diagnostic imaging study that records the relative distribution of pulmonary arterial blood flow in each lung (left, right), and within comparable areas within each lung (eg, upper, middle and lower thirds). Under the supervision of the physician, the technologist administers the radiopharmaceutical. The study consists of acquisition of timed imaging data from both the anterior and posterior projections, and may include comparable lateral projections. Measurements of relative radioactivity are made and the results expressed as percentages of the whole. The physician verifies the adequacy of the imaging data before completion of the study, and directs the technologist to obtain additional views or re-process data, when necessary. The data are formatted for film and/or digital display and analysis. The physician reviews the study for artifacts and abnormal distribution. Quantitative evaluation of the images, including but not limited to anterior, posterior, and the geometric mean(s) for global and regional perfusion is (are) calculated and recorded. The processed and raw images when performed (eg, upright or supine, posterior, anterior, etc) are compared to a current chest X ray and any additional relevant prior studies, and formally interpreted, ie, a report is dictated for the medical record.

 Clinical Example (78598)

A 64-year-old female with chronic obstructive pulmonary disease is scheduled to have surgery for a non-small cell lung cancer. There is concern for postoperative residual lung function. A quantitative perfusion and ventilation study is ordered.

Description of Procedure (78598)

Quantitative lung ventilation and perfusion scintigraphy is a combination of two radionuclide diagnostic imaging studies that measure the bronchopulmonary distribution of an inhaled radioactive aerosol or gas and the relative distribution of pulmonary arterial blood flow in each lung (left, right) and within comparable areas within each lung (eg, upper, middle and lower thirds). Under the supervision of the physician, the technologist gives specific breathing instructions to the patient while administering the radiopharmaceuticals. The study consists of multiple acquisitions of timed imaging data from both the anterior and posterior projections, and may include comparable lateral projections. Measurements of relative radioactivity are made and the results expressed as percentages of the whole. The physician verifies the adequacy of the imaging data before completion of the study, and directs the technologist to obtain additional views or reprocess data, when necessary. The data are formatted for film and/or digital display and analysis. The physician reviews the study for artifacts and abnormal distribution.

Quantitative evaluation of the images, including but not limited to anterior, posterior and the geometric mean(s) for global and regional perfusion is/are calculated and recorded. The processed and raw images when performed (eg, upright or supine, posterior, etc) are compared to a current chest X ray and any additional relevant prior studies, and formally interpreted, ie, a report is dictated for the medical record.

Pathology and Laboratory

There have been numerous changes made to the Pathology and Laboratory section in the CPT code set. A major change to this section is the addition of a new Molecular Pathology subsection, which is further subdivided into two subsections (Tier 1 and Tier 2 Molecular Pathology Procedures) with accompanying guidelines and definitions to clarify the use of the 101 new codes that were added under these subsections. In addition, two codes have been deleted, five codes have been revised, and two additional codes have been added in addition to the 101 new codes mentioned earlier.

Pathology and Laboratory

Urinalysis

81099   Unlisted urinalysis procedure

▶Molecular Pathology◀

 Rationale

A new Molecular Pathology section has been added to CPT 2012 to describe molecular pathology procedures. Molecular pathology procedures are medical laboratory procedures involving the analyses of nucleic acid to detect variants in genes that may be indicative of germline (eg, constitutional disorders) or somatic (eg, neoplasia) conditions, or to test for histocompatibility antigens (eg, HLA). This section includes new guidelines and definitions to provide proper reporting of these codes.

The molecular pathology codes are split into two tiers. Tier 1 contains 92 codes (81200-81383) and describes gene-specific and genomic procedures. Tier 2 contains nine codes (81400-81408) and describes molecular pathology procedures that are not listed in the Tier 1 molecular pathology codes (81200-81383). The Tier 2 codes are arranged by level of technical resources and interpretive professional work required. There are instructional parenthetical notes as well as cross-references added throughout this section to provide additional instructions for the appropriate reporting of these codes.

▶Molecular pathology procedures are medical laboratory procedures involving the analyses of nucleic acid to detect variants in genes that may be indicative of germline (eg, constitutional disorders) or somatic (eg, neoplasia) conditions, or to test for histocompatibility antigens (eg, HLA). Code selection is typically based on the specific gene(s) that is being analyzed. Genes are described using Human Genome Organization (HUGO) approved gene names and are italicized in the code descriptors. Gene names were taken from tables of the HUGO Gene Nomenclature Commmittee (HGNC) at the time the CPT codes were developed. For the most part, Human Genome Variation Society (HGVS) recommendations were followed for the names of specific molecular variants. The familiar name is used for some variants because defined criteria were not in place when the variant was first described or because HGVS recommendations were changed over time (eg, intronic variants, processed proteins). When the gene name is represented by an abbreviation, the abbreviation is listed first, followed by the full gene name italicized in parentheses (eg, "F5 [coagulation Factor V]"), except for the HLA series of codes. Proteins or diseases commonly associated with the genes are listed as examples in the code descriptors. The examples do not represent all conditions in which testing of the gene may be indicated.

Codes that describe tests to assess for the presence of gene variants (see definitions) use common gene variant names. Typically, all of the listed variants would be tested. However, these lists are not exclusive. If other variants are also tested in the analysis, they would be included in the procedure and not reported separately. Full gene sequencing should not be reported using codes that assess for the presence of gene variants unless specifically stated in the code descriptor.

The molecular pathology codes include all analytical services performed in the test (eg, cell lysis, nucleic acid stabilization, extraction, digestion, amplification, and detection). Any procedures required prior to cell lysis (eg, microdissection, codes 88380 and 88381) should be reported separately.

The results of the procedure may require interpretation by a physician or other qualified health care professional. When only the interpretation and report are performed, modifier 26 may be appended to the specific molecular pathology code.

All analyses are qualitative unless otherwise noted.

For microbial identification, see 87149-87153 and 87470-87801, and 87900-87904. For in situ hybridization analyses, see 88271-88275 and 88365-88368.

Molecular pathology procedures that are not specified in 81200-81350 should be reported using either the appropriate Tier 2 code (81400-81408) or the appropriate methodology codes in the 83890-83914 and 88384-88386 series.

Definitions

For purposes of CPT reporting, the following definitions apply:

Abnormal allele: an alternative form of a gene that contains a disease-related variation from the normal sequence.

Breakpoint: the region at which a chromosome breaks during a translocation (defined elsewhere). These regions are often consistent for a given translocation.

Codon: a discrete unit of three nucleotides of a DNA or mRNA sequence that encodes a specific amino acid within, or signals the termination of, a polypeptide.

Common variants: variants (as defined elsewhere) that are associated with compromised gene function and are interrogated in a single round of laboratory testing (in a single, typically multiplex, assay format or using more than one assay to encompass all variants to be tested). These variants typically fit the definition of a "mutation," and are usually the predominant ones causing disease. Testing for additional uncommon variants may provide additional limited value in assessment of a patient. Often there are professional society recommendations or guidelines for which variants are most appropriate to test (eg, American College of Medical Genetics/American College of Obstetrics and Gynecology guidelines for variants used in population screening for cystic fibrosis).

Constitutional: synonymous with germline, often used in reference to the genetic code that is present at birth.

Cytogenomic: chromosome analysis using molecular techniques.

Duplication/Deletion(Dup/Del): terms that are usually used together with the '/' to refer to molecular testing, which assesses the dosage of a particular genomic region. The region tested is typically of modest to substantial size—from several dozen to several million or more nucleotides.

⊘=Modifier 51 Exempt   ⊙=Moderate Sedation   ✚=Add-on Code   𝑵=FDA approval pending

Normal gene dosage is two copies per cell, except for the sex chromosomes (X and Y). Thus, zero or one copy represents a deletion, and three (or more) copies represent a duplication.

Dynamic mutation: polynucleotide (eg, trinucleotide) repeats that are in or associated with genes that can undergo disease-producing increases or decreases in the numbers of repeats within tissues and across generations.

Exon: typically, one of multiple nucleic acid sequences used to encode information for a gene product (polypeptide or protein). Exons are separated from each other by non-protein-coding sequences known as introns. Exons at the respective ends of a gene also contain nucleic acid sequence that does not code for the gene's protein product.

Gene: a nucleic acid sequence that typically contains information for coding a protein as well as for the regulated expression of that protein. Human genes usually contain multiple protein coding regions (exons) separated by non-protein coding regions (introns). See also *exon, intron,* and *polypeptide.*

Intron: a nucleic acid sequence found between exons in human genes. An intron contains essential sequences for its proper removal (by a process known as *splicing*) to join exons together and thus facilitate production of a functional protein from a gene. An intron is sometimes referred to as an intervening sequence (IVS).

Microarray: surface(s) on which multiple specific nucleic acid sequences are attached in a known arrangement. Sometimes referred to as a 'gene chip'. Examples of uses of microarrays include evaluation of a patient specimen for gains or losses of DNA sequences (copy number variants, CNVs), identification of the presence of specific nucleotide sequence variants (also known as single nucleotide polymorphisms, SNPs), mRNA expression levels, or DNA sequence analysis.

Mutations: typically are variants associated with altered gene function that lead to functional deficits or disease (pathogenic).

Mutation scanning: a technique (eg, single strand conformation polymorphism, temperature gradient gel electrophoresis, etc.) typically employed on multiple PCR amplicons to indicate the presence of DNA sequence variants by differences in physical properties compared to normal. Variants are then further characterized by DNA sequence analysis only in amplicons which demonstrate differences.

Polymorphisms: typically are variants that do not compromise gene function or produce disease (benign).

Polypeptide: a sequence of amino acids covalently linked in a specified order. Polypeptides alone or in combination with other polypeptide subunits are the building blocks of proteins.

Short Tandem Repeat (STR): a region of DNA where a pattern of two or more nucleotides are repeated. The number of repeating segments can be used as genetic markers for human identity testing.

Single-nucleotide polymorphism (SNP): a DNA sequence variation existing at a significant frequency in the population, in which a single nucleotide (A, T, C, or G) differs between individuals and/or within an individual's paired chromosomes,

Somatic: synonymous with acquired, referring to genetic code alterations that develop after birth (eg, occurring in neoplastic cells)

Translocation: an abnormality resulting from the breakage of a chromosome and the relocation of a portion of that chromosome's DNA sequence to the same or another chromosome. Most common translocations involve a reciprocal exchange of DNA sequences between two differently numbered (ie, non-homologous) chromosomes, with or without a clinically significant loss of DNA.

Variant: a nucleotide sequence difference from the "normal" (predominant) sequence for a given region. Variants are typically of two types: substitutions of one nucleotide for another, and deletions or insertions of nucleotides. Occasionally, variants reflect several nucleotide sequence changes in reasonably close proximity on the same chromosomal strand of DNA (a haplotype). These nucleotide sequence variants often result in amino acid changes in the protein made by the gene. The term *variant* does not itself carry a functional implication for those protein changes.

Variants in introns are typically described in one of two ways. The altered nucleotide(s) within a defined intervening sequence (eg, IVS3-2A>G) of a gene is listed with a "+" or "-" sign, which indicates the position relative to the first or last nucleotide of the intron. Or, the variant position is indicated relative to the last nucleotide of the preceding exon or first nucleotide of the following exon (eg, c.171+1G>A c.172-1G>T are single nucleotide changes at the first and last nucleotide of a given intron for a specific gene).

The majority of the variants described here are listed by the amino acid change using the single letter amino acid code for the original amino acid followed by the numerical position in the protein product and the amino acid substitution, eg, for ASPA E285A, Glutamic acid (E) at position 285 is replaced with an alanine (A). A few of the variants are described by the DNA change using the numerical position followed by the original nucleotide, a greater than sign (>) and the new nucleotide, eg, *MTHFR.* 677C>T.

A known familial variant is a specific mutation that has previously been identified within a patient's family.◄

►Tier 1 Molecular Pathology Procedures◄

►The following codes represent gene-specific and genomic procedures:◄

●**81200**   *ASPA (aspartoacylase)* (eg, Canavan disease) gene analysis, common variants (eg, E285A, Y231X)

●**81205**   *BCKDHB (branched-chain keto acid dehydrogenase E1, beta polypeptide)* (eg, Maple syrup urine disease) gene analysis, common variants (eg, R183P, G278S, E422X)

●**81206**   *BCR/ABL1 (t(9;22))* (eg, chronic myelogenous leukemia) translocation analysis; major breakpoint, qualitative or quantitative

●**81207**   minor breakpoint, qualitative or quantitative

●**81208**   other breakpoint, qualitative or quantitative

●**81209**   *BLM (Bloom syndrome, RecQ helicase-like)* (eg, Bloom syndrome) gene analysis, 2281del6ins7 variant

●**81210**   *BRAF (v-raf murine sarcoma viral oncogene homolog B1)* (eg, colon cancer), gene analysis, V600E variant

●**81211**   *BRCA1, BRCA2 (breast cancer 1 and 2)* (eg, hereditary breast and ovarian cancer) gene analysis; full sequence analysis and common duplication/deletion variants in BRCA1 (ie, exon 13 del 3.835kb, exon 13 dup 6kb, exon 14-20 del 26kb, exon 22 del 510bp, exon 8-9 del 7.1kb)

●**81212**   185delAG, 5385insC, 6174delT variants

●**81213**   uncommon duplication/deletion variants

●**81214**   *BRCA1 (breast cancer 1)* (eg, hereditary breast and ovarian cancer) gene analysis; full sequence analysis and common duplication/deletion variants (ie, exon 13 del 3.835kb, exon 13 dup 6kb, exon 14-20 del 26kb, exon 22 del 510bp, exon 8-9 del 7.1kb)

    ►(When performing *BRCA1* full sequence analysis with *BRCA2* full sequence analysis, use 81211)◄

●**81215**   known familial variant

●**81216**   *BRCA2 (breast cancer 2)* (eg, hereditary breast and ovarian cancer) gene analysis; full sequence analysis

    ►(When performing *BRCA2* full sequence analysis with *BRCA1* full sequence analysis, use 81211)◄

●**81217**   known familial variant

●**81220**   *CFTR (cystic fibrosis transmembrane conductance regulator)* (eg, cystic fibrosis) gene analysis; common variants (eg, ACMG/ACOG guidelines)

    ►(When Intron 8 poly-T analysis is performed in conjunction with 81220 in a R117H positive patient, do not report 81224)◄

●**81221**   known familial variants

●**81222**   duplication/deletion variants

●**81223**   full gene sequence

●**81224**   intron 8 poly-T analysis (eg, male infertility)

●**81225**   *CYP2C19 (cytochrome P450, family 2, subfamily C, polypeptide 19)* (eg, drug metabolism), gene analysis, common variants (eg, *2, *3, *4, *8, *17)

●**81226**   *CYP2D6 (cytochrome P450, family 2, subfamily D, polypeptide 6)* (eg, drug metabolism), gene analysis, common variants (eg, *2, *3, *4, *5, *6, *9, *10, *17, *19, *29, *35, *41, *1XN, *2XN, *4XN)

●**81227**   *CYP2C9 (cytochrome P450, family 2, subfamily C, polypeptide 9)* (eg, drug metabolism), gene analysis, common variants (eg, *2, *3, *5, *6)

●**81228**   Cytogenomic constitutional (genome-wide) microarray analysis; interrogation of genomic regions for copy number variants (eg, Bacterial Artificial Chromosome [BAC] or oligo-based comparative genomic hybridization [CGH] microarray analysis)

●**81229**   interrogation of genomic regions for copy number and single nucleotide polymorphism (SNP) variants for chromosomal abnormalities

    ►(Do not report 81228 in conjunction with 81229)◄

●**81240**   *F2 (prothrombin, coagulation factor II)* (eg, hereditary hypercoagulability) gene analysis, 20210G>A variant

●**81241**   *F5 (coagulation Factor V)* (eg, hereditary hypercoagulability) gene analysis, Leiden variant

●**81242**   *FANCC (Fanconi anemia, complementation group C)* (eg, Fanconi anemia, type C) gene analysis, common variant (eg, IVS4+4A>T)

●81243   *FMR1 (Fragile X mental retardation 1)* (eg, fragile X mental retardation) gene analysis; evaluation to detect abnormal (eg, expanded) alleles

▶(For evaluation to detect and characterize abnormal alleles, see 81243, 81244)◀

▶(For evaluation to detect and characterize abnormal alleles using a single assay [eg, PCR], use 81243)◀

●81244   characterization of alleles (eg, expanded size and methylation status)

●81245   *FLT3 (fms-related tyrosine kinase 3)* (eg, acute myeloid leukemia), gene analysis, internal tandem duplication (ITD) variants (ie, exons 14, 15)

●81250   *G6PC (glucose-6-phosphatase, catalytic subunit)* (eg, Glycogen storage disease, Type 1a, von Gierke disease) gene analysis, common variants (eg, R83C, Q347X)

●81251   *GBA (glucosidase, beta, acid)* (eg, Gaucher disease) gene analysis, common variants (eg, N370S, 84GG, L444P, IVS2+1G>A)

●81255   *HEXA (hexosaminidase A [alpha polypeptide])* (eg, Tay-Sachs disease) gene analysis, common variants (eg, 1278insTATC, 1421+1G>C, G269S)

●81256   *HFE (hemochromatosis)* (eg, hereditary hemochromatosis) gene analysis, common variants (eg, C282Y, H63D)

●81257   *HBA1/HBA2 (alpha globin 1 and alpha globin 2)* (eg, alpha thalassemia, Hb Bart hydrops fetalis syndrome, HbH disease), gene analysis, for common deletions or variant (eg, Southeast Asian, Thai, Filipino, Mediterranean, alpha3.7, alpha4.2, alpha20.5, and Constant Spring)

●81260   *IKBKAP (inhibitor of kappa light polypeptide gene enhancer in B-cells, kinase complex-associated protein)* (eg, familial dysautonomia) gene analysis, common variants (eg, 2507+6T>C, R696P)

●81261   *IGH@ (Immunoglobulin heavy chain locus)* (eg, leukemias and lymphomas, B-cell), gene rearrangement analysis to detect abnormal clonal population(s); amplified methodology (eg, polymerase chain reaction)

●81262   direct probe methodology (eg, Southern blot)

●81263   *IGH@ (Immunoglobulin heavy chain locus)* (eg, leukemia and lymphoma, B-cell), variable region somatic mutation analysis

●81264   *IGK@ (Immunoglobulin kappa light chain locus)* (eg, leukemia and lymphoma, B-cell), gene rearrangement analysis, evaluation to detect abnormal clonal population(s)

▶(For immunoglobulin lambda gene *[IGL@]* rearrangement or immunoglobulin kappa deleting element, [IGKDEL] analysis, report the appropriate methodology code[s] in the 83890-83914 series)◀

●81265   Comparative analysis using Short Tandem Repeat (STR) markers; patient and comparative specimen (eg, pre-transplant recipient and donor germline testing, post-transplant non-hematopoietic recipient germline [eg, buccal swab or other germline tissue sample] and donor testing, twin zygosity testing, or maternal cell contamination of fetal cells)

+●81266   each additional specimen (eg, additional cord blood donor, additional fetal samples from different cultures, or additional zygosity in multiple birth pregnancies) (List separately in addition to code for primary procedure)

    ⊘=Modifier 51 Exempt   ⊙=Moderate Sedation   ✚=Add-on Code   ✔=FDA approval pending

►(Use 81266 in conjunction with 81265)◄

●**81267** Chimerism (engraftment) analysis, post transplantation specimen (eg, hematopoietic stem cell), includes comparison to previously performed baseline analyses; without cell selection

●**81268**   with cell selection (eg, CD3, CD33), each cell type

►(If comparative STR analysis of recipient [using buccal swab or other germline tissue sample] and donor are performed after hematopoietic stem cell transplantation, report 81265, 81266 in conjunction with 81267, 81268 for chimerism testing)◄

●**81270** *JAK2 (Janus kinase 2)* (eg, myeloproliferative disorder) gene analysis, p.Val617Phe (V617F) variant

●**81275** *KRAS (v-Ki-ras2 Kirsten rat sarcoma viral oncogene)* (eg, carcinoma) gene analysis, variants in codons 12 and 13

●**81280** Long QT syndrome gene analyses *(eg, KCNQ1, KCNH2, SCN5A, KCNE1, KCNE2, KCNJ2, CACNA1C, CAV3, SCN4B, AKAP, SNTA1, and ANK2)*; full sequence analysis

●**81281**   known familial sequence variant

●**81282**   duplication/deletion variants

●**81290** *MCOLN1 (mucolipin 1)* (eg, Mucolipidosis, type IV) gene analysis, common variants (eg, IVS3-2A>G, del6.4kb)

●**81291** *MTHFR (5,10-methylenetetrahydrofolate reductase)* (eg, hereditary hypercoagulability) gene analysis, common variants (eg, 677T, 1298C)

●**81292** *MLH1 (mutL homolog 1, colon cancer, nonpolyposis type 2)* (eg, hereditary non-polyposis colorectal cancer, Lynch syndrome) gene analysis; full sequence analysis

●**81293**   known familial variants

●**81294**   duplication/deletion variants

●**81295** *MSH2 (mutS homolog 2, colon cancer, nonpolyposis type 1)* (eg, hereditary non-polyposis colorectal cancer, Lynch syndrome) gene analysis; full sequence analysis

●**81296**   known familial variants

●**81297**   duplication/deletion variants

●**81298** *MSH6 (mutS homolog 6 [E. coli])* (eg, hereditary non-polyposis colorectal cancer, Lynch syndrome) gene analysis; full sequence analysis

●**81299**   known familial variants

●**81300**   duplication/deletion variants

●**81301** Microsatellite instability analysis (eg, hereditary non-polyposis colorectal cancer, Lynch syndrome) of markers for mismatch repair deficiency (eg, BAT25, BAT26), includes comparison of neoplastic and normal tissue, if performed

●**81302** *MECP2 (methyl CpG binding protein 2)* (eg, Rett syndrome) gene analysis; full sequence analysis

●**81303**   known familial variant

●**81304**   duplication/deletion variants

●81310   *NPM1 (nucleophosmin)* (eg, acute myeloid leukemia) gene analysis, exon 12 variants

●81315   *PML/RARalpha, (t(15;17)), (promyelocytic leukemia/retinoic acid receptor alpha)* (eg, promyelocytic leukemia) translocation analysis; common breakpoints (eg, intron 3 and intron 6), qualitative or quantitative

●81316   single breakpoint (eg, intron 3, intron 6 or exon 6), qualitative or quantitative

         ▶(For intron 3 and intron 6 [including exon 6 if performed] analysis, use 81315)◀

         ▶(If both intron 6 and exon 6 are analyzed, without intron 3, use one unit of 81316)◀

●81317   *PMS2 (postmeiotic segregation increased 2 [S. cerevisiae])* (eg, hereditary non-polyposis colorectal cancer, Lynch syndrome) gene analysis; full sequence analysis

●81318   known familial variants

●81319   duplication/deletion variants

●81330   *SMPD1(sphingomyelin phosphodiesterase 1, acid lysosomal)* (eg, Niemann-Pick disease, Type A) gene analysis, common variants (eg, R496L, L302P, fsP330)

●81331   *SNRPN/UBE3A (small nuclear ribonucleoprotein polypeptide N and ubiquitin protein ligase E3A)* (eg, Prader-Willi syndrome and/or Angelman syndrome), methylation analysis

●81332   *SERPINA1 (serpin peptidase inhibitor, clade A, alpha-1 antiproteinase, antitrypsin, member 1)* (eg, alpha-1-antitrypsin deficiency), gene analysis, common variants (eg, *S and *Z)

●81340   *TRB@ (T cell antigen receptor, beta)* (eg, leukemia and lymphoma), gene rearrangement analysis to detect abnormal clonal population(s); using amplification methodology (eg, polymerase chain reaction)

●81341   using direct probe methodology (eg, Southern blot)

●81342   *TRG@ (T cell antigen receptor, gamma)* (eg, leukemia and lymphoma), gene rearrangement analysis, evaluation to detect abnormal clonal population(s)

         ▶(For T cell antigen alpha *[TRA@]* gene rearrangement analysis, report the appropriate methodology code(s) in the 83890-83914 series)◀

         ▶(For T cell antigen delta *[TCD@]* gene rearrangement analysis, report 81401)◀

●81350   *UGT1A1 (UDP glucuronosyltransferase 1 family, polypeptide A1)* (eg, irinotecan metabolism), gene analysis, common variants (eg, *28, *36, *37)

●81355   *VKORC1 (vitamin K epoxide reductase complex, subunit 1)* (eg, warfarin metabolism), gene analysis, common variants (eg, -1639/3673)

         ▶Human Leukocyte Antigen (HLA) typing is performed to assess compatibility of recipients and potential donors as a part of solid organ and hematopoietic stem cell pretransplant testing. HLA testing is also performed to identify HLA alleles and allele groups (antigen equivalents) associated with specific diseases and individualized responses to drug therapy (eg, HLA-B*27 and ankylosing spondylitis and HLA-B*57:01 and abacavir hypersensitivity), as well as other clinical uses. One or more HLA genes may be tested in specific clinical situations (eg, HLA-DQB1 for narcolepsy and HLA-A, -B, -C, -DRB1 and -DQB1 for kidney transplantation). Each HLA gene typically has multiple variant alleles or allele groups that can be identified by typing. For HLA result reporting, a low resolution HLA type is denoted by a two digit HLA name (eg, A*02) and intermediate resolution typing by a string of alleles or an NMDP (National Marrow Donor Program) code (eg, B*14:01/07N/08/12/14, B*39CKGN). Both low and intermediate resolution are considered low resolution for code assignment. High resolution typing resolves the common well defined (CWD) alleles and is usually denoted by at least 4 digits (eg, A*02:02, *03:01:01:01, A*26:01:01G, and C*03:04P), however, high resolution typing may include some ambiguities for rare alleles, which may be reported as a string of alleles or an NMDP code.

If additional testing is required to resolve ambiguous allele combinations for high resolution typing, this is included in the base HLA typing codes below. The gene names have been italicized similar to the other molecular pathology codes.◄

▶(For HLA antigen typing by non-molecular pathology techniques, see 86812-86822)◄

●**81370** HLA Class I and II typing, low resolution (eg, antigen equivalents); *HLA-A, -B, -C, -DRB1/3/4/5, and -DQB1*

●**81371** *HLA-A, -B, and -DRB1/3/4/5* (eg, verification typing)

●**81372** HLA Class I typing, low resolution (eg, antigen equivalents); complete *(ie, HLA-A, -B, and -C)*

▶(When performing both Class I and II low resolution *HLA typing for HLA-A,-B,-C, -DRB1/3/4/5,* and *-DQB1,* use 81370)◄

●**81373** one locus *(eg, HLA-A, -B, or -C)*, each

▶(When performing a complete Class I *[HLA-A,-B, and -C]* low resolution HLA typing, use 81372)◄

▶(When the presence or absence of a single antigen equivalent is reported using low resolution testing, use 81374)◄

●**81374** one antigen equivalent (eg, *B*27*), each

▶(When testing for presence or absence of more than 2 antigen equivalents at a locus, use 81373 for each locus tested)◄

●**81375** HLA Class II typing, low resolution (eg, antigen equivalents); *HLA-DRB1/3/4/5 and -DQB1*

▶(When performing both Class I and II low resolution HLA typing for *HLA-A,-B,-C, -DRB1/3/4/5,* and *–DQB1,* use 81370)◄

●**81376** one locus (eg, *HLA-DRB1/3/4/5, -DQB1, -DQA1, -DPB1, or -DPA1*), each

▶(When low resolution typing is performed for *HLA-DRB1/3/4/5 and -DQB1,* use 81375)◄

▶(For low resolution typing, *HLA-DRB1/3/4/5* should be treated as a single locus)◄

●**81377** one antigen equivalent, each

▶(When testing for presence or absence of more than 2 antigen equivalents at a locus, use 81376 for each locus)◄

●**81378** HLA Class I and II typing, high resolution (ie, alleles or allele groups), *HLA-A, -B, -C, and -DRB1*

●**81379** HLA Class I typing, high resolution (ie, alleles or allele groups); complete (ie, *HLA-A, -B, and -C*);

●**81380** one locus (eg, *HLA-A, -B, or -C*), each

▶(When a complete Class I high resolution typing for *HLA-A,-B,* and *-C* is performed, use 81379)◄

►(When the presence or absence of a single allele or allele group is reported using high resolution testing, use 81381)◄

●**81381**   one allele or allele group (eg, *B*57:01P*), each

►(When testing for the presence or absence of more than 2 alleles or allele groups at a locus, use 81380 for each locus)◄

●**81382**   HLA Class II typing, high resolution (ie, alleles or allele groups); one locus (eg, *HLA-DRB1, -DRB3, -DRB4, -DRB5, -DQB1, -DQA1, -DPB1, or -DPA1*), each

►(When only the presence or absence of a single allele or allele group is reported using high resolution testing, use 81383)◄

●**81383**   one allele or allele group (eg, *HLA-DQB1*06:02P*), each

►(When testing for the presence or absence of more than 2 alleles or allele groups at a locus, use 81382 for each locus)◄

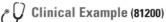

Clinical Example (81200)

A 25-year-old female is seen by her obstetrician for prenatal care. During an office visit, the physician learns that she is of Jewish ancestry, but has not previously been tested to determine if she carries a mutation for Canavan disease. A sample of anticoagulated peripheral blood is submitted to the laboratory to test for two variants in the ASPA gene common in the Ashkenazi Jewish population.

Description of Procedure (81200)

Upon receipt of the specimen, high quality genomic DNA is isolated and subjected to multiplex PCR. Following exonuclease I and shrimp alkaline phosphatase treatment, a second reaction using allele specific primer extension (ASPE) amplifies either the normal or mutant allele sequences. Extension products are hybridized to color-coded microspherical beads specific for normal and mutant alleles. The fluorescent signal ratio of mutant to normal alleles is calculated, and the pathologist or other qualified health care professional examines the allelic ratios to determine zygosity status. The pathologist or other qualified health care professional composes a report that specifies the patient's mutation status. The report is edited and signed, and the results are communicated to appropriate caregivers.

Clinical Example (81205)

A 25-year-old female is seen by her obstetrician for prenatal care. During an office visit, the physician learns that she is of Jewish ancestry, but has not previously been tested to determine if she carries a mutation for Maple Syrup urine disease. A sample of anticoagulated peripheral blood is submitted to the laboratory to test for three variants in the BCKDHB gene common in the Ashkenazi Jewish population.

Description of Procedure (81205)

Upon receipt of the specimen, high quality genomic DNA is isolated and subjected to multiplex PCR. Following exonuclease I and shrimp alkaline phosphatase treatment, a second reaction using allele specific primer extension (ASPE) amplifies either the normal or mutant allele sequences. Extension products are hybridized to

⊘=Modifier 51 Exempt   ⊙=Moderate Sedation   ✚=Add-on Code   𝑁=FDA approval pending color-coded microspherical beads specific for normal and mutant alleles. The fluorescent signal ratio of mutant to normal alleles is calculated, and the pathologist or other qualified health care professional examines the allelic ratios to determine zygosity status. The pathologist or other qualified health care professional composes a report that specifies the patient's mutation status. The report is edited and signed, and the results are communicated to appropriate caregivers.

Clinical Example (81206)

A 54-year-old male diagnosed with chronic myelogenous leukemia (CML) on maintenance therapy with imatinib mesylate sees his oncologist for a routine follow-up visit. Molecular studies at diagnosis confirmed the presence of a Philadelphia chromosome with the major breakpoint translocation joining the BCR and ABL1 genes. The patient feels well and has no complaints, and a hemogram in the office demonstrates normal white cell, red cell, and platelet counts. A sample of anticoagulated peripheral blood is submitted to the laboratory for quantitative assessment of BCR/ABL1 major breakpoint transcript level.

Description of Procedure (81206)

Upon receipt of the specimen, high quality total cellular RNA is isolated and stored under RNase-free conditions. Working in duplicate from this point, reverse transcriptase is used to convert RNA to cDNA followed by quantitative real-time PCR amplification using primers for both the BCR/ABL1 major breakpoint translocation as well as a "housekeeping gene" necessary to normalize BCR/ABL1 expression levels. The pathologist or other qualified health care professional reviews the real-time PCR tracings to determine the status of the of BCR/ABL1 major breakpoint transcripts, that the assay is performing at acceptable sensitivity, and whether RNA degradation or inhibitors of PCR are present. The pathologist or other qualified health care professional reviews duplicate values as well as the ratio of BCR/ABL1 to housekeeping gene expression for patient and control samples. Values are converted to an international reporting standard using a previously determined correction factor for the laboratory's assay. The pathologist or other qualified health care professional composes a report that describes the transcript status and copy number, and compares these results with the patient's previous results. The report is edited and signed, and the results are communicated to appropriate caregivers.

Clinical Example (81207)

A 64-year-old female diagnosed with acute lymphocytic leukemia (ALL) treated with imatinib mesylate and hyper-CVAD therapy sees her oncologist for a routine follow-up visit. Molecular studies at diagnosis confirmed the presence of a Philadelphia chromosome with the minor breakpoint translocation joining the BCR and ABL1 genes. The patient feels well and has no complaints, and a hemogram in the office demonstrates normal white cell, red cell, and platelet counts. A sample of anticoagulated bone marrow is submitted to the laboratory for quantitative assessment of BCR/ABL1 minor breakpoint transcript level.

Description of Procedure (81207)

Upon receipt of the specimen, high quality total cellular RNA is isolated and stored under RNase-free conditions. Working in duplicate from this point, reverse transcriptase is used to convert RNA to cDNA followed by quantitative real-time PCR amplification using primers for both the BCR/ABL1 minor breakpoint translocation as well as a "housekeeping gene" necessary to normalize BCR/ABL1 expression levels. The pathologist or other qualified health care professional reviews the real-time PCR tracings to determine the status of BCR/ABL1 minor breakpoint transcripts, that the assay is performing at acceptable sensitivity, and whether RNA degradation or inhibitors of PCR are present. The pathologist or other qualified health care professional reviews duplicate values as well as the ratio of BCR/ABL1 to housekeeping gene expression for patient and control samples. The pathologist or other qualified health care professional composes a report that describes the transcript status and whether disease level appears to be stable, increasing, or decreasing. The report is edited and signed, and the results are communicated to appropriate caregivers.

Clinical Example (81208)

A 52-year-old female visits her primary care physician complaining of abdominal discomfort. Splenomegaly is identified on physical examination. A hemogram demonstrates leukocytosis with a left shift along with modest anemia and thrombocytopenia. Cytogenetic analysis demonstrates a classic Philadelphia chromosome, but studies for BCR/ABL1 major and minor breakpoints are negative. A sample of anticoagulated peripheral blood is submitted to the laboratory for assessment of the uncommon BCR/ABL1 "micro"(u) translocation breakpoint.

Description of Procedure (81208)

Upon receipt of the specimen, high quality total cellular RNA is isolated and stored under RNase-free conditions. Working in duplicate from this point, reverse transcriptase is used to convert RNA to cDNA followed by qualitative real-time PCR amplification using primers specific for the BCR/ABL1 micro(u) breakpoint translocation as well as a "housekeeping gene." The pathologist or other qualified health care professional reviews the real-time PCR tracings to the status of a BCR/ABL1 micro breakpoint translocation and whether RNA degradation or inhibitors of PCR are present. The pathologist or other qualified health care professional composes a report that specifies the status of the translocation. The report is edited and signed, and the results are communicated to appropriate caregivers.

Clinical Example (81209)

A 25-year-old female is seen by her obstetrician for prenatal care. During an office visit, the physician learns that she is of Jewish ancestry, but has not previously been tested to determine if she carries a mutation for Bloom syndrome. A sample of anticoagulated peripheral blood is submitted to the laboratory to test for a variant in the BLM gene common in the Ashkenazi Jewish population to determine her carrier status.

⊘=Modifier 51 Exempt   ⊙=Moderate Sedation   ✚=Add-on Code   ⊿=FDA approval pending

Description of Procedure (81209)

Upon receipt of the specimen, high quality genomic DNA is isolated and subjected to multiplex PCR. Following exonuclease I and shrimp alkaline phosphatase treatment, a second reaction using allele specific primer extension (ASPE) amplifies either the normal or mutant allele sequences. Extension products are hybridized to color-coded microspherical beads specific for normal and mutant alleles. The fluorescent signal ratio of mutant to normal alleles is calculated, and the pathologist or other qualified health care professional examines the allelic ratios to determine the mutation and zygosity status. The pathologist or other qualified health care professional composes a report that specifies the patient's mutation status. The report is edited and signed, and the results are communicated to appropriate caregivers.

 ## Clinical Example (81210)

A 54-year-old male with metastatic colorectal carcinoma is being considered for targeted therapy with anti-epidermal growth factor receptor (EGFR) monoclonal antibodies. Initial molecular studies indicate the tumor does not contain any of 12 common KRAS mutations at codons 12 or 13. A tumor-rich tissue sample is submitted for BRAF gene mutation testing.

Description of Procedure (81210)

Paraffin is removed, and high quality DNA is isolated from the patient's tumor tissue. DNA is subjected to PCR amplification for exon 15 of the BRAF gene. The PCR products undergo bidirectional dideoxynucleotide chain termination sequencing on a capillary electrophoresis instrument. The pathologist or other qualified health care professional evaluates the electropherograms to identify nucleotide sequence variants. The pathologist or other qualified health care professional composes a report that specifies the patient's mutation status. The report is edited and signed, and the results are communicated to appropriate caregivers.

 ## Clinical Example (81211)

A small left breast lump is detected in a pre-menopausal 36-year-old female of Norwegian and Irish Catholic ancestry with a family history significant for breast and ovarian cancer during an annual physical examination by her family physician. She is referred to a general surgeon for further evaluation. A biopsy of the patient's left breast lump reveals invasive ductal carcinoma. An anticoagulated peripheral blood specimen is submitted for full gene sequence analysis and large genomic rearrangement analysis of BRCA1 gene variants as well as full gene sequence analysis of BRCA2 gene variants associated with hereditary breast and ovarian cancer.

Description of Procedure (81211)

High quality DNA is isolated from whole blood and subjected to 35 individual PCR amplification reactions for BRCA1 and 47 individual PCR amplification reactions for BRCA2. The PCR products from each reaction undergo bidirectional dideoxynucleotide chain termination sequencing using a capillary electrophoresis instrument. The potential presence of five specific large BRCA1 gene rearrangements is also assessed using recombination-specific PCR amplification. Sequence data analysis is performed by computer software, followed by visual inspection and confirmation under the direction of a certified laboratory director. Genetic variants are identified by comparison with a consensus wild-type reference sequence. A system-generated report is prepared that specifies the patient's mutation status to include information from an internal database and the literature regarding the significance of variants identified. The report is reviewed and signed by a pathologist or other health care provider. The results are communicated to the appropriate health care provider.

Clinical Example (81212)

A 43-year-old female of Ashkenazi Jewish descent whose 37-year-old sister was recently diagnosed with breast cancer asks her internist whether she should have genetic testing for hereditary breast cancer. The internist advises screening for common BRCA1 and BRCA2 gene variants associated with hereditary breast and ovarian cancer in Ashkenazi Jews. An anticoagulated peripheral blood specimen is submitted for BRCA1 and BRCA2 common (Ashkenazi Jewish) variant gene testing.

Description of Procedure (81212)

High quality DNA is isolated from the patient specimen and subjected to three individual PCR amplification reactions. The PCR products from each reaction undergo bidirectional dideoxynucleotide chain termination sequencing using a capillary electrophoresis instrument. Sequence data analysis is performed by computer software, followed by visual inspection and confirmation under the direction of a certified laboratory director. Genetic variants are identified by comparison with a consensus wild-type reference sequence. A system-generated report is prepared that specifies the patient's mutation status. The report is reviewed and signed by a pathologist or other health care provider. The results are communicated to the appropriate health care provider.

Clinical Example (81213)

A 36-year-old premenopausal female of Norwegian and Irish Catholic ancestry with a history of invasive ductal carcinoma was recently tested with full gene BRCA1 full gene sequence analysis, BRCA1 common duplication/deletion variant analysis, and BRCA2 full gene sequence analysis. Results of this testing are negative (no deleterious mutation is identified). Because of a family history strongly suggestive of hereditary breast cancer, an anticoagulated peripheral blood specimen is submitted for analysis of uncommon duplication/deletion variants in the BRCA1 and BRCA2 genes associated with hereditary breast and ovarian cancer.

Description of Procedure (81213)

High quality DNA is isolated from peripheral blood and subjected to multiplexed quantitative PCR all coding exons and the promoter regions of the BRCA1 and BRCA2 genes. Data analysis is performed by computer software, followed by visual inspection and confirmation under the direction of a certified laboratory director. Duplication/deletion variants are identified by comparison with a consensus wild-type reference sequence. A system-generated report is prepared that specifies the patient's mutation status to include information from an internal database and the

⊘=Modifier 51 Exempt ⊙=Moderate Sedation ✚=Add-on Code 𝘕=FDA approval pending

literature regarding the significance of variants identified. The report is reviewed and signed by a pathologist or other health care provider. The results are communicated to the appropriate health care provider.

Clinical Example (81214)

A small left breast lump is detected in a premenopausal 36-year-old female of Norwegian and Irish Catholic ancestry with a family history significant for breast and ovarian cancer during an annual physical examination by her family physician. She is referred to a general surgeon for further evaluation. A biopsy of the patient's left breast lump reveals invasive ductal carcinoma. An anticoagulated peripheral blood specimen is submitted for full gene sequence analysis and large genomic rearrangement analysis of BRCA1 gene variants associated with hereditary breast and ovarian cancer.

Description of Procedure (81214)

High quality DNA is isolated from whole blood and subjected to 35 individual PCR amplification reactions. The PCR products from each reaction undergo bidirectional dideoxynucleotide chain termination sequencing using a capillary electrophoresis instrument. The potential presence of five specific large BRCA1 gene rearrangements is also assessed using recombination-specific PCR amplification. Sequence data analysis is performed by computer software, followed by visual inspection and confirmation under the direction of a certified laboratory director. Genetic variants are identified by comparison with a consensus wild-type reference sequence. A system-generated report is prepared that specifies the patient's mutation status to include information from an internal database and the literature regarding the significance of variants identified. The report is reviewed and signed by a pathologist or other health care provider. The results are communicated to the appropriate health care provider.

Clinical Example (81215)

The 45-year-old sister of a 39-year old woman who recently was found by DNA sequence analysis to carry a BRCA1 gene mutation requests genetic testing, to see if she also carries the familial mutation. An anti-coagulated peripheral blood specimen is submitted for targeted gene sequence analysis of the relevant region of the BRCA1 gene.

Description of Procedure (81215)

High quality DNA is isolated from whole blood and subjected to PCR amplification for the BRCA1 exon which contains the known familial mutation. The PCR product undergoes bidirectional dideoxynucleotide chain termination sequencing using a capillary electrophoresis instrument. Sequence data analysis is performed by computer software, followed by visual inspection and confirmation under the direction of a certified laboratory director. Genetic variants are detected by comparison with a consensus wild-type reference sequence. A system-generated report is prepared that specifies the patient's mutation status. The report is reviewed and signed by a pathologist or other health care provider. The results are communicated to the appropriate health care provider.

A small left breast lump is detected in a premenopausal 36-year-old female of Norwegian and Irish Catholic ancestry with a family history significant for breast and ovarian cancer during an annual physical examination by her family physician. She is referred to a general surgeon for further evaluation. A biopsy of the patient's left breast lump reveals invasive ductal carcinoma. An anticoagulated peripheral blood sample is submitted for full gene sequence analysis and large genomic rearrangement analysis of BRCA2 gene variants associated with hereditary breast and ovarian cancer.

Description of Procedure (81216)

High quality DNA is isolated from whole blood and subjected to 47 individual PCR amplification reactions. The PCR products from each reaction undergo bidirectional dideoxynucleotide chain termination sequencing by capillary electrophoresis instrument. Sequence data analysis is performed by computer software, followed by visual inspection and confirmation under the direction of a certified laboratory director. Genetic variants are identified by comparison with a consensus wild-type reference sequence. A system-generated report is prepared that specifies the patient's mutation status to include information from an internal database and the literature regarding the significance of variants identified. The report is reviewed and signed by a pathologist or other health care provider. The results are communicated to the appropriate health care provider.

🩺 **Clinical Example** (81217)

The 45-year-old sister of a 39-year-old woman who recently was found by DNA sequence analysis to carry a BRCA2 gene mutation requests genetic testing, to see if she also carries the familial mutation. An anticoagulated peripheral blood specimen is submitted for targeted gene sequence analysis of the relevant region of the BRCA2 gene.

Description of Procedure (81217)

High quality DNA is isolated from whole blood and subjected to PCR amplification for the BRCA2 gene exon which contains the known familial mutation. The PCR product undergoes bidirectional dideoxynucleotide chain termination sequencing using a capillary electrophoresis instrument. Sequence data analysis is performed by computer software, followed by visual inspection and confirmation under the direction of a certified laboratory director. Genetic variants are identified by comparison with a consensus wild-type reference sequence. A system-generated report is prepared that specifies the patient's mutation status to include information from an internal database and the literature regarding the significance of variants identified. The report is reviewed and signed by a pathologist or other health care provider. The results are communicated to the appropriate health care provider.

🩺 **Clinical Example** (81220)

A 26-year-old Caucasian female, approximately eight weeks pregnant and otherwise in good health, visits her obstetrician for a first prenatal visit. After discussing advantages and limitations of prenatal cystic fibrosis carrier screening with her obstetrician, an anticoagulated peripheral blood sample is sent to the laboratory to be tested for common mutations and variants associated with cystic fibrosis.

Description of Procedure (81220)

Upon receipt of the specimen, high quality genomic DNA is isolated and subjected to multiplex PCR. Following exonuclease I and shrimp alkaline phosphatase treatment, a second reaction using allele specific primer extension (ASPE) amplifies either the normal or mutant allele sequences. Extension products are hybridized to color-coded microspherical beads specific for normal and mutant alleles. The fluorescent signal ratio of mutant to normal alleles is calculated, and the pathologist or other qualified health care professional examines the allelic ratios to determine the mutation and zygosity status. The pathologist or other qualified health care professional composes a report that specifies the patient's mutation status and residual risk based on ethnic background. The report is edited and signed, and the results are communicated to appropriate caregivers.

Clinical Example (81221)

A 1-year-old Caucasian male, whose 6-year-old brother was previously diagnosed with cystic fibrosis is brought by his mother to the pediatrician for genetic testing. The brother was previously demonstrated to be a compound heterozygote carrying one copy each of the common CFTR DeltaF508 mutation as well as a rare variant not included in assays which test for common variants of CFTR but known to cause cystic fibrosis. An anticoagulated peripheral blood sample is sent to the laboratory for testing of these known mutations.

Description of Procedure (81221)

Upon receipt of the specimen, high quality DNA is isolated from whole blood and subjected to PCR amplification for the respective CFTR gene exons which contain the known familial mutations. Following exonuclease I and shrimp alkaline phosphatase treatment, each PCR product undergoes bidirectional Sanger dideoxynucleotide chain termination sequencing using appropriate forward and reverse primers. Sequencing products are analyzed on a capillary electrophoresis instrument and electropherograms are printed for visual inspection and are transferred to a software program to identify potential nucleotide sequence changes. The pathologist or other qualified health care professional composes a report specifying the patient's mutation status. The report is edited and signed, and the results are communicated to appropriate caregivers.

Clinical Example (81222)

A 17-year-old Caucasian female, previously diagnosed with cystic fibrosis based on convincing clinical criteria and two elevated sweat chloride results, visits her pediatrician with her father to discuss potential additional genetic testing. Previous tests with a screening assay for common mutations and variants followed by CFTR full gene sequence analysis revealed only heterozygosity for the DeltaF508 mutation. An anticoagulated peripheral blood sample is forwarded to a reference laboratory for deletion/duplication analysis for an uncommon CFTR mutation.

Description of Procedure (81222)

Upon receipt of the specimen, high quality DNA is isolated from whole blood and subjected to multiplex ligation probe ligation analysis (MLPA) which involves hybridization and ligation of multiple pairs of oligonucleotide probes specific for the 27 exons of the CFTR gene to assess dosage of each exon. The pathologist or other qualified health care provider examines peak heights and calculated ratios of individual exons to control gene sequences to determine dosage status for all exons tested in the CFTR gene. The pathologist or other qualified health care professional composes a report specifying the patient's mutation status. The report is edited and signed, and the results are communicated to appropriate caregivers.

Clinical Example (81223)

A 17-year-old Caucasian female with chronic rhino-sinusitis, idiopathic bronchiectasis, and two sweat chloride measurements in the intermediate range (40-60 meq/L) is suspected by her pediatrician of having an atypical form of cystic fibrosis. A tube of anticoagulated peripheral blood is submitted to the laboratory for full CFTR gene sequence analysis.

Description of Procedure (81223)

Upon receipt of the specimen, high quality DNA is isolated from whole blood and subjected to 29 individual PCR amplification reactions whose products encompass the entire coding sequence, exon-intron boundaries, and portions of 5'- and 3'-untranslated regions of the CFTR gene. Following exonuclease I and shrimp alkaline phosphatase treatment, each PCR product undergoes bidirectional Sanger dideoxynucleotide chain termination sequencing using appropriate forward and reverse primers. Sequencing products are analyzed on a capillary electrophoresis instrument and electropherograms are printed for visual inspection and are transferred to a software program to identify potential nucleotide sequence changes. The pathologist or other qualified health care professional composes a report specifying the patient's mutation status to include information from a literature and database search regarding the significance of variants identified. The report is edited and signed, and the results are communicated to appropriate caregivers.

Clinical Example (81224)

Following recent consultation with his family physician regarding his wife's difficulty in conceiving a child, a 34-year-old Caucasian male is referred to a urologist for infertility workup. Physical Further examination and testing reveals bilateral absence of the vas deferens. The urologist recommends genetic analysis of the CFTR gene to look for common CFTR mutations and assess the intron 8 poly-T region frequently associated with male infertility. An anticoagulated peripheral blood sample is forwarded to the laboratory for testing.

Description of Procedure (81224)

Upon receipt of the specimen, high quality genomic DNA is isolated and subjected to multiplex PCR. Following exonuclease I and shrimp alkaline phosphatase treatment, a second reaction using allele specific primer extension (ASPE) amplifies either normal or mutant allele sequences including poly-T length variants. Extension products are hybridized to color-coded microspherical beads specific

⊘=Modifier 51 Exempt   ⊙=Moderate Sedation   ✚=Add-on Code   ✒=FDA approval pending

for normal and mutant alleles as well as poly-T length variants in intron 8. The fluorescent signal ratio of mutant, normal, and poly-T alleles is calculated, and the pathologist or other qualified health care professional examines the allelic ratios to determine the mutation, zygosity, and specific poly-T allele status. The pathologist or other qualified health care professional composes a report that specifies the patient's mutation and poly-T status. The report is edited and signed, and the results are communicated to appropriate caregivers.

🩺 Clinical Example (81225)

A 60-year-old Caucasian male is seen by a cardiologist after experiencing an acute myocardial infarct. The physician is considering percutaneous coronary intervention for this patient and needs to place the patient on an antiplatelet drug (clopidogrel) to prevent clotting. To determine whether the standard 300 mg loading dose of clopidogrel should be altered, a sample of anticoagulated peripheral blood is submitted to the laboratory to test for common variants in the CYP2C19 gene.

Description of Procedure (81225)

High quality genomic DNA is isolated and subjected to two amplification reactions (PCR). Pooled PCR amplicons are enzymatically fragmented, labeled with biotin, and hybridized to a microarray containing oligonucleotide probes. After staining with a streptavidin-conjugated fluorescent dye, the array is scanned to detect signal from the hybridized DNA fragments. The pathologist or other qualified health care professional evaluates the allelic ratios and data supporting the recommended identification of specific CYP2C19 variants. The pathologist or other qualified health care professional composes a report that specifies the patient's CYP2C19 allele status. The report is edited and signed, and the results are communicated to appropriate caregivers.

🩺 Clinical Example (81226)

A premenopausal 47-year-old female is seen by an oncologist for breast cancer. Her tumor was positive for estrogen and progesterone receptors. The oncologist is considering treatment with tamoxifen rather than an aromatase inhibitor. To aid in this decision, the oncologist desires to predict the patient's ability to metabolize tamoxifen to the more active drug, endoxifen. A sample of anticoagulated peripheral blood is submitted to the laboratory to test for common variants in the CYP2D6 gene.

Description of Procedure (81226)

High quality genomic DNA is isolated and subjected to two amplification reactions (PCR). Pooled PCR amplicons are enzymatically fragmented, labeled with biotin, and hybridized to a microarray containing oligonucleotide probes. After staining with a streptavidin-conjugated fluorescent dye, the array is scanned to detect signal from the hybridized DNA fragments. The pathologist or other qualified health care professional evaluates the allelic ratios and data supporting the recommended identification of specific CYP2D6 variants. The pathologist or other qualified health care professional composes a report that specifies the patient's CYP2D6 allele status. The report is edited and signed, and the results are communicated to appropriate caregivers.

Clinical Example (81227)

A 60-year-old male presents to his physician with complaints of fatigue, lightheadedness, and palpitations. Diagnostic workup revealed atrial fibrillation, for which the physician would like to prescribe warfarin. In order to facilitate rapid achievement of the proper dose, the physician orders warfarin sensitivity genotyping for common variants of the CYP2C9 gene, which have been shown to significantly influence the dose of warfarin needed to achieve appropriate therapeutic levels. A sample of peripheral blood is submitted to the laboratory for genotypic analysis of the CYP2C9 gene.

Description of Procedure (81227)

High quality genomic DNA is isolated and subjected to a multiplexed PCR reaction, using primers specific for the most common variants, CYP2C9(*2) and CYP2C9(*3). The amplified target DNA is hybridized to a ferrocene signal probe and to an allele-specific capture probe, which is immobilized on an oligoarray. The captured target DNA generates a specific electrochemical signal that identifies the target DNA sequence. The pathologist or other qualified health care professional examines the data and analytic system controls, and determines whether CYP2C9 variants are present in the patient's sample. The pathologist or other qualified health care professional composes a report that specifies the patient's genotype. The report is edited and signed, and the results are communicated to appropriate caregivers.

Clinical Example (81228)

An 18-month-old male presents to his physician with unexplained developmental delay. The patient has a normal karyotype, and his diagnostic evaluation is otherwise unrevealing. A sample of anticoagulated peripheral blood is submitted to the laboratory for cytogenomic constitutional (genome-wide) microarray analysis.

Description of Procedure (81228)

A large quantity of high quality genomic DNA is isolated from a peripheral blood sample. Equal aliquots of patient DNA and normal female control DNA are enzymatically digested and labeled with different fluorescent dyes. The labeled DNA specimens are mixed and hybridized to a microarray slide containing hundreds of thousands of oligonucleotide probes and scanned. A pathologist or other qualified health care professional evaluates parameters such as signal-to-noise ratio, numbers and locations of variations from the reference sequence, and the signal ratios of the patient and opposite sex control for consistency and appropriateness. He or she evaluates graphically displayed patterns for copy number variants throughout the genome with the assistance of computer software. The pathologist or other qualified health care professional composes a report that specifies the patient's copy number variant status using established nomenclature, to include information from a search of internal and publicly accessible databases and published medical literature. The report is edited and signed, and the results are communicated to the appropriate caregivers.

⊘=Modifier 51 Exempt   ⊙=Moderate Sedation   ✚=Add-on Code   ✔=FDA approval pending

⚕ Clinical Example (81229)

A newborn female is determined to have multiple congenital anomalies by the attending physician. The patient has a normal karyotype, and her diagnostic evaluation is otherwise unrevealing. The parents indicate they are both from the same ethnic background. A sample of anticoagulated peripheral blood is submitted to the laboratory for cytogenomic constitutional (genome-wide) microarray analysis.

Description of Procedure (81229)

A large quantity of high quality genomic DNA is isolated from a peripheral blood sample. The patient's DNA is enzymatically digested, PCR amplified, fragmented, and labeled. The labeled DNA is hybridized to a microarray chip containing hundreds of thousands of oligonucleotide probes to detect copy number variants and hundreds of thousands of single nucleotide polymorphism (SNP) probes to determine zygosity status. After scanning the microarray chip, a pathologist or other qualified health care professional assesses parameters such as signal-to-noise ratio, numbers and locations of variations from the reference sequence, and the signal ratios of the patient and a normal reference library for consistency and appropriateness. He or she evaluates graphically displayed patterns for copy number variants and large regions of homozygosity throughout the genome with the assistance of computer software. The pathologist or other qualified health care professional composes a report that specifies the patient's copy number variant and zygosity status using established nomenclature, to include information from a search of internal and publicly accessible databases and published medical literature. The report is edited and signed, and the results are communicated to the appropriate caregivers.

⚕ Clinical Example (81240)

A 45-year-old male with anxiety and kidney stones presented with a two-week history of shortness of breath and pleuritic chest pain. Diagnostic workup revealed multiple bilateral pulmonary emboli. There was a vague history of other family members having "clotting problems." A sample of anticoagulated peripheral blood is submitted to the laboratory for F2 (Prothrombin, coagulation factor II) mutation testing for the 20210G>A variant.

Description of Procedure (81240)

Upon receipt of the specimen, high quality genomic DNA is isolated. The genomic region containing the site of the F2 20210G>A mutation site is amplified by PCR and the amplicon is then subjected to melting curve analysis. The pathologist or other qualified health care professional examines the melting curve plot of red fluorescent signal vs temperature, as well as the plot of the negative first derivative of red fluorescent signal vs temperature. Based on the analysis of these curves, and comparison to the results obtained with wild type and mutant controls, the pathologist or other qualified health care professional determines the F2 20210G>A mutation and zygosity status. He or she composes a report that specifies the patient's mutation status. The report is edited and signed, and the results are communicated to appropriate caregivers.

Clinical Example (81241)

A 25-year-old female developed a right femoral venous thrombosis following a three-hour airplane flight and subsequently developed pulmonary emboli. She had been on oral contraception. There was a vague history of other family members having "clotting problems." A functional, clot-based screening test for resistance to activated protein C (ie, activated protein C resistance assay, APCR) was positive. A sample of anticoagulated peripheral blood is submitted to the laboratory for F5 Leiden mutation testing.

Description of Procedure (81241)

Upon receipt of the specimen, high quality genomic DNA is isolated. The genomic region containing the site of the F5 Leiden mutation site is amplified by PCR, and the amplicon is then subjected to melting curve analysis. The pathologist or other qualified health care professional examines the melting curve plot of red fluorescent signal vs temperature, as well as the plot of the negative first derivative of red fluorescent signal vs temperature. Based on the analysis of these curves, and comparison to the results obtained with wild type and mutant controls, the pathologist or other qualified health care professional determines the F5 Leiden mutation and zygosity status. He or she composes a report that specifies the patient's mutation status. The report is edited and signed, and the results are communicated to appropriate caregivers.

Clinical Example (81242)

A 25-year-old female is seen by her obstetrician for prenatal care. During an office visit, the physician learns that she is of Jewish ancestry, but has not previously been tested to determine if she carries a mutation for Fanconi anemia. A sample of anticoagulated peripheral blood is submitted to the laboratory to test for a variant in the FANCC gene common in the Ashkenazi Jewish population.

Description of Procedure (81242)

Upon receipt of the specimen, high quality genomic DNA is isolated and subjected to multiplex PCR. Following exonuclease I and shrimp alkaline phosphatase treatment, a second reaction using allele specific primer extension (ASPE) amplifies either the normal or mutant allele sequences. Extension products are hybridized to color-coded microspherical beads specific for normal and mutant alleles. The fluorescent signal ratio of mutant to normal alleles is calculated, and the pathologist or other qualified health care professional examines the allelic ratios to determine zygosity status. The pathologist or other qualified health care professional composes a report that specifies the patient's mutation status. The report is edited and signed, and the results are communicated to appropriate caregivers.

Clinical Example (81243)

A 17-year-old male with moderate mental retardation (IQ 50 - 60) of above average height with a long narrow face, close-set eyes, a highly arched palate, a prominent mandible, joint laxity in his fingers, and macroorchidism, presents to a physician for evaluation for the etiology of his mental retardation. Although his mother was of normal intelligence, his family history was remarkable for having an 18-year-old sister with a mild learning disability, a maternal aunt with premature ovarian

⃠=Modifier 51 Exempt   ⊙=Moderate Sedation   ✚=Add-on Code   ✦=FDA approval pending failure, and a 68-year-old maternal grandfather with a progressive neurological illness characterized by development of a tremor, followed by difficulties with balance and occasional falling. A previously performed karyotype was normal. A sample of anticoagulated peripheral blood is submitted to the laboratory for FMR1 gene testing.

Description of Procedure (81243)

Upon receipt of the specimen, high quality genomic DNA is isolated. The genomic region containing the site of the CGG trinucleotide repeat region that is expanded in fragile X syndrome is amplified by using a PCR technique. The amplicons are then subjected to analysis using fluorescent capillary electrophoresis. The pathologist or other qualified health care professional examines the electropherogram and compares it to a sizing ladder to determine the number of CGG repeats within the amplicon. Based on this analysis, the pathologist or other qualified health care professional determines the patient's FMR1 allele status and whether additional characterization of alleles is necessary. He or she composes a report that specifies the patient's allele status. The report is edited and signed, and the results are communicated to appropriate caregivers.

Clinical Example (81244)

During a routine pediatric office visit, the mother of a 10-year-old female describes what she considers to be unusual shyness leading to apparent social isolation, as well as occasional stereotypic behaviors such as hand wringing. The child attends regular school classes and her performance is somewhat below average. There is no family history of mental retardation or other neurologic problems. Both parents are healthy and of average intelligence and the patient has a 13-year-old brother who is otherwise healthy and performs well in school. The patient had a normal karyotype and array CGH study. FMR1 gene testing performed by gel-based PCR analysis revealed a single allele of normal CGG repeat size, but did not definitely show the presence of a second allele. A sample of anticoagulated peripheral blood is sent to the laboratory for Southern blot testing for fragile X syndrome utilizing a methylation specific enzyme.

Description of Procedure (81244)

Upon receipt of the specimen, a large quantity of high quality genomic DNA is isolated. Gel electrophoresis of the extracted DNA is performed to assess DNA integrity. The DNA specimen undergoes double restriction digestion with the methylation-sensitive restriction enzyme EagI and the methylation-insensitive restriction enzyme EcoRI. The genomic fragments are separated by gel electrophoresis, transferred to a nylon membrane by capillary action, and hybridized to a labeled probe. The hybridization pattern is visualized on X-ray film by autoradiography. The pathologist or other qualified health care professional examines the image, compares the observed fragments to a sizing ladder to estimate CGG repeat numbers, and analyzes the patterns generated to assess the methylation status of the promoter region of the expanded FMR1 allele. Based on this analysis the pathologist or other qualified health care professional determines the patient's allele status, presence of expanded allele(s), and methylation status of the FMR1 promoter. He or she composes a report that specifies the patient's allele status, approximate allele sizes, and promoter methylation status. The report is edited and signed, and the results are communicated to the appropriate caregivers.

Clinical Example (81245)

A 55-year-old male presents to his primary care physician complaining of fatigue, dyspnea on exertion, and easy bruising. The patient's hemogram demonstrates leukocytosis with 30% blasts, anemia, and thrombocytopenia. The peripheral blood smear shows decreased platelets and red blood cells along with large blasts with prominent nucleoli and Auer rods. The bone marrow contains 80% blasts which demonstrate an aberrant immunophenotype (CD33/CD13-positive with some cells expressing CD34 and CD117). The karyotype of the malignant cells is normal. An anticoagulated bone marrow specimen is submitted to the laboratory for FLT3 internal tandem duplication (ITD) mutation analysis.

Description of Procedure (81245)

High quality genomic DNA is isolated from the bone marrow sample and subjected to a single PCR amplification encompassing the region which normally contains FLT3 internal tandem duplications. The fluorescent PCR products are separated by capillary electrophoresis. The pathologist or other qualified health care professional evaluates the electropherogram comparing the relative sizes of the PCR product(s) to a control peak to determine FLT3/ITD mutation status. The pathologist or other qualified health care professional composes a report that specifies the FLT3 ITD mutation status of the patient's leukemic cells. The report is edited and signed, and the results are communicated to appropriate caregivers.

Clinical Example (81250)

A 25-year-old female is seen by her obstetrician for prenatal care. During an office visit, the physician learns that she is of Jewish ancestry, but has not previously been tested to determine if she carries a mutation for glycogen storage disease, type 1a (glucose-6-phosphatase deficiency). A sample of anticoagulated peripheral blood is submitted to the laboratory to test for two variants in the G6PC gene common in the Ashkenazi Jewish population.

Description of Procedure (81250)

Upon receipt of the specimen, high quality genomic DNA is isolated and subjected to multiplex PCR. Following exonuclease I and shrimp alkaline phosphatase treatment, a second reaction using allele specific primer extension (ASPE) amplifies either the normal or mutant allele sequences. Extension products are hybridized to color-coded microspherical beads specific for normal and mutant alleles. The fluorescent signal ratio of mutant to normal alleles is calculated, and the pathologist or other qualified health care professional examines the allelic ratios to determine zygosity status. The pathologist or other qualified health care professional composes a report that specifies the patient's mutation status. The report is edited and signed, and the results are communicated to appropriate caregivers.

Clinical Example (81251)

A 25-year-old female is seen by her obstetrician for prenatal care. During an office visit, the physician learns that she is of Jewish ancestry, but has not previously

⊘ =Modifier 51 Exempt   ⊙ =Moderate Sedation   ✚ =Add-on Code   𝒩 =FDA approval pending

been tested to determine if she carries a mutation for Gaucher disease. A sample of anticoagulated peripheral blood is submitted to the laboratory to test for four variants in the GBA gene common in the Ashkenazi Jewish population.

Description of Procedure (81251)

Upon receipt of the specimen, high quality genomic DNA is isolated and subjected to multiplex PCR. Following exonuclease I and shrimp alkaline phosphatase treatment, a second reaction using allele specific primer extension (ASPE) amplifies either the normal or mutant allele sequences. Extension products are hybridized to color-coded microspherical beads specific for normal and mutant alleles. The fluorescent signal ratio of mutant to normal alleles is calculated, and the pathologist or other qualified health care professional examines the allelic ratios to determine zygosity status. The pathologist or other qualified health care professional composes a report that specifies the patient's mutation status. The report is edited and signed, and results are communicated to appropriate caregivers.

Clinical Example (81255)

A 25-year-old female is seen by her obstetrician for prenatal care. During an office visit, the physician learns that she is of Jewish ancestry, but has not previously been tested to determine if she carries a mutation for Tay-Sachs disease. A sample of anticoagulated peripheral blood is submitted to the laboratory to test for three variants in the HEXA gene common in the Ashkenazi Jewish population.

Description of Procedure (81255)

Upon receipt of the specimen, high quality genomic DNA is isolated and subjected to multiplex PCR. Following exonuclease I and shrimp alkaline phosphatase treatment, a second reaction using allele specific primer extension (ASPE) amplifies either the normal or mutant allele sequences. Extension products are hybridized to color-coded microspherical beads specific for normal and mutant alleles. The fluorescent signal ratio of mutant to normal alleles is calculated, and the pathologist or other qualified health care professional examines the allelic ratios to determine zygosity status. The pathologist or other qualified health care professional composes a report that specifies the patient's mutation status. The report is edited and signed, and results are communicated to appropriate caregivers.

Clinical Example (81256)

A 38-year-old male is found to have elevated transferrin saturation (65%) and ferritin (800 ng/mL) on routine testing. The patient is otherwise healthy, and his family history is unremarkable. A sample of anticoagulated peripheral blood is submitted to the laboratory for testing for the HFE p. C282Y (c.845G>A) and p. H63D (c.187 C>G) hereditary hemochromatosis mutations.

Description of Procedure (81256)

Upon receipt of the specimen, high quality genomic DNA is isolated. The genomic regions containing the sites of the HFE p. C282Y (c.845G>A) and p. H63D (c.187 C>G) mutations are amplified by PCR and the amplicons are then subjected to melting curve analysis. The pathologist or other qualified health care professional examines the melting curve plot of red and green fluorescent signals vs temperature, as well as the plot of the negative first derivatives of red and green fluorescent signals vs temperature. Based on the analysis of these curves, and comparison to the results obtained with wild type and mutant controls, the pathologist or other qualified health care professional determines the status of the p. C282Y (c.845G>A) and p. H63D (c.187 C>G) mutations and determines the patient's status as homozygous, heterozygous, or compound heterozygous for each of these mutations. He or she composes a report that specifies the patient's mutation status. The report is edited and signed, and the results are communicated to appropriate caregivers.

Clinical Example (81257)

A 26-year-old G1P0 female of Vietnamese descent presents to her obstetrician for a first prenatal visit after missing a menstrual cycle and obtaining a positive home pregnancy test result. Both the patient and her partner have been identified as alpha thalassemia carriers by hemoglobin electrophoresis. An anticoagulated peripheral blood sample is submitted to the laboratory for testing to identify the specific type of alpha thalassemia mutation the patient carries.

Description of Procedure (81257)

High quality genomic DNA is isolated from whole blood and subjected to multiplex PCR amplification utilizing primers for seven commonly occurring alpha thalassemia deletions. The PCR products, a molecular weight marker, and an allelic ladder are separated by gel electrophoresis. The pathologist or other qualified health care professional evaluates the patterns of the PCR products on the gel in order to identify the patient's specific deletion. The pathologist or other qualified health care professional composes a report specifying the patient's mutation status and the respective chromosomal locations (eg, cis, trans). The report is edited and signed, and the results are communicated to appropriate caregivers.

Clinical Example (81260)

A 25-year-old female is seen by her obstetrician for prenatal care. During an office visit, the physician learns that she is of Jewish ancestry, but has not previously been tested to determine if she carries a mutation for familial dysautonomia. A sample of anticoagulated peripheral blood is submitted to the laboratory to test for two variants in the IKBKAP gene common in the Ashkenazi Jewish population.

Description of Procedure (81260)

Upon receipt of the specimen, high quality genomic DNA is isolated and subjected to multiplex PCR. Following exonuclease I and shrimp alkaline phosphatase treatment, a second reaction using allele specific primer extension (ASPE) amplifies either the normal or mutant allele sequences. Extension products are hybridized to color-coded microspherical beads specific for normal and mutant alleles. The fluorescent signal ratio of mutant to normal alleles is calculated, and the pathologist or other qualified health care professional examines the allelic ratios to determine zygosity status. The pathologist or other qualified health care professional composes a report that specifies the patient's mutation status. The report is edited and signed, and the results are communicated to appropriate caregivers.

⊘=Modifier 51 Exempt ⊙=Moderate Sedation ✚=Add-on Code ✎=FDA approval pending

Clinical Example (81261)

An enlarged supraclavicular lymph node is identified during physical examination of a 62-year-old male at a routine physician visit. A biopsy of the supraclavicular node is taken; initial morphologic and immunologic studies demonstrate a B-cell population that is suspicious for malignancy. A lymph node sample is submitted for immunoglobulin heavy chain gene rearrangement analysis for further evidence of a clonal B-lymphoid population.

Description of Procedure (81261)

High quality genomic DNA is isolated from the lymph node sample and subjected to five multiplex PCR amplification reactions using fluorescently-tagged primers directed at various framework, diversity, and joining regions of the immunoglobulin heavy chain gene. Following amplification, the reaction products from each tube are separately subjected to capillary electrophoresis. The pathologist or other qualified health care professional evaluates the electrophoretic tracings for one or two predominant fragments of discrete size against background polyclonal or oligoclonal peaks for evidence of clonality. The pathologist or other qualified health care professional composes a report that specifies the clonality status of the B-cell population in the patient sample. The report is edited and signed, and the results are communicated to appropriate caregivers.

Clinical Example (81262)

An enlarged inguinal lymph node and splenomegaly was found on physical examination of a 54-year-old Caucasian male who visited his internist complaining of increasing abdominal discomfort. The enlarged inguinal lymph node is excised and initial morphologic and immunologic studies demonstrate a B-cell population that is suspicious for malignancy. A lymph node sample retained frozen is submitted for immunoglobulin heavy chain gene rearrangement Southern blot analysis.

Description of Procedure (81262)

A large quantity of high quality genomic DNA is isolated from the lymph node sample, and gel electrophoresis is performed to assess integrity of the extracted DNA. The DNA undergoes digestion with the three restriction enzymes. The genomic fragments are separated by gel electrophoresis, transferred to a nylon membrane by capillary action, and hybridized to radiolabeled probes directed toward sequences in the immunoglobulin heavy chain joining region. The pathologist or other qualified health care professional evaluates the autoradiographically generated hybridization patterns of the digestion fragments in relation to marker and control lanes for evidence of clonal rearrangements or polymorphisms. The pathologist or other qualified health care professional composes a report specifying the clonality status of the B-cell population. The report is edited and signed, and the results are communicated to appropriate caregivers.

Clinical Example (81263)

A 60-year-old male presents to his primary care physician complaining of recent fatigue, early satiety, and a 5 to 10 lbs. weight loss. The patient has generalized lymphadenopathy and a palpable spleen tip. The complete blood count demonstrates lymphocytosis with anemia and thrombocytopenia. The peripheral blood smear shows an excess of small lymphocytes, occasional prolymphocytes, and smudge cells. Flow cytometry confirms a diagnosis of chronic lymphocytic leukemia. A blood specimen is submitted for IgVH sequencing to assess for somatic hypermutation in the leukemic cells.

Description of Procedure (81263)
High quality genomic DNA is isolated from whole blood and subjected to two multiplex PCR reactions utilizing primers directed at the leader, framework 1, and junctional regions of the immunoglobulin heavy chain gene. PCR products are separated by gel electrophoresis. After purification, clonal PCR products are subjected to dideoxynucleotide sequencing. The pathologist or other qualified health care professional evaluates the degree of divergence from an appropriately selected reference sequence in order to determine somatic hypermutation status. The pathologist or other qualified health care professional composes a report that specifies the patient's IvGH mutation status. The report is edited and signed, and the results are communicated to appropriate caregivers.

Clinical Example (81264)

An enlarged supraclavicular lymph node is identified during physical examination of a 62-year-old male patient at a routine physician visit. A biopsy of the enlarged node is taken and initial morphologic and immunologic studies demonstrate a B-cell population that is suspicious for malignancy. A lymph node sample is submitted for immunoglobulin kappa light chain gene rearrangement analysis for further evidence of a clonal B-lymphoid population.

Description of Procedure (81264)
High quality genomic DNA is isolated from the lymph node sample and subjected to two multiplex PCR amplification reactions using fluorescently-tagged primers directed at various framework, intronic, joining, and kappa-deletion regions of the immunoglobulin kappa light chain gene. Following amplification, the reaction products from each tube are separately subjected to capillary electrophoresis. The pathologist or other qualified health care professional evaluates the electrophoretic tracings for one or two predominant fragments of discrete size against background polyclonal or oligoclonal peaks for evidence of clonality. The pathologist or other qualified health care professional composes a report that specifies the rearrangement and clonality status of the B-cell population in the patient sample. The report is edited and signed, and the results are communicated to appropriate caregivers.

Clinical Example (81265)

A 55-year-old male presents to his physician complaining of fatigue, dyspnea on exertion, and easy bruising. The patient's complete blood count, peripheral blood smear, flow cytometry analysis, and bone marrow examination support a diagnosis of acute myeloid leukemia. Normal cytogenetic findings and the presence of a FLT3 internal tandem duplication mutation place him at high risk for relapse following initial treatment. The patient achieves remission with induction chemotherapy, and he is referred for peripheral blood stem cell transplantation. A matched related donor is found. Stem cells are collected from the donor, and blood

⊘=Modifier 51 Exempt   ⊙=Moderate Sedation   ✚=Add-on Code   𝒩=FDA approval pending

specimens from the patient and the donor are submitted for pretransplant testing to identify informative short tandem repeat (STR) markers for posttransplant chimerism testing.

Description of Procedure (81265)

High quality genomic DNA is isolated from the recipient and donor whole blood samples. The individual DNA isolates are each subjected to a single multiplex PCR amplification reaction that utilizes a combination of 16 primer sets directed toward 15 polymorphic STRs and the gender marker amelogenin. The donor and recipient fluorescent PCR products are separated by capillary electrophoresis. The pathologist or other qualified health care professional compares the relative sizes of the PCR products from the respective electropherograms, and identifies informative alleles that can be used for posttransplant engraftment monitoring. The pathologist or other qualified health care professional composes a report specifying the informative STRs for future chimerism testing. The report is edited and signed, and the results are communicated to appropriate caregivers.

 Clinical Example (81266)

A 55-year-old male presents to his physician complaining of fatigue, dyspnea on exertion, and easy bruising. The patient's complete blood count, peripheral blood smear, flow cytometry analysis, and bone marrow examination support a diagnosis of acute myeloid leukemia. Normal cytogenetic findings and the presence of a FLT3 internal tandem duplication mutation place him at high risk for relapse following initial treatment. The patient achieves remission with induction chemotherapy, and he is referred for peripheral blood stem cell transplantation. Because a matched donor cannot be identified, the patient will undergo a double cord blood transplant. A blood specimen from the patient and samples of each donor cord blood are submitted for pretransplant testing to identify informative short tandem repeat (STR) markers for posttransplant chimerism testing.

Description of Procedure (81266)

High quality genomic DNA is isolated from the recipient whole blood and both cord blood samples. The individual DNA isolates are each subjected to a single multiplex PCR amplification reaction that utilizes a combination of 16 primer sets directed toward 15 polymorphic STRs and the gender marker amelogenin. The fluorescent PCR products from the donors and recipient are separated by capillary electrophoresis. The pathologist or other qualified health care professional compares the relative sizes of the PCR products from the respective electropherograms, and identifies informative alleles that can be used for posttransplant engraftment monitoring. The pathologist or other qualified health care professional composes a report that specifies the informative STRs for future chimerism testing. The report is edited and signed, and the results are communicated to appropriate caregivers.

Clinical Example (81267)

A 55-year-old male who presents with normal karyotype acute myeloid leukemia (AML) undergoes a peripheral blood stem cell transplant after achieving remission with cytarabine and anthracycline chemotherapy. Thirty days posttransplant a blood specimen from the patient is submitted for engraftment (chimerism) testing.

Description of Procedure (81267)

High quality genomic DNA is isolated and subjected to a single multiplex PCR amplification reaction that utilizes a combination of 16 primer sets directed toward 15 polymorphic STRs and the gender marker amelogenin. The fluorescent PCR products are separated by capillary electrophoresis. The pathologist or other qualified health care professional compares electropherogram to the pretransplant recipient and donor electropherograms, and analyzes the informative alleles for the relative proportions of donor and recipient DNA. The pathologist or other qualified health care professional composes a report that states the percentages of donor and recipient alleles present. The report is edited and signed, and the results are communicated to appropriate caregivers.

 Clinical Example (81268)

A 55-year-old male who presents with normal karyotype acute myeloid leukemia (AML) undergoes a peripheral blood stem cell transplant after achieving remission with cytarabine and anthracycline chemotherapy. Thirty days post-transplant a blood specimen from the patient is submitted for engraftment (chimerism) testing.

Description of Procedure (81268)

CD3-positive and CD33-positive cells are isolated using fluorescent antibody-based flow cytometry. High quality genomic DNA is isolated from each of these cellular fractions and subjected to a single multiplex PCR amplification reaction that utilizes a combination of 16 primer sets directed toward 15 polymorphic STRs and the gender marker amelogenin. The fluorescent PCR products are separated by capillary electrophoresis. The pathologist or other qualified health care professional compares the electropherograms to the pretransplant recipient and donor electropherograms, and analyzes the informative alleles for the relative proportions of donor and recipient DNA for each cellular component. The pathologist or other qualified health care professional composes a report that states the percentages of donor and recipient alleles present for each cellular component. The report is edited and signed, and the results are communicated to appropriate caregivers.

Clinical Example (81270)

A 56-year-old male presents with headache, dizziness, and hypertension. A CBC reveals hemoglobin of 20 g/dL and platelet count of 600 000/μL. The physician is concerned that the patient may have a myeloproliferative disorder such as polycythemia vera. A sample of anticoagulated peripheral blood is submitted to the laboratory for JAK2 V617F mutation detection.

Description of Procedure (81270)

Upon receipt of the specimen, high quality DNA is isolated. Allele-specific, real time PCR utilizing hydrolysis probes is performed to amplify a short region spanning the mutation site. Following amplification, genotyping is performed by allelic discrimination, using a mixture of two probes, one of which is specific for the wild type gene, and the other specific for the mutant gene. The pathologist or other qualified health care professional examines a graphical display of the fluorescence signal for the patient's sample, compares the results to mutant and wild type controls, and determines the status of the JAK2 mutant allele. He or she composes a

⃠=Modifier 51 Exempt   ⊙=Moderate Sedation   ✚=Add-on Code   ⊮=FDA approval pending

report that specifies the patient's mutation status. The report is edited and signed, and the results are communicated to appropriate caregivers.

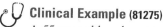

Clinical Example (81275)

A 55-year-old male patient presents with fatigue and weight loss. A full history and physical was performed and blood is discovered in the stool. Gastrointestinal endoscopic examination is performed and a large mass lesion in the sigmoid colon is found. Biopsies are taken and demonstrate a moderately differentiated adenocarcinoma of colonic origin. Subsequent radiologic studies identify possible enlarged lymph nodes in the region of the mass lesion. A resection is performed and metastases are identified. KRAS mutation testing is ordered as the patient is a potential candidate for targeted therapy.

Description of Procedure (81275)

DNA is extracted from a tumor tissue sample. PCR is performed to detect KRAS mutations in a background of wild-type DNA in eight separate reactions utilizing fluorescent probe-linked primers specific for each of the seven most common mutations in codons 12 and 13 of exon 2 of the KRAS gene, as well as a control reaction that amplifies a region of KRAS exon 4. The pathologist or other qualified health care professional analyzes the fluorescent curves that are produced as the PCR products are generated for each reaction. The pathologist or other qualified health care professional assesses the amplification of internal controls in each reaction and compares the difference between the crossing thresholds of the mutation assay and the control assay to the established mutation status. The pathologist or other qualified health care professional composes a report that specifies the mutation status of the patient's tumor and includes a comment on the implications of the lower limit of detection of the test relative to the tumor content of the sample. The report is edited and signed, and the results are communicated to appropriate caregivers.

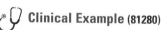

Clinical Example (81280)

A 41-year-old female with no significant cardiac history was eating pizza with her boyfriend when she slumped over and became unresponsive. The patient was transported to the Emergency Department where she was found to be in asystole. She was converted to a normal cardiac rhythm after two rounds of defibrillation. Her QT interval was noted to be markedly prolonged and remained so after stabilization of hypokalemia. The patient was subsequently seen in the outpatient clinic, and an anticoagulated blood sample was submitted for genetic analysis of possible long QT syndrome.

Description of Procedure (81280)

High quality genomic DNA is isolated and the entire coding regions of 12 genes (KCNQ1, KCNH2, SCN5A, KCNE1, KCNE2, KCNJ2, CACNA1C, CAV3, SCN4B, AKAP9, SNTA1, and ANK2) (~224 exons) are examined using a "next generation/massive parallel" sequencing-process that interrogates a large number of amplicons simultaneously. The DNA sequence is assembled using computer software. The pathologist or other health care professional assesses the sequence data, evaluates sequence variants against genomic reference sequences, and identifies any potential mutations. Potential mutations are further subjected to conventional dideoxynucleotide termination DNA sequence analysis. The pathologist or other qualified health care professional evaluates the sequencing electropherograms for the potential mutations. The pathologist or other qualified health care professional composes a report that specifies the patient's mutation status to include comparison to a regularly updated library of novel sequence variants. The report is edited and signed, and the results are communicated to appropriate caregivers.

Clinical Example (81281)

A 34-year-old Caucasian male is referred to a cardiologist by his family physician for evaluation and possible genetic testing. His 38-year-old sister recently underwent testing for a panel of 12 genes associated with long QT syndrome and was diagnosed with a known pathogenic variant in the CACNA1C gene. A blood sample is submitted for targeted gene sequence analysis of the relevant region of the CACNA1C gene.

Description of Procedure (81281)

High quality genomic DNA is isolated from whole blood and subjected to PCR amplification for the CACNA1C gene exon which contains the known familial mutation. The PCR products undergo bidirectional dideoxynucleotide chain termination sequencing using capillary electrophoresis. The pathologist or other qualified health care professional evaluates the sequencing electropherograms for the known familial mutation and any other variants that may be present. The pathologist or other health care professional composes a report that specifies the patient's mutation status. The report is edited and signed, and the results are communicated to appropriate caregivers.

Clinical Example (81282)

A previously asymptomatic 41-year-old Caucasian female who had a recent unexpected occurrence of asystole at which a markedly prolonged QT interval was noted on EKG returns to her cardiologist's office to discuss the results of genetic testing for 12 genes associated with long QT syndrome. No mutations were found. After discussion of those results and given the history and cardiac findings, additional testing for duplication/deletion mutations which are found in ~10% of patients with long QT syndrome is requested.

Description of Procedure (81282)

Using high quality genomic DNA isolated from a previously submitted sample, the laboratory performs deletion/duplication analysis by array comparative genomic hybridization (aCGH) using a custom-designed microarray with probes that detect large and small deletions or duplications in 12 long QT syndrome genes (KCNQ1, KCNH2, SCN5A, KCNE1, KCNE2, KCNJ2, CACNA1C, CAV3, SCN4B, AKAP9, SNTA1, and ANK2). The pathologist or other health care provider evaluates the performance characteristics of hybridization files with the assistance of computer software. The pathologist or other qualified health care professional then evaluates hybridization data for all regions of the 12 interrogated genes. Any positive test results for duplication or deletion are subjected to quantitative PCR

⊘=Modifier 51 Exempt   ⊙=Moderate Sedation   ✚=Add-on Code   𝒩=FDA approval pending

amplification analysis of the involved region(s). The pathologist or other qualified health care professional evaluates the performance characteristics and sample behavior. The pathologist or other qualified health care professional assesses the fluorescent signals generated, normalizing those from the individual amplicons against those from a control gene with the assistance of computer software to determine gene copy number. The pathologist or other qualified health care professional composes a report specifying the patient's mutation status. The report is edited and signed, and the results are communicated to appropriate caregivers.

Clinical Example (81290)

A 25-year-old female is seen by her obstetrician for prenatal care. During an office visit, the physician learns that she is of Jewish ancestry, but has not previously been tested to determine if she carries a mutation for Type IV Mucolipidosis. A sample of anticoagulated peripheral blood is submitted to the laboratory to test for two variants in the MCOLN1gene common in the Ashkenazi Jewish population.

Description of Procedure (81290)

Upon receipt of the specimen, high quality genomic DNA is isolated and subjected to multiplex PCR. Following exonuclease I and shrimp alkaline phosphatase treatment, a second reaction using allele specific primer extension (ASPE) amplifies either the normal or mutant allele sequences. Extension products are hybridized to color-coded microspherical beads specific for normal and mutant alleles. The fluorescent signal ratio of mutant to normal alleles is calculated, and the pathologist or other qualified health care professional examines the allelic ratios to determine zygosity status. The pathologist or other qualified health care professional composes a report that specifies the patient's mutation status. The report is edited and signed, and results are communicated to appropriate caregivers.

Clinical Example (81291)

A 43-year-old male developed a right femoral venous thrombosis following a three-hour airplane flight and subsequently developed pulmonary emboli. There was a vague history of other family members having "clotting problems." His plasma homocysteine level was mildly elevated. A sample of anticoagulated peripheral blood is submitted to the laboratory for MTHFR c.677C>T and c.1298A>C mutation testing.

Description of Procedure (81291)

Upon receipt of the specimen, high quality genomic DNA is isolated. The genomic regions containing the sites of the MTHFR c.677C>T and c.1298A>C variants are amplified by multiplex PCR and the resulting amplicons subjected to melting curve analysis. The pathologist or other qualified health care professional examines the melting curve plots of red and green fluorescent signals vs temperature, as well as the negative first derivative plots of the melting curves. Based on this analysis and comparison of results with appropriate controls, the pathologist or other qualified health care professional determines the zygosity status of the c.677C>T and c.1298A>C variants and composes a report specifying the patient's genotype. The report is edited and signed, and the results are communicated to appropriate caregivers.

Clinical Example (81292)

A 45-year-old male patient presents with fatigue and weight loss. On physical examination, occult blood is discovered in the stool. The patient's family history is positive for colon cancer in several relatives. The patient undergoes a right hemicolectomy after a large, poorly differentiated adenocarcinoma with lymphocytic infiltration is found in the right colon. Microsatellite instability testing performed on the tumor demonstrates high level instability (MSI-H). Immunohistochemical staining reveals a loss of MLH1 protein expression. Mutation testing of the tumor for the BRAF V600E mutation and MLH1 hypermethylation are negative. An anticoagulated peripheral blood sample is submitted for MLH1 gene sequencing to assess the patient for the presence of an HNPCC-related mutation.

Description of Procedure (81292)

High quality genomic DNA is isolated from whole blood and subjected to 19 individual PCR amplification reactions whose products encompass the entire coding sequence, exon-intron boundaries, and portions of 5'- and 3'-untranslated regions of the MLH1 gene. The PCR products from each reaction undergo bidirectional dideoxynucleotide chain termination sequencing using a capillary electrophoresis instrument. The pathologist or other qualified health care professional evaluates the sequencing electropherograms for potential nucleotide sequence variants, insertions, deletions, or other changes. The pathologist or other qualified health care professional compares this evaluation with possible variants suggested by computer software to ensure that all abnormalities are identified. The pathologist or other health care professional composes a report that specifies the patient's mutation status to include information from a database and literature search regarding the significance of variants identified. The report is edited and signed, and the results are communicated to appropriate caregivers.

Clinical Example (81293)

A 40-year-old asymptomatic female whose 45-year-old brother was recently diagnosed with colon cancer and Lynch Syndrome presents to her physician for genetic testing. The brother has a disease-associated mutation in the MLH1 gene. An anticoagulated peripheral blood sample from the asymptomatic woman is submitted for testing for this known familial mutation.

Description of Procedure (81293)

High quality genomic DNA is isolated from whole blood and subjected to PCR amplification for the respective MLH1 exon that contains the known familial mutation. The PCR products undergo bidirectional dideoxynucleotide chain termination sequencing using a capillary electrophoresis instrument. The pathologist or other qualified health care professional evaluates the sequencing electropherograms for the known familial mutation and any other variants that may be present. The pathologist or other health care professional composes a report that specifies the patient's mutation status. The report is edited and signed, and the results are communicated to appropriate caregivers.

⊘=Modifier 51 Exempt   ⊙=Moderate Sedation   ✚=Add-on Code   ⊮=FDA approval pending

Clinical Example (81294)

A 40-year-old male with a family history of colon cancer undergoes a right hemicolectomy to remove a poorly differentiated colonic adenocarcinoma with lymphocytic infiltration. The tumor demonstrates high level microsatellite instability (MSI-H). Immunohistochemistry staining reveals a loss of MLH1 protein expression. Mutation testing on the tumor for the BRAF V600E mutation and MLH1 hypermethylation are negative. Prior MLH1 sequencing performed to assess the patient for the presence of an HNPCC-related mutation was negative. Deletion/duplication analysis of the MLH1 gene is performed.

Description of Procedure (81294)

High quality genomic DNA previously isolated from whole blood is subjected to multiplex ligation probe ligation analysis (MLPA), which involves hybridization and ligation of multiple pairs of oligonucleotide probes specific for the 19 exons of the MLH1 gene to assess dosage of each exon. The pathologist or other qualified health care provider examines peak heights and calculated ratios of individual exons to control gene sequences to determine dosage status for all exons tested in the MLH1 gene. The pathologist or other qualified health care professional composes a report that specifies the patient's mutation status. The report is edited and signed, and the results are communicated to appropriate caregivers.

Clinical Example (81295)

A 45-year-old male patient presents with fatigue and weight loss. On physical examination, occult blood is discovered in the stool. The patient's family history is positive for colon cancer in several relatives. The patient undergoes a right hemicolectomy after a large, poorly differentiated adenocarcinoma with lymphocytic infiltration is found in the right colon. Microsatellite instability testing performed on the tumor demonstrates high level instability (MSI-H). Immunohistochemical staining reveals a loss of MSH2 protein expression. An anticoagulated peripheral blood sample is submitted for MSH2 gene sequencing to assess the patient for the presence of an HNPCC-related mutation.

Description of Procedure (81295)

High quality genomic DNA is isolated from whole blood and subjected to 16 individual PCR amplification reactions. The PCR products from each reaction undergo bidirectional dideoxynucleotide chain termination sequencing using a capillary electrophoresis instrument. The pathologist or other qualified health care professional evaluates the sequencing electropherograms for potential nucleotide sequence variants, insertions, deletions, or other changes. The pathologist or other qualified health care professional compares this evaluation with possible variations suggested by computer software to ensure that all abnormalities are identified. The pathologist or other health care professional composes a report specifying the patient's mutation status to include information from a database and literature search regarding the significance of variants identified. The report is edited and signed, and the results are communicated to appropriate caregivers.

Clinical Example (81296)

A 40-year-old asymptomatic female whose 45-year-old brother was recently diagnosed with colon cancer and Lynch Syndrome presents to her primary care physician for genetic testing. The brother has a disease-associated mutation in the MSH2 gene. An anticoagulated peripheral blood sample from the asymptomatic woman is submitted for testing for this known familial mutation.

Description of Procedure (81296)

High quality genomic DNA is isolated from whole blood and subjected to PCR amplification for the respective MSH2 exon that contains the known familial mutation. The PCR products undergo bidirectional dideoxynucleotide chain termination sequencing using a capillary electrophoresis instrument. The pathologist or other qualified health care professional evaluates the sequencing electropherograms for the known familial mutation and any other variants that may be present. The pathologist or other health care professional composes a report that specifies the patient's mutation status. The report is edited and signed, and the results are communicated to appropriate caregivers.

Clinical Example (81297)

A 40-year-old male with a family history of colon cancer undergoes a right hemicolectomy to remove a poorly differentiated colonic adenocarcinoma with lymphocytic infiltration. The tumor demonstrates high level microsatellite instability (MSI-H). Immunohistochemistry staining reveals a loss of MSH2 protein expression. Prior MLH2 sequencing performed to assess the patient for the presence of an HNPCC-related mutation was negative. Deletion/duplication analysis of the MSH2 gene is performed.

Description of Procedure (81297)

High quality genomic DNA previously isolated from whole blood is subjected to multiplex ligation probe ligation analysis (MLPA), which involves hybridization and ligation of multiple pairs of oligonucleotide probes specific for the 16 exons of the MSH2 gene to assess dosage of each exon. The pathologist or other qualified health care provider examines peak heights and calculated ratios of individual exons to control gene sequences to determine dosage status for all exons tested in the MSH2 gene. The pathologist or other qualified health care professional composes a report that specifies the patient's mutation status. The report is edited and signed, and the results are communicated to appropriate caregivers.

Clinical Example (81298)

A 45-year-old male patient presents with fatigue and weight loss. On physical examination, occult blood is discovered in the stool. The patient's family history is positive for colon cancer in several relatives. The patient undergoes a right hemicolectomy after a large, poorly differentiated adenocarcinoma with lymphocytic infiltration is found in the right colon. Microsatellite instability testing performed on the tumor demonstrates high level instability (MSI-H). Immunohistochemical staining reveals a loss of MSH6 protein expression. An anticoagulated peripheral blood sample is submitted for MSH6 gene sequencing to assess the patient for the presence of an HNPCC-related mutation.

⊘=Modifier 51 Exempt   ⊙=Moderate Sedation   ✚=Add-on Code   ✐=FDA approval pending

Description of Procedure (81298)

High quality genomic DNA is isolated from whole blood and subjected to 10 individual PCR amplification reactions whose products encompass the entire coding sequence, exon-intron boundaries, and portions of 5'- and 3'-untranslated regions of the MSH6 gene. The PCR products from each reaction undergo bidirectional dideoxynucleotide chain termination sequencing using a capillary electrophoresis instrument. The pathologist or other qualified health care professional evaluates the sequencing electropherograms for potential nucleotide sequence variants, insertions, deletions, or other changes. The pathologist or other qualified health care professional compares this evaluation with possible variations suggested by computer software to ensure that all abnormalities are identified. The pathologist or other health care professional composes a report that specifies the patient's mutation status to include information from a database and literature search regarding the significance of variants identified. The report is edited and signed, and the results are communicated to appropriate caregivers.

 ## Clinical Example (81299)

A 40-year-old asymptomatic female whose 45-year-old brother was recently diagnosed with colon cancer and Lynch Syndrome presents to her primary care physician for genetic testing. The brother was found to have a disease-associated mutation in the MSH6 gene. An anticoagulated peripheral blood sample from the asymptomatic woman is submitted to test for an MSH6 gene known familial mutation.

Description of Procedure (81299)

Upon receipt of the specimen, high quality genomic DNA is isolated from whole blood and subjected to PCR amplification for the respective MSH6 exon that contains the known familial mutation. The PCR products undergo bidirectional dideoxynucleotide chain termination sequencing using a capillary electrophoresis instrument. The pathologist or other qualified health care professional evaluates the sequencing electropherograms for the known familial mutation and any other variants that may be present. The pathologist or other health care professional composes a report that specifies the patient's mutation status. The report is edited and signed, and the results are communicated to appropriate caregivers.

Clinical Example (81300)

A 40-year-old male with a family history of colon cancer undergoes a right hemicolectomy to remove a poorly differentiated colonic adenocarcinoma with lymphocytic infiltration. The tumor demonstrates high level microsatellite instability (MSI-H). Immunohistochemical staining reveals a loss of MSH6 protein expression. Prior MLH6 gene sequencing performed to assess the patient for the presence of an HNPCC-related mutation was negative. Deletion/duplication analysis of the MSH6 gene is performed.

Description of Procedure (81300)

High quality genomic DNA previously isolated from whole blood is subjected to multiplex ligation probe ligation analysis (MLPA), which involves hybridization and ligation of multiple pairs of oligonucleotide probes specific for the 10 exons of the MSH6 gene to assess dosage of each exon. The pathologist or other qualified health care professional examines peak heights and calculated ratios of individual exons to control gene sequences to determine dosage status for all exons tested in the MSH6 gene. The pathologist or other qualified health care professional composes a report that specifies the patient's mutation status. The report is edited and signed, and the results are communicated to appropriate caregivers.

Clinical Example (81301)

A 45-year-old male patient presents with fatigue and weight loss. On physical examination, occult blood is discovered in the stool. The patient's family history is positive for colon cancer in several relatives. The patient undergoes a right hemicolectomy after a large, poorly differentiated adenocarcinoma with lymphocytic infiltration is found in the right colon. Microsatellite instability (MSI) testing is performed on the tumor and adjacent normal tissue.

Description of Procedure (81301)

Paraffin is removed, and DNA is isolated from the patient's tumor and normal tissue. Each DNA isolate is subjected to a multiplex PCR amplification reaction that utilizes a combination of seven fluorescently-labeled primer sets directed toward five mononucleotide repeat markers (BAT-25, BAT-26, NR-21, NR-24, and MONO-27), and two pentanucleotide repeat markers (Penta C and Penta D). The fluorescent PCR products from the tumor and normal tissue are each separated by capillary electrophoresis. The pathologist or other qualified health care professional determines the MSI status of the tumor by comparing the electrophoretic patterns generated by the PCR products from tumor and normal tissue DNA in relation to a sizing standard for each of the repeat markers, and assessing the proportion of unstable markers. The pathologist or other qualified health care professional composes a report that specifies the MSI status of the tumor. The report is edited and signed, and the results are communicated to appropriate caregivers.

Clinical Example (81302)

A 2-½ year-old female born to a G2P2 mother following an unremarkable pregnancy presents to her pediatrician with regression in her language and motor skills over several months. On physical examination, the patient is small, with a head circumference in the fifth percentile. She has mildly decreased muscle tone in her limbs and slight truncal ataxia. She displays occasional abnormal limb posturing, as well as repetitive hand wringing. Rett syndrome is suspected. An anticoagulated peripheral blood sample is submitted for MECP2 sequencing to assess the patient's MECP2 mutation status.

Description of Procedure (81302)

High quality genomic DNA is isolated from whole blood and subjected to four individual PCR amplification reactions, the products of which encompass the entire coding sequence, intron-exon boundaries, and portions of 5'- and 3'-untranslated regions of the MECP2 gene. The PCR products from each reaction undergo bidirectional dideoxynucleotide chain termination sequencing using a capillary electrophoresis instrument. The pathologist or other qualified health care professional evaluates the sequencing electropherograms for potential nucleotide

⊘=Modifier 51 Exempt   ⊙=Moderate Sedation   ✛=Add-on Code   ℵ=FDA approval pending

sequence variants, insertions, deletions, or other changes. The pathologist or other qualified health care professional compares this evaluation with possible variations suggested by computer software to ensure that all abnormalities are identified. The pathologist or other health care professional composes a report that specifies the patient's mutation status. The report is edited and signed, and the results are communicated to appropriate caregivers.

Clinical Example (81303)

A 14-month-old female born to a G2P2 mother who has a known MECP2 mutation presents to her pediatrician with developmental delay. The patient's older sister was diagnosed with Rett syndrome two years previously, and a mutation in the MECP2 gene was identified. At that time, the patient's mother was tested and was found to carry the identical MECP2 mutation. An anticoagulated peripheral blood sample is submitted for MECP2 sequencing to assess the patient for the known familial MECP2 mutation.

Description of Procedure (81303)

High quality genomic DNA is isolated from whole blood and subjected to PCR amplification reaction of the exon that contains the known familial MECP2 mutation. The PCR products undergo bidirectional dideoxynucleotide chain termination sequencing using a capillary electrophoresis instrument. The pathologist or other qualified health care professional evaluates the sequencing electropherograms for the known familial mutation and any other variants that may be present. The pathologist or other health care professional composes a report that specifies the patient's mutation status. The report is edited and signed, and the results are communicated to appropriate caregivers.

Clinical Example (81304)

A 2-½ year-old female born to a G2P2 mother following an unremarkable pregnancy presents to her pediatrician with regression in her language and motor skills over several months. On physical examination, the patient is small with a head circumference in the fifth percentile. She has mildly decreased muscle tone in her limbs and slight truncal ataxia. She displays occasional abnormal limb posturing, as well as repetitive hand wringing. Rett syndrome is suspected. An anticoagulated peripheral blood sample was submitted to the laboratory for MECP2 sequencing, and a mutation was not detected. Deletion/duplication analysis of the MECP2 gene is performed.

Description of Procedure (81304)

High quality genomic DNA previously isolated from whole blood is subjected to multiplex ligation probe ligation analysis (MLPA), which involves hybridization and ligation of oligonucleotide probes specific for the four exons of the MECP2 gene to assess dosage of each exon. The pathologist or other qualified health care provider examines peak heights and calculated ratios of individual exons to control gene sequences to determine dosage status for all exons tested in the MECP2 gene. The pathologist or other qualified health care professional composes a report that specifies the patient's mutation status. The report is edited and signed, and the results are communicated to appropriate caregivers.

Clinical Example (81310)

A 55-year-old male presents to his primary care physician complaining of fatigue, dyspnea on exertion, and easy bruising. The patient's hemogram demonstrates leukocytosis with 30% blasts, anemia, and thrombocytopenia. The peripheral blood smear shows decreased platelets and red blood cells along with large blasts with prominent nucleoli and Auer rods. The bone marrow contains 80% blasts which demonstrate an aberrant immunophenotype (CD33/CD13-positive with some cells expressing CD34 and CD117). The karyotype of the malignant cells is normal. A sample of anticoagulated bone marrow is submitted for NPM1 exon 12 tetranucleotide insertion mutation testing.

Description of Procedure (81310)

Upon receipt of the specimen high quality genomic DNA is isolated. A single PCR amplification is performed encompassing the region which normally contains NPM1 tetranucleotide insertion mutations. The fluorescent PCR products are separated by capillary electrophoresis. The pathologist or other qualified health care professional evaluates the electropherogram comparing the relative sizes of the PCR product(s) in relation to a control peak to determine the NPM1 exon 12 mutation status. The pathologist or other qualified health care professional composes a report describing the NPM1 exon 12 mutation status of the patient's leukemic cells. The report is edited and signed, and the results are communicated to appropriate caregivers.

Clinical Example (81315)

A 45-year-old previously healthy male presented to his physician complaining of fatigue, weakness, dyspnea, and easy bruising. He was found to have an elevated white blood count, anemia, and severe thrombocytopenia. The peripheral blood smear demonstrated large numbers of promyelocytes. Laboratory studies indicated DIC was present. The patient was emergently started on all transretinoic acid, an anthracycline, and supportive therapy for his coagulopathy. Bone marrow aspiration was performed, cytogenetic studies were ordered, and anticoagulated marrow was immediately sent to the laboratory for PML/RARalpha translocation testing by quantitative real-time PCR.

Description of Procedure (81315)

Upon receipt of the specimen, total RNA is isolated and assessed for quality. Quantitative real-time reverse transcriptase PCR is performed in three separate tubes to detect and quantify the bcr1, bcr2, and bcr3 breakpoints as well as the Abelson gene (ABL1) in each tube. The pathologist or other qualified health care professional analyzes the blue fluorescent curves that are produced as the PCR products are generated to determine the status of the translocation. He or she relates the crossing threshold to previously generated standard curves for the PML-RARA and ABL transcripts to determine the normalized and absolute copy numbers of the PML-RARA transcripts present in the specimen at the time of testing. The pathologist or other qualified health care professional composes a report that describes the transcript status, the specific isoform, and the normalized copy number. The report is edited and signed, and the results are communicated to appropriate caregivers.

⊘=Modifier 51 Exempt ⊙=Moderate Sedation ✚=Add-on Code 𝒩=FDA approval pending

Clinical Example (81316)

Quantitative PCR testing is requested on a 45-year-old male with an established diagnosis of acute promyelocytic leukemia to assess for treatment effectiveness and disease relapse. Anticoagulated marrow is sent to the laboratory for PML/RARalpha translocation testing for the previously identified breakpoint by quantitative real-time PCR.

Description of Procedure (81316)

Upon receipt of the specimen, total RNA is isolated and assessed for quality. Quantitative real-time reverse transcriptase PCR is performed to detect and quantify the patient's specific breakpoint and the Abelson gene (ABL1). The pathologist or other qualified health care professional analyzes the blue fluorescent curves that are produced as the PCR products are generated to determine the status of the translocation. He or she relates the crossing threshold to previously generated standard curves for the PML-RARA and ABL transcripts to determine the normalized and absolute copy numbers of the PML-RARA transcript present in the specimen at the time of testing. The pathologist or other qualified health care professional composes a report that describes the transcript status and the normalized copy number, and compares these breakpoint specific results with the patient's previous results. The report is edited and signed, and the results are communicated to appropriate caregivers.

Clinical Example (81317)

A 45-year-old male patient presents with fatigue and weight loss. On physical examination, occult blood is discovered in the stool. The patient's family history is positive for colon cancer in several relatives. The patient undergoes a right hemicolectomy after a large, poorly differentiated adenocarcinoma with lymphocytic infiltration is found in the right colon. Microsatellite instability testing performed on the tumor demonstrates high level instability (MSI-H). Immunohistochemical staining reveals a loss of PMS2 protein expression. An anticoagulated peripheral blood sample is submitted for PMS2 sequencing to assess the patient for the presence of an HNPCC-related mutation.

Description of Procedure (81317)

High quality genomic DNA is isolated from whole blood and subjected to 15 individual PCR amplification reactions. The PCR products from each reaction undergo bidirectional dideoxynucleotide chain termination sequencing using a capillary electrophoresis instrument. The pathologist or other qualified health care professional evaluates the sequencing electropherograms for potential nucleotide sequence variants, insertions, deletions, or other changes. The pathologist or other qualified health care professional compares this evaluation with possible variations suggested by computer software to ensure that all abnormalities are identified. The pathologist or other health care professional composes a report that specifies the patient's mutation status to include information from a database and literature search regarding the significance of variants identified. The report is edited and signed, and the results are communicated to appropriate caregivers.

Clinical Example (81318)

A 40-year-old asymptomatic female whose 45-year-old brother was recently diagnosed with colon cancer and Lynch Syndrome presents to her primary care physician for genetic testing. The brother has a disease-associated mutation in the PMS2 gene. An anticoagulated peripheral blood sample from the asymptomatic woman is submitted for testing for this known familial mutation.

Description of Procedure (81318)

High quality genomic DNA is isolated from whole blood and subjected to PCR amplification for the respective PMS2 gene exon that contains the known familial mutation. The PCR products undergo bidirectional dideoxynucleotide chain termination sequencing using a capillary electrophoresis instrument. The pathologist or other qualified health care professional evaluates the sequencing electropherograms for the known familial mutation and any other variants that may be present. The pathologist or other health care professional composes a report that specifies the patient's mutation status. The report is edited and signed, and the results are communicated to appropriate caregivers.

Clinical Example (81319)

A 40-year-old male with a family history of colon cancer undergoes a right hemicolectomy to remove a poorly differentiated colonic adenocarcinoma with lymphocytic infiltration. The tumor demonstrates high level microsatellite instability. Immunohistochemistry staining reveals a loss of PMS2 protein expression. Prior PMS2 gene sequencing performed to assess the patient for the presence of an HNPCC-related mutation was negative. Deletion/duplication analysis of the PMS2 gene is performed.

Description of Procedure (81319)

High quality genomic DNA previously isolated from whole blood is subjected to multiplex ligation probe ligation analysis (MLPA) which involves hybridization and ligation of multiple pairs of oligonucleotide probes specific for 13 of the 15 exons of the PMS2 gene to assess dosage of each exon. The pathologist or other qualified health care provider examines peak heights and calculated ratios of individual exons to control gene sequences to determine dosage status for all exons tested in the PMS2 gene. The pathologist or other qualified health care professional composes a report that specifies the patient's mutation status. The report is edited and signed, and the results are communicated to appropriate caregivers.

Clinical Example (81330)

A 25-year-old female is seen by her obstetrician for prenatal care. During an office visit, the physician learns that she is of Jewish ancestry, but has not previously been tested to determine if she carries a mutation for Niemann-Pick disease. A sample of anticoagulated peripheral blood is submitted to the laboratory to test for three variants in the SMPD1gene common in the Ashkenazi Jewish population.

Description of Procedure (81330)

Upon receipt of the specimen, high quality genomic DNA is isolated and subjected to multiplex PCR. Following exonuclease I and shrimp alkaline phosphatase treatment, a second reaction using allele specific primer extension (ASPE) amplifies

⊘=Modifier 51 Exempt   ⊙=Moderate Sedation   ✚=Add-on Code   ✗=FDA approval pending

either the normal or mutant allele sequences. Extension products are hybridized to color-coded microspherical beads specific for normal and mutant alleles. The fluorescent signal ratio of mutant to normal alleles is calculated, and the pathologist or other qualified health care professional examines the allelic ratios to determine zygosity status. The pathologist or other qualified health care professional composes a report that specifies the patient's mutation status. The report is edited and signed, and results are communicated to appropriate caregivers.

Clinical Example (81331)

A 2-year-old female is brought to a pediatrician for evaluation. She has consistently been in the 5th to 10th percentile on growth charts, is somewhat developmentally delayed, and is a voracious eater. The pediatrician discusses the possibility of Prader-Willi syndrome with the parents. A sample of anticoagulated peripheral blood is submitted for SNRPN/UBE3A methylation analysis.

Description of Procedure (81331)

High quality genomic DNA is isolated from the blood sample and undergoes bisulfite modification to convert unmethylated cytosine nucleotides to uracil. Following PCR amplification using primers specific for sequences on the maternal (methylated) and paternal (unmethylated) chromosomes, the PCR products are separated on agarose gels. The pathologist or other qualified health care professional evaluates the electrophoretic patterns to determine whether normal biparental inheritance is demonstrated. The pathologist or other qualified health care professional composes a report that specifies the patient's SNRPN/UBE3A mutation status. The report is edited and signed, and the results are communicated to appropriate caregivers.

Clinical Example (81332)

A 53-year-old female with an extensive smoking history complains to her family physician that she has been experiencing modest but increasing shortness of breath. Pulmonary function studies suggest mild airflow obstruction consistent with chronic obstructive pulmonary disease. Liver enzyme studies are normal. Alpha-1-antitrypsin deficiency is part of the differential diagnosis. An anticoagulated peripheral blood sample is submitted for SERPINA1 genotype determination of the "Z" and "S" alleles.

Description of Procedure (81332)

High quality genomic DNA is isolated and subjected to two separate PCR amplification reactions encompassing the regions of the SERPIN1A gene which code for the "Z" and "S" alleles. PCR amplification products are digested with different restriction endonucleases, and the digestion products are visualized separately by ethidium bromide staining following agarose gel electrophoresis. The pathologist or other qualified health care professional evaluates the patterns of restriction endonuclease digestion products on gel photographs to determine the patient's mutation status for the normal "M" as well as mutant "Z" and "S" alleles. The pathologist or other qualified health care professional composes a report that specifies the patient's SERPINA1 mutation status. The report is edited and signed, and the results are communicated to the appropriate caregivers.

Clinical Example (81340)

A 55-year-old male patient presents with fever, episodic night sweats, weight loss, and lymphadenopathy. A biopsy of an enlarged supraclavicular node is taken; initial morphologic and immunologic studies demonstrate a T-cell population that is suspicious for malignancy. A frozen sample of the lymph node is submitted for T-cell antigen receptor gene and beta rearrangement studies as part of a pathologic evaluation for lymphoma.

Description of Procedure (81340)

High quality genomic DNA is extracted from a lymph node sample. In order to detect a clonally rearranged population of T-cells against a background of polyclonal T-cells, three multiplex PCR reactions are performed using fluorescent-linked primers directed at the variable, joining, and diversity regions of the T-cell receptor beta chain genes. The resulting PCR products are separated using capillary electrophoresis. The pathologist or other qualified health care professional evaluates the capillary tracing for a predominant fragment of discrete size and appropriate morphology against background polyclonal or oligoclonal peaks for evidence of clonality. The pathologist or other qualified health care professional composes a report that specifies the clonality status of the T-cell population. The report is edited and signed, and the results are communicated to appropriate caregivers.

Clinical Example (81341)

A 55-year-old male patient presents with fever, episodic night sweats, weight loss, and lymphadenopathy. Biopsy of an enlarged supraclavicular node is taken; initial morphologic and immunologic studies demonstrate a T-cell population that is suspicious for malignancy. T-cell gene rearrangement studies performed using PCR analysis are indeterminate. A frozen sample of the lymph node is submitted to the laboratory for Southern blot analysis to further assess for a clonally rearranged population of T-cells.

Description of Procedure (81341)

A large quantity of high quality genomic DNA is isolated from the lymph node sample. Gel electrophoresis of the extracted DNA is performed to assess DNA integrity. The DNA undergoes digestion with three restriction enzymes. The genomic fragments are separated by gel electrophoresis, transferred to a nylon membrane by capillary action, and hybridized to radiolabeled probes directed toward the TCRB joining regions (Jβ1 and 2). The pathologist or other qualified health care professional evaluates the autoradiographically generated hybridization patterns of the digestion fragments in relation to marker and control lanes to determine T-cell clonality status. The pathologist or other qualified health care professional composes a report that specifies the clonality status of the T-cell population. The report is edited and signed, and the results are communicated to appropriate caregivers.

Clinical Example (81342)

A 55-year-old male patient presents with fever, episodic night sweats, weight loss, and lymphadenopathy. A biopsy of an enlarged supraclavicular node is taken;

⊘=Modifier 51 Exempt   ⊙=Moderate Sedation   ✚=Add-on Code   ✗=FDA approval pending

initial morphologic and immunologic studies demonstrate a T-cell population that is suspicious for malignancy. A frozen sample of the lymph node is submitted for T-cell antigen receptor gene and gamma rearrangement studies as part of a pathologic evaluation for lymphoma.

Description of Procedure (81342)

High quality genomic DNA is extracted from a lymph node sample. In order to detect a clonally rearranged population of T-cells against a background of polyclonal T-cells, two multiplex PCR reactions are performed using fluorescent linked primers directed toward the variable and joining regions of the T-cell receptor gamma genes. The resulting PCR products are separated using capillary electrophoresis. The pathologist or other qualified health care professional evaluates the capillary tracing for a predominant fragment of discrete size and appropriate shape against background polyclonal or oligoclonal peaks for evidence of clonality. The pathologist or other qualified health care professional composes a report that specifies the clonality status of the T-cell population. The report is edited and signed, and the results are communicated to appropriate caregivers.

Clinical Example (81350)

A 60-year-old male patient presents with fatigue and weight loss. The patient is found to have poorly differentiated adenocarcinoma of the colon with unresectable metastases to the liver. Despite 5-FU, leucovorin, and oxaliplatin (FLOFOX) therapy, the patient's disease progresses, and irinotecan therapy is recommended. Prior to beginning irinotecan treatment, an anticoagulated peripheral blood sample is submitted to test the patient's UGT1A1 promoter TA repeat numbers.

Description of Procedure (81350)

High quality genomic DNA is isolated from whole blood and subjected to PCR amplification for the region containing the UGT1A1 promoter TA repeat segment. The fluorescent products are subjected to analysis using capillary electrophoresis. The pathologist or other qualified health care professional evaluates the electropherogram and compares it to a sizing ladder to determine the patient's genotype. Based on this analysis, the pathologist or other qualified health care professional composes a report that specifies the patient's genotype. The report is edited and signed, and the results are communicated to appropriate caregivers.

Clinical Example (81355)

A 60-year-old male presents to his physician with complaints of fatigue, light-headedness, and palpitations. A diagnostic workup revealed atrial fibrillation, for which the physician would like to prescribe warfarin. In order to facilitate rapid achievement of the proper dose, the physician orders warfarin sensitivity genotyping for common variants of the VKORC1 gene, which have been shown to significantly influence the dose of warfarin needed to achieve appropriate therapeutic levels. A sample of peripheral blood is submitted for genotypic analysis of the VKORC1 gene.

Description of Procedure (81355)

High quality genomic DNA is isolated and subjected to a multiplexed PCR reaction, using primers specific for the most common variants, VKORC1 (-1639A).

The amplified target DNA is hybridized to a ferrocene signal probe and to an allele-specific capture probe, which is immobilized on an oligoarray. The captured target DNA generates a specific electrochemical signal that identifies the target DNA sequence. The pathologist or other qualified health care professional examines the patient's results and analytic system controls, and determines whether VKORC1 variants are present in the patient's sample. The pathologist or other qualified health care professional composes a report that specifies the patient's genotype. The report is edited and signed, and the results are communicated to appropriate caregivers.

Clinical Example (81370)

A 55-year-old male with insulin dependent diabetes mellitus has end stage renal disease for which he is receiving dialysis treatment. The patient is found to be a suitable renal transplant candidate, and HLA typing is requested for listing on the UNOS kidney registry for potential recipients. A sample of anticoagulated peripheral blood is submitted to the laboratory for low resolution HLA-A, -B, -C, -DRB1/3/4/5, and -DQB1 testing.

Description of Procedure (81370)

High quality genomic DNA is isolated from whole blood. The genomic regions containing the HLA-A, -B, -C, -DRB1/3/4/5 and -DQB1 loci are amplified by PCR using a series of 142 sequence-specific primer sets. The amplicons produced are separated by size via gel electrophoresis. The pathologist or other qualified health care professional examines a digitized image or photograph of the ethidium bromide stained gel to assess the presence or absence of amplicons produced for the allele group-specific reactions in comparison to positive and negative controls. Based on the manual analysis of amplicon patterns and with the assistance of computer software, the pathologist or other qualified health care professional determines the HLA type for the HLA-A, -B, -C, DRB1/3/4/5, and High quality genomic DNA is isolated from whole blood. The genomic region containing the HLA-DQB1 locus is PCR amplified using sets of sequence-specific primers to detect HLA-DQB1*06 group alleles and to distinguish among DQB1*06 alleles. The amplicons produced are separated by size via gel electrophoresis. The pathologist or other qualified health care professional examines the digitized images or photographs of the ethidium bromide stained gels to assess the presence or absence of amplicons produced for the specific reactions in comparison to positive and negative controls. Based on the manual analysis of the amplicon patterns and with the assistance of computer software, the pathologist or other qualified health care professional determines whether the HLA-DQB1*06:02 allele is present. The pathologist or other qualified health care professional composes a report that specifies the patient's HLA-DQB1*06:02 allele status. The report is edited and signed, and the results are communicated to appropriate caregivers. The pathologist or other qualified health care professional composes a report that specifies the patient's HLA type at the low resolution level. The report is edited and signed, and the results are communicated to appropriate caregivers.

Clinical Example (81371)

A 45-year-old male with acute myelogenous leukemia with unfavorable cytogenetics is in his first remission. The patient will require a hematopoietic stem cell transplant. A potential HLA-matched unrelated donor has been identified through the National Marrow Donor Program. Prior to final donor selection, a sample of anticoagulated peripheral blood is submitted to the laboratory for low resolution typing for HLA-A, -B, -DRB1/3/4/5 to confirm the recipient's typing and donor match.

Description of Procedure (81371)

High quality genomic DNA is isolated from whole blood. The genomic regions containing the HLA-A, -B, -DRB1/3/4/5 loci are amplified by PCR using a series of 95 sequence-specific primer sets. The amplicons produced are separated by size via gel electrophoresis. The pathologist or other qualified health care professional examines a digitized image or photograph of the ethidium bromide stained gel to assess the presence or absence of amplicons produced for the allele group-specific reactions in comparison to positive and negative controls. Based on the manual analysis of the amplicon patterns and with the assistance of computer software, the pathologist or other qualified health care professional determines the HLA type for the HLA-A, -B, and -DRB1/3/4/5 loci, and compares the results to the original high resolution typing used for the donor search to verify the original typing result. The pathologist or other qualified health care professional composes a report that specifies the patient's HLA type from both analyses. The report is edited and signed, and the results are communicated to appropriate caregivers.

Clinical Example (81372)

A 40-year-old female has a history of diffuse large cell lymphoma. The patient has undergone chemotherapy and has been multiply transfused. She has become refractory to platelet transfusion as a result of antibodies to Class I HLA antigens. A sample of anticoagulated peripheral blood is submitted to the laboratory for low resolution HLA-A, -B, -C testing to initiate a search for an HLA matched platelet unit for transfusion.

Description of Procedure (81372)

High quality genomic DNA is isolated from whole blood. The genomic regions containing the HLA-A, -B, -C loci are amplified by PCR using a series of 95 sequence-specific primer sets. The amplicons produced are separated by size via gel electrophoresis. The pathologist or other qualified health care professional examines a digitized image or photograph of the ethidium bromide stained gel to assess the presence or absence of amplicons produced for the allele group-specific reactions in comparison to positive and negative controls. Based on the manual analysis of the amplicon patterns and with the assistance of computer software, the pathologist or other qualified health care professional determines the HLA type for the HLA-A, -B, and -C loci. The pathologist or other qualified health care professional composes a report that specifies the patient's HLA type at the low resolution level. The report is edited and signed, and the results are communicated to appropriate caregivers.

Clinical Example (81373)

A 32-year-old female has a complex array of symptoms and signs that indicate the presence of an autoimmune disorder. Several disorders with HLA-B associations are considered. A sample of anticoagulated peripheral blood is submitted to the laboratory for HLA-B typing.

Description of Procedure (81373)

High quality genomic DNA is isolated from whole blood. The genomic region containing the HLA-B locus is amplified by PCR using 47 sequence-specific primers sets. The amplicons produced are separated by size via gel electrophoresis. The pathologist or other qualified health care professional examines a digitized image or photograph of the ethidium bromide stained gel to assess the presence or absence of amplicons produced for the allele group-specific reactions in comparison to positive and negative controls. Based on the manual analysis of the amplicon patterns and with the assistance of computer software, the pathologist or other qualified health care professional determines the HLA type for the HLA-B locus. The pathologist or other qualified health care professional composes a report that specifies the patient's HLA-B type at the low resolution level. The report is edited and signed, and the results are communicated to appropriate caregivers.

Clinical Example (81374)

A 37-year-old male has suspected ankylosing spondylitis. A sample of anticoagulated peripheral blood is submitted to the laboratory for HLA-B*27 testing.

Description of Procedure (81374)

High quality genomic DNA is isolated from whole blood. The genomic region containing the HLA-B locus is amplified with the PCR using a set of primers specific for HLA-B27. The amplicons produced are separated by size via gel electrophoresis. The pathologist or other qualified health care professional examines a digitized image or photograph of the ethidium bromide stained gel to assess the presence or absence of amplicons produced for the allele group-specific reactions in comparison to positive and negative controls. Based on the manual analysis of the amplicon patterns and with the assistance of computer software, the pathologist or other qualified health care professional determines the HLA-B*27 status. The pathologist or other qualified health care professional composes a report that specifies the patient's HLA-B*27 status. The report is edited and signed, and the results communicated to appropriate caregivers.

Clinical Example (81375)

A 28-year-old male is being considered as a potential hematopoietic stem cell donor for his sister who has been diagnosed with acute myelogenous leukemia. He and the other asymptomatic siblings were initially typed for Class I HLA (HLA-A,-B,-C). He was found to be a full match for his sister at these loci. A sample of anticoagulated peripheral blood is submitted to the laboratory for low resolution HLA-DRB1/3/4/5 and -DQB1 typing.

⊘=Modifier 51 Exempt   ⊙=Moderate Sedation   ✚=Add-on Code   ⟋=FDA approval pending

Description of Procedure (81375)

High quality genomic DNA is isolated from whole blood. The genomic region containing the HLA-DRB1/3/4/5 and -DQB1 loci are amplified by PCR using 48 sequence-specific primer sets. The amplicons produced are separated by size via gel electrophoresis. The pathologist or other qualified health care professional examines a digitized image or photograph of the ethidium bromide stained gel to assess the presence or absence of amplicons produced for the allele group-specific reactions in comparison to positive and negative controls. Based on the manual analysis of the amplicon patterns and with the assistance of computer software, the pathologist or other qualified health care professional determines the HLA type for the HLA-DRB1/3/4/5, and -DQB1 loci. The pathologist or other qualified health care professional composes a report that specifies the donor's HLA-DRB1/3/4/5 and -DQB1 type at the low resolution level and assesses the match with the recipient. The report is edited and signed, and the results are communicated to appropriate caregivers.

Clinical Example (81376)

A 45-year-old male is being considered as a potential kidney donor for a friend with end-stage renal disease. The potential recipient has antibodies against multiple HLA-DQ antigens and will be incompatible with 85% of the donor pool. The physician wishes to screen the potential donor for HLA-DQB1 before proceeding with a full donor work-up. A sample of anticoagulated peripheral blood from the potential donor is submitted to the laboratory for HLA-DQB1 typing.

Description of Procedure (81376)

High quality genomic DNA is isolated from whole blood. The genomic region containing the HLA -DQB1 loci is amplified by PCR using 24 sequence-specific primer sets. The amplicons produced are separated by size via gel electrophoresis. The pathologist or other qualified health care professional examines a digitized image or photograph of the ethidium bromide stained gel to assess the presence or absence of amplicons produced for the allele group-specific reactions in comparison to positive and negative controls. Based on the manual analysis of the amplicon patterns and with the assistance of computer software, the pathologist or other qualified health care professional determines the HLA type for the HLA-DQB1 locus. The pathologist or other qualified health care professional composes a report that specifies the patient's HLA-DQB1 type at the low resolution level. The report is edited and signed, and the results are communicated to appropriate caregivers.

Clinical Example (81377)

A 50-year-old female presents to an ophthalmologist for ocular pain and photophobia. She has been suffering headaches and dizziness for several weeks. Upon examination, the doctor finds signs of posterior uveitis and observes vitiligo on her face and her arms. He suspects Vogt-Koyanagi-Harada (VKH), an autoimmune disease strongly associated with HLA-DR4. A sample of anticoagulated peripheral blood is submitted to the laboratory for HLA-DR4 typing.

Description of Procedure (81377)

High quality genomic DNA is isolated and subjected to PCR amplification using a set of primers specific for the HLA-DRB1*04 allele group. A series of negative and positive control DNA samples are run in parallel. The amplicons produced are separated by size via gel electrophoresis. The pathologist or other qualified health care professional examines a digitized image or photograph of the ethidium bromide stained gel to assess the presence or absence of amplicons produced for the allele group-specific reactions in comparison to positive and negative controls. Based on the manual analysis of the amplicon patterns and with the assistance of computer software, the pathologist or other qualified health care professional determines the HLA-DRB1*04 status. The pathologist or other qualified health care professional composes a report that specifies the patient's HLA-DRB1*04 status. The report is edited and signed, and the results are communicated to appropriate caregivers.

 Clinical Example (81378)

A 45-year-old male with acute myelogenous leukemia with unfavorable cytogenetics is in his first remission. The patient will require a hematopoietic stem cell transplant and has no siblings. A sample of anticoagulated peripheral blood is submitted to the laboratory for high resolution HLA-A, -B, -C and -DRB1 testing to search for an HLA matched donor through the National Marrow Donor Program.

Description of Procedure (81378)

High quality genomic DA is isolated from whole blood. The genomic regions containing the HLA-A, -B, -C and DRB1 genes are amplified by PCR using locus specific primers. For each locus, the PCR products are sequenced with a series of forward and reverse primers. The pathologist or other qualified health care professional visually analyzes the DNA sequences obtained and assesses their alignment against a consensus sequence and comparison with a database of all known alleles with the assistance of software. Ambiguities are resolved using sequence-specific primers. Based on these analyses, the pathologist or other qualified health care professional assigns an HLA type for HLA-A, -B, -C and DRB1 at the allele level. The pathologist or other qualified health care professional composes a report that specifies the patient's HLA type. The report is edited and signed, and the results are communicated to appropriate caregivers.

Clinical Example (81379)

A 45-year-old male with acute myelogenous leukemia is being considered for a hematopoietic stem cell transplant from an unrelated donor. The potential recipient has been previously typed by high resolution for HLA Class II and low resolution for HLA-A, -B, and -C in an unsuccessful attempt to identify a related donor. To select the best unrelated donor, high resolution typing of the patient is necessary. A sample of anticoagulated peripheral blood is submitted to the laboratory for high resolution HLA-A, -B, and -C allele identification.

Description of Procedure (81379)

High quality genomic DNA is isolated from whole blood. The genomic regions containing the HLA-A, -B, and -C genes are amplified by PCR using locus specific

⊘=Modifier 51 Exempt   ⊙=Moderate Sedation   ✚=Add-on Code   ✗=FDA approval pending

primers. For each locus, the PCR products are sequenced with a series of forward and reverse primers. The pathologist or other qualified health care professional evaluates the DNA sequences obtained, assesses their alignment against a consensus sequence, and compares results against a database of all known alleles with the assistance of computer software. Ambiguities are resolved using sequence-specific primers. Based on these analyses, the pathologist or other qualified health care professional assigns an HLA type for HLA-A, -B, and -C at the allele level. The pathologist or other qualified health care professional composes a report that specifies the patient's HLA type. The report is edited and signed, and the results are communicated to appropriate caregivers.

Clinical Example (81380)

A 34-year-old female with acute myelogenous leukemia is being considered for a hematopoietic stem cell transplant from a related donor. Low resolution HLA typing of the patient and several family members identifies a brother who is a potential 2 haplotype match. However, four closely related HLA-B allele groups are segregating in the family, calling into question whether the patient and her brother have inherited identical HLA-B alleles. High resolution typing of the B locus of the patient and her brother is required to resolve this ambiguity. A sample of anticoagulated peripheral blood from the patient is submitted to the laboratory for high resolution HLA-B locus testing to assess her HLA-B allele type for comparison to her brother's type.

Description of Procedure (81380)

High quality genomic DNA is isolated from whole blood. The genomic regions containing the HLA-B gene are amplified by PCR using locus-specific primers. The resulting PCR products are sequenced with a series of forward and reverse primers. The pathologist or other qualified health care professional evaluates the DNA sequences obtained, assesses their alignment against a consensus sequence and compares results against a database of all known alleles with the assistance of computer software. Ambiguities are resolved using sequence-specific primers. Based on these analyses, the pathologist or other qualified health care professional assigns an HLA type for HLA-B at the allele level. The pathologist or other qualified health care professional composes a report that specifies the patient's HLA type and assesses the match with the potential donor. The report is edited and signed, and the results are communicated to appropriate caregivers.

Clinical Example (81381)

An antiretroviral regimen including the drug abacavir is planned for a 35-year-old male with a diagnosis of HIV-1. Prior to beginning abacavir treatment, a sample of anticoagulated peripheral blood is submitted to the laboratory for HLA-B*57:01 allele testing.

Description of Procedure (81381)

High quality genomic DNA is isolated from whole blood. The genomic region containing the HLA-B locus is amplified by PCR, and the amplicons are interrogated in hybridization reactions with 100 oligonucleotide probes immobilized on fluorescent microscopic beads. Fluorescence is then assessed in a fluorescent bead array assay. The pathologist or other qualified health care professional examines the fluorescent intensities seen with each probe and determines the status of the HLA-B*57 allele group with the assistance of computer software. Testing with additional probes to distinguish HLA-B*57:01 from other B*57 alleles is performed if necessary. Based on these analyses, the pathologist or other qualified health care professional determines the status of the HLA-B*57:01 allele. The pathologist or other qualified health care professional composes a report that specifies the patient's HLA-B*57:01 allele status. The report is edited and signed, and the results are communicated to appropriate caregivers.

 Clinical Example (81382)

A 45-year-old male with acute myelogenous leukemia with unfavorable cytogenetics is in his first remission. The patient will require a hematopoietic stem cell transplant and has no siblings. In addition to high resolution HLA-A, -B, -C and DRB1 testing, the physician requests that HLA-DQB1 be included in the search for an HLA matched donor through the National Marrow Donor Program. A sample of anticoagulated peripheral blood is submitted to the laboratory for HLA-DQB1 allele typing.

Description of Procedure (81382)

High quality genomic DNA is isolated from whole blood. The genomic region containing the HLA Class II gene is amplified by PCR using locus-specific primers. The PCR products are sequenced with a series of forward and reverse primers. The pathologist or other qualified health care professional evaluates the DNA sequences obtained, assesses their alignment against a consensus sequence and compares results against a database of all known alleles with the assistance of computer software. Ambiguities are resolved using sequence-specific primers. Based on these analyses, the pathologist or other qualified health care professional assigns an HLA type at the allele level. The pathologist or other qualified health care professional composes a report that specifies the patient's HLA-DQB1 alleles. The report is edited and signed, and the results are communicated to appropriate caregivers.

Clinical Example (81383)

A 30-year-old female describes excessive daytime sleepiness over the past two months and a recent single episode of transient weakness resulting in her collapse to the floor while discussing a family member's recent death. The results of a polysomnogram and a multiple sleep latency test are indeterminate in helping reach a diagnosis of narcolepsy. A sample of anticoagulated peripheral blood is submitted to the laboratory for HLA-DQB1*06:02 allele identification.

Description of Procedure (81383)

High quality genomic DNA is isolated from whole blood. The genomic region containing the HLA-DQB1 locus is PCR amplified using sets of sequence-specific primers to detect HLA-DQB1*06 group alleles and to distinguish among DQB1*06 alleles. The amplicons produced are separated by size via gel electrophoresis. The pathologist or other qualified health care professional examines the digitized images or photographs of the ethidium bromide stained gels to assess the presence

⊘=Modifier 51 Exempt ⊙=Moderate Sedation ✚=Add-on Code ⚡=FDA approval pending or absence of amplicons produced for the specific reactions in comparison to positive and negative controls. Based on the manual analysis of the amplicon patterns and with the assistance of computer software, the pathologist or other qualified health care professional determines whether the HLA-DQB1*06:02 allele is present. The pathologist or other qualified health care professional composes a report that specifies the patient's HLA-DQB1*06:02 allele status. The report is edited and signed, and the results are communicated to appropriate caregivers.

▶Tier 2 Molecular Pathology Procedures◀

▶The following molecular pathology procedure (Tier 2) codes are used to report procedures not listed in the Tier 1 molecular pathology codes (81200-81350). They represent medically useful procedures that are generally performed in lower volumes than Tier 1 procedures (eg, the incidence of the disease being tested is rare). They are arranged by level of technical resources and interpretive work by the physician or other qualified health care professional. The individual analyses listed under each code (ie, level of procedure) utilize the definitions and coding principles as described in the introduction preceding the Tier 1 molecular pathology codes. The parenthetical examples of methodologies presented near the beginning of each code provide general guidelines used to group procedures for a given level and are not all-inclusive.

Use the appropriate molecular pathology procedure level code that includes the specific analyte listed after the code descriptor. If the analyte tested is not listed under one of the Tier 2 codes or is not represented by a Tier 1 code, use the appropriate methodology codes in the 83890-83914 and 88384-88386 series.◀

●81400   Molecular pathology procedure, Level 1 (eg, identification of single germline variant [eg, SNP] by techniques such as restriction enzyme digestion or melt curve analysis)

ACADM (acyl-CoA dehydrogenase, C-4 to C-12 straight chain, MCAD) (eg, medium chain acyl dehydrogenase deficiency), K304E variant

ACE (angiotensin converting enzyme) (eg, hereditary blood pressure regulation), insertion/deletion variant

AGTR1 (angiotensin II receptor, type 1) (eg, essential hypertension), 1166A>C variant

CCR5 (chemokine C-C motif receptor 5) (eg, HIV resistance), 32-bp deletion mutation/794 825del32 deletion

DPYD (dihydropyrimidine dehydrogenase) (eg, 5-fluorouracil/5-FU and capecitabine drug metabolism), IVS14+1G>A variant

F2 (coagulation factor 2) (eg, hereditary hypercoagulability), 1199G>A variant

F5 (coagulation factor V) (eg, hereditary hypercoagulability), HR2 variant

F7 (coagulation factor VII [serum prothrombin conversion accelerator]) (eg, hereditary hypercoagulability), R353Q variant

F13B (coagulation factor XIII, B polypeptide) (eg, hereditary hypercoagulability), V34L variant

FGB (fibrinogen beta chain) (eg, hereditary ischemic heart disease), -455G>A variant

Human Platelet Antigen 1 genotyping (HPA-1), *ITGB3 (integrin, beta 3 [platelet glycoprotein IIIa], antigen CD61 [GPIIIa])* (eg, neonatal alloimmune thrombocytopenia [NAIT], post-transfusion purpura), HPA-1a/b (L33P)

Human Platelet Antigen 2 genotyping (HPA-2), *GP1BA (glycoprotein Ib [platelet], alpha polypeptide [GPIba])* (eg, neonatal alloimmune thrombocytopenia [NAIT], post-transfusion purpura), HPA-2a/b (T145M)

Human Platelet Antigen 3 genotyping (HPA-3), *ITGA2B (integrin, alpha 2b [platelet glycoprotein IIb of IIb/IIIa complex], antigen CD41 [GPIIb])* (eg, neonatal alloimmune thrombocytopenia [NAIT], post-transfusion purpura), HPA-3a/b (I843S)

Human Platelet Antigen 4 genotyping (HPA-4), *ITGB3 (integrin, beta 3 [platelet glycoprotein IIIa], antigen CD61 [GPIIIa])* (eg, neonatal alloimmune thrombocytopenia [NAIT], post-transfusion purpura), HPA-4a/b (R143Q)

Human Platelet Antigen 5 genotyping (HPA-5), *ITGA2 (integrin, alpha 2 [CD49B, alpha 2 subunit of VLA-2 receptor] [GPIa])* (eg, neonatal alloimmune thrombocytopenia [NAIT], post-transfusion purpura), HPA-5a/b (K505E)

Human Platelet Antigen 6 genotyping (HPA-6w), *ITGB3 (integrin, beta 3 [platelet glycoprotein IIIa, antigen CD61] [GPIIIa])* (eg, neonatal alloimmune thrombocytopenia [NAIT], post-transfusion purpura), HPA-6a/b (R489Q)

Human Platelet Antigen 9 genotyping (HPA-9w), *ITGA2B (integrin, alpha 2b [platelet glycoprotein IIb of IIb/IIIa complex, antigen CD41] [GPIIb])* (eg, neonatal alloimmune thrombocytopenia [NAIT], post-transfusion purpura), HPA-9a/b (V837M)

Human Platelet Antigen 15 genotyping (HPA-15), *CD109 (CD109 molecule)* (eg, neonatal alloimmune thrombocytopenia [NAIT], post-transfusion purpura), HPA-15a/b(S682Y)

SERPINE1 (serpine peptidase inhibitor clade E, member 1, plasminogen activator inhibitor -1, PAI-1) (eg, thrombophilia), 4G variant

●**81401**   Molecular pathology procedure, Level 2 (eg, 2-10 SNPs, 1 methylated variant, or 1 somatic variant [typically using nonsequencing target variant analysis], or detection of a dynamic mutation disorder/ triplet repeat)

ABL (c-abl oncogene 1, receptor tyrosine kinase) (eg, acquired imatinib resistance), T315I variant

ACADM (acyl-CoA dehydrogenase, C-4 to C-12 straight chain, MCAD) (eg, medium chain acyl dehydrogenase deficiency), commons variants (eg, K304E, Y42H)

ADRB2 (adrenergic beta-2 receptor surface) (eg, drug metabolism), common variants (eg, G16R, Q27E)

APOE (apolipoprotein E) (eg, hyperlipoproteinemia type III, cardiovascular disease, Alzheimer disease), common variants (eg, *2, *3, *4)

CBFB/MYH11 (inv(16)) (eg, acute myeloid leukemia), qualitative, and quantitative, if performed

CCND1/IGH (BCL1/IgH, t(11;14)) (eg, mantle cell lymphoma) translocation analysis, major breakpoint, qualitative, and quantitative, if performed

CFH/ARMS2 (complement factor H/age-related maculopathy susceptibility 2) (eg, macular degeneration), common variants (eg, Y402H [CFH], A69S [ARMS2])

⊘=Modifier 51 Exempt   ⊙=Moderate Sedation   ✚=Add-on Code   ⋏=FDA approval pending

CYP3A4 (cytochrome P450, family 3, subfamily A, polypeptide 4) (eg, drug metabolism), common variants (eg, *2, *3, *4, *5, *6)

CYP3A5 (cytochrome P450, family 3, subfamily A, polypeptide 5) (eg, drug metabolism), common variants (eg, *2, *3, *4, *5, *6)

DMPK (dystrophia myotonica-protein kinase) (eg, myotonic dystrophy, type 1), evaluation to detect abnormal (eg, expanded) alleles

F11 (coagulation factor XI) (eg, coagulation disorder), common variants (eg, E117X [Type II], F283L [Type III], IVS14del14, and IVS14+1G>A [Type I])

FGFR3 (fibroblast growth factor receptor 3) (eg, achondroplasia), common variants (eg, 1138G>A, 1138G>C)

FIP1L1/PDGFRA (del[4q12]) (eg, imatinib-sensitive chronic eosinophilic leukemia), qualitative, and quantitative, if performed

GALT (galactose-1-phosphate uridylyltransferase) (eg, galactosemia), common variants (eg, Q188R, S135L, K285N, T138M, L195P, Y209C, IVS2-2A>G, P171S, del5kb, N314D, L218L/N314D)

HBB (hemoglobin, beta) (eg, sickle cell anemia, hemoglobin C, hemoglobin E), common variants (eg, HbS, HbC, HbE)

HTT (huntingtin) (eg, Huntington disease), evaluation to detect abnormal (eg, expanded) alleles

RUNX1/RUNX1T1 (t(8;21)) (eg, acute myeloid leukemia) translocation analysis, qualitative, and quantitative, if performed

SEPT9 (Septin 9) (eg, colon cancer), methylation analysis

TPMT (thiopurine S-methyltransferase) (eg, drug metabolism), common variants (eg, *2, *3)

VWF (von Willebrand factor) (eg, von Willebrand disease type 2N), common variants (eg, T791M, R816W, R854Q)

●**81402**   Molecular pathology procedure, Level 3 (eg, >10 SNPs, 2-10 methylated variants, or 2-10 somatic variants [typically using non-sequencing target variant analysis], immunoglobulin and T-cell receptor gene rearrangements, duplication/deletion variants 1 exon)

CYP21A2 (cytochrome P450, family 21, subfamily A, polypeptide 2) (eg, congenital adrenal hyperplasia, 21-hydroxylase deficiency), common variants (eg, IVS2-13G, P30L, I172N, exon 6 mutation cluster [I235N, V236E, M238K], V281L, L307FfsX6, Q318X, R356W, P453S, G110VfsX21, 30-kb deletion variant)

ESR1/PGR (receptor 1/progesterone receptor) ratio (eg, breast cancer)

KIT (v-kit Hardy-Zuckerman 4 feline sarcoma viral oncogene homolog) (eg, mastocytosis), common variants (eg, D816V, D816Y, D816F)

MEFV (Mediterranean fever) (eg, familial Mediterranean fever), common variants (eg, E148Q, P369S, F479L, M680I, I692del, M694V, M694I, K695R, V726A, A744S, R761H)

MPL (myeloproliferative leukemia virus oncogene, thrombopoietin receptor, TPOR) (eg, myeloproliferative disorder), common variants (eg, W515A, W515K, W515L, W515R)

TCD@ (T cell antigen receptor, delta) (eg, leukemia and lymphoma), gene rearrangement analysis, evaluation to detect abnormal clonal population

●81403   Molecular pathology procedure, Level 4 (eg, analysis of single exon by DNA sequence analysis, analysis of >10 amplicons using multiplex PCR in 2 or more independent reactions, mutation scanning or duplication/deletion variants of 2-5 exons)

ABL1 (c-abl oncogene 1, receptor tyrosine kinase) (eg, acquired imatinib tyrosine kinase inhibitor resistance), variants in the kinase domain

DAZ/SRY (deleted in azoospermia and sex determining region Y) (eg, male infertility), common deletions (eg, AZFa, AZFb, AZFc, AZFd)

GJB1 (gap junction protein, beta 1) (eg, Charcot-Marie-Tooth X-linked), full gene sequence

JAK2 (Janus kinase 2) (eg, myeloproliferative disorder), exon 12 sequence and exon 13 sequence, if performed

KRAS (v-Ki-ras2 Kirsten rat sarcoma viral oncogene) (eg, carcinoma), gene analysis, variant(s) in exon 2

MPL (myeloproliferative leukemia virus oncogene, thrombopoietin receptor, TPOR) (eg, myeloproliferative disorder), exon 10 sequence

VHL (von Hippel-Lindau tumor suppressor) (eg, von Hippel-Lindau familial cancer syndrome), deletion/duplication analysis

VWF (von Willebrand factor) (eg, von Willebrand disease types 2A, 2B, 2M), targeted sequence analysis (eg, exon 28)

●81404   Molecular pathology procedure, Level 5 (eg, analysis of 2-5 exons by DNA sequence analysis, mutation scanning or duplication/deletion variants of 6-10 exons, or characterization of a dynamic mutation disorder/triplet repeat by Southern blot analysis)

BTD (biotinidase) (eg, biotinidase deficiency), full gene sequence

CYP1B1 (cytochrome P450, family 1, subfamily B, polypeptide 1) (eg, primary congenital glaucoma), full gene sequence

DMPK (dystrophia myotonica-protein kinase) (eg, myotonic dystrophy type 1), characterization of abnormal (eg, expanded) alleles

EGR2 (early growth response 2) (eg, Charcot-Marie-Tooth), full gene sequence

FKRP (Fukutin related protein) (eg, congenital muscular dystrophy type 1C [MDC1C], limb-girdle muscular dystrophy [LGMD] type 2I), full gene sequence

FOXG1 (forkhead box G1) (eg, Rett syndrome), full gene sequence

FSHMD1A (facioscapulohumeral muscular dystrophy 1A) (eg, facioscapulohumeral muscular dystrophy), evaluation to detect abnormal (eg, deleted) alleles

FSHMD1A (facioscapulohumeral muscular dystrophy 1A) (eg, facioscapulohumeral muscular dystrophy), characterization of haplotype(s) (ie, chromosome 4A and 4B haplotypes)

HBB (hemoglobin, beta, Beta-Globin) (eg, thalassemia), full gene sequence

⊘=Modifier 51 Exempt   ⊙=Moderate Sedation   ✚=Add-on Code   ✗=FDA approval pending

KIT (C-kit) (v-kit Hardy-Zuckerman 4 feline sarcoma viral oncogene homolog) (eg, GIST, acute myeloid leukemia, melanoma), targeted gene analysis (eg, exons 8, 11, 13, 17, 18)

LITAF (lipopolysaccharide-induced TNF factor) (eg, Charcot-Marie-Tooth), full gene sequence

MEFV (Mediterranean fever) (eg, familial Mediterranean fever), full gene sequence

NRAS (neuroblastoma RAS viral oncogene homolog) (eg, colorectal carcinoma), exon 1 and exon 2 sequences

PDGFRA (platelet-derived growth factor receptor alpha polypeptide) (eg, gastrointestinal stromal tumor), targeted sequence analysis (eg, exons 12, 18)

RET (ret proto-oncogene) (eg, multiple endocrine neoplasia, type 2B and familial medullary thyroid carcinoma), common variants (eg, M918T, 2647_2648delinsTT, A883F)

SDHD (succinate dehydrogenase complex, subunit D, integral membrane protein) (eg, hereditary paraganglioma), full gene sequence

VHL (von Hippel-Lindau tumor suppressor) (eg, von Hippel-Lindau familial cancer syndrome), full gene sequence

VWF (von Willebrand factor) (eg, von Willebrand disease type 1C), targeted sequence analysis (eg, exons 26, 27, 37)

●**81405**   Molecular pathology procedure, Level 6 (eg, analysis of 6-10 exons by DNA sequence analysis, mutation scanning or duplication/deletion variants of 11-25 exons)

CYP21A2 (cytochrome P450, family 21, subfamily A, polypeptide2) (eg, steroid 21-hydroxylase isoform, congenital adrenal hyperplasia), full gene sequence

FKTN (fukutin) (eg, limb-girdle muscular dystrophy [LGMD] type 2M or 2L), full gene sequence

MPZ (myelin protein zero) (eg, Charcot-Marie-Tooth), full gene sequence

NEFL (neurofilament, light polypeptide) (eg, Charcot-Marie-Tooth), full gene sequence

RET (ret proto-oncogene) (eg, multiple endocrine neoplasia, type 2A and familial medullary thyroid carcinoma), targeted sequence analysis (eg, exons 10, 11, 13-16)

SDHB (succinate dehydrogenase complex, subunit B, iron sulfur) (eg, hereditary paraganglioma), full gene sequence

TGFBR1 (transforming growth factor, beta receptor 1) (eg, Marfan syndrome), full gene sequence

TGFBR2 (transforming growth factor, beta receptor 2) (eg, Marfan syndrome), full gene sequence

THRB (thyroid hormone receptor, beta) (eg, thyroid hormone resistance, thyroid hormone beta receptor deficiency), full gene sequence or targeted sequence analysis of >5 exons

TP53 (tumor protein 53) (eg, Li-Fraumeni syndrome, tumor samples), full gene sequence or targeted sequence analysis of >5 exons

VWF (von Willebrand factor) (eg, von Willebrand disease type 2N), targeted sequence analysis (eg, exons 18-20, 23-25)

● **81406** Molecular pathology procedure, Level 7 (eg, analysis of 11-25 exons by DNA sequence analysis, mutation scanning or duplication/deletion variants of 26-50 exons, cytogenomic array analysis for neoplasia)

CAPN3 (Calpain 3) (eg, limb-girdle muscular dystrophy [LGMD] type 2A, calpainopathy), full gene sequence

Cytogenomic microarray analysis, neoplasia (eg, interrogation of copy number, and loss-of-heterozygosity via single nucleotide polymorphism [SNP]-based comparative genomic hybridization [CGH] microarray analysis)

GALT (galactose-1-phosphate uridylyltransferase) (eg, galactosemia), full gene sequence

HEXA (hexosaminidase A, alpha polypeptide) (eg, Tay-Sachs disease), full gene sequence

LMNA (lamin A/C) (eg, Emery-Dreifuss muscular dystrophy [EDMD1, 2 and 3] limb-girdle muscular dystrophy [LGMD] type 1B, dilated cardiomyopathy [CMD1A], familial partial lipodystrophy [FPLD2]), full gene sequence

PAH (phenylalanine hydroxylase) (eg, phenylketonuria), full gene sequence

POLG (polymerase [DNA directed], gamma) (eg, Alpers-Huttenlocher syndrome, autosomal dominant progressive external ophthalmoplegia), full gene sequence

POMGNT1 (protein O-linked mannose beta1,2-N acetylglucosaminyltransferase) (eg, muscle-eye-brain disease, Walker-Warburg syndrome), full gene sequence

POMT1 (protein-O-mannosyltransferase 1) (eg, limb-girdle muscular dystrophy [LGMD] type 2K, Walker-Warburg syndrome), full gene sequence

POMT2 (protein-O-mannosyltransferase 2) (eg, limb-girdle muscular dystrophy [LGMD] type 2N, Walker-Warburg syndrome), full gene sequence

RYR1 (ryanodine receptor 1, skeletal) (eg, malignant hyperthermia), targeted sequence analysis of exons with functionally-confirmed mutations

VWF (von Willebrand factor) (von Willebrand disease type 2A), extended targeted sequence analysis (eg, exons 11-16, 24-26, 51, 52)

● **81407** Molecular pathology procedure, Level 8 (eg, analysis of 26-50 exons by DNA sequence analysis, mutation scanning or duplication/deletion variants of >50 exons, sequence analysis of multiple genes on one platform)

SCN1A (sodium channel, voltage-gated, type 1, alpha subunit) (eg, generalized epilepsy with febrile seizures), full gene sequence

● **81408** Molecular pathology procedure, Level 9 (eg, analysis of >50 exons in a single gene by DNA sequence analysis)

FBN1 (fibrillin 1) (eg, Marfan syndrome), full gene sequence

NF1 (neurofibromin 1) (eg, neurofibromatosis, type 1), full gene sequence

RYR1 (ryanodine receptor 1, skeletal) (eg, malignant hyperthermia), full gene sequence

VWF (von Willebrand factor) (eg, von Willebrand disease types 1 and 3), full gene sequence

⊘=Modifier 51 Exempt   ⊙=Moderate Sedation   ✚=Add-on Code   ⫫=FDA approval pending

Clinical Example (81400)

An asymptomatic newborn female of Northern European descent is suspected to have medium chain acyl dehydrogenase deficiency (MCAD) on the basis of newborn screening. A sample of anticoagulated peripheral blood is submitted for genetic testing for the common ACADM gene K304E variant.

Description of Procedure (81400)

High quality genomic DNA is isolated. The genomic region containing the site of the K304E variant is amplified by PCR using primers that in the presence of the K304E variant, introduce an additional restriction endonuclease site into the amplicon. The PCR products undergo digestion with a restriction endonuclease, and the resulting fragments are separated using gel electrophoresis. The pathologist or other qualified health care professional evaluates the patterns of the digestion fragments in relation to marker and control lanes to determine the patient's mutation and zygosity status. The pathologist or other qualified health care professional composes a report that specifies the patient's mutation and zygosity status. The report is edited and signed, and the results are communicated to appropriate caregivers.

Clinical Example (81401)

A 30-year-old asymptomatic male with a family history of Huntington disease presents to his physician for predictive genetic testing for Huntington disease. A sample of anticoagulated peripheral blood is submitted for HTT mutation testing.

Description of Procedure (81401)

High quality genomic DNA is isolated. The genomic region containing the site of the CAG trinucleotide repeat region that is expanded in Huntington Disease syndrome is then PCR-amplified and the fluorescently-labeled products subjected to capillary electrophoresis. The pathologist or other qualified health care professional examines the electropherogram and compares the amplicon peaks to a sizing ladder to determine the number of CAG repeats within each allele. Based on this analysis, the pathologist or other qualified health care professional determines the patient's HTT mutation status. The pathologist or other qualified health care professional composes a report that specifies the patient's mutation status. The report is edited and signed, and the results are communicated to appropriate caregivers.

Clinical Example (81402)

A 14-year-old female of Turkish descent is seen by her physician for her third episode of fever accompanied by pleuritic chest pain, abdominal discomfort, and pain in the lower extremity joints. Her physical examination demonstrates a temperature of 38.5C and dullness to percussion at the left lung base. Her abdomen is rigid with apparent rebound tenderness and diminished bowel sounds, and her left knee is warm and swollen with pain upon passive motion. Her white blood count, erythrocyte sedimentation rate, and fibrinogen level are elevated. Familial Mediterranean fever is suspected, and a sample of anticoagulated peripheral blood is submitted for genetic testing for common variants in the MEFV gene.

Description of Procedure (81402)

High quality genomic DNA is isolated and subjected to multiplex PCR. Following exonuclease I and shrimp alkaline phosphatase treatment, a second reaction using allele specific primer extension (ASPE) amplifies either the normal or mutant allele sequences for 11 common MEFV variants. The fluorescently-tagged PCR products are separated by capillary electrophoresis. The pathologist or other qualified health care professional evaluates the electropherogram comparing the relative sizes and peak heights of the PCR products to determine mutation and zygosity status. The pathologist or other qualified health care professional composes a report that specifies the patient's mutation status. The report is edited and signed, and the results are communicated to appropriate caregivers.

 Clinical Example (81403)

A 72-year-old male with chronic myelogenous leukemia (CML) of several years duration on maintenance therapy with imatinib mesylate, experiences a greater than 1 log increase in his BCR/ABL1 transcript levels on repeat measurements. He reports adherence to his therapeutic regimen, and his imatinib level was found to be within the therapeutic range. Because of an apparent loss of response to imatinib, a sample of anticoagulated peripheral blood is submitted for ABL1 tyrosine kinase domain sequencing to assess for imatinib resistance mutations.

Description of Procedure (81403)

High quality total cellular RNA is isolated and stored under RNase-free conditions. Reverse transcriptase is used to convert RNA to cDNA. PCR amplification using primers for the BCR/ABL1 major breakpoint translocation is performed, followed by nested PCR amplification using internal primers flanking the tyrosine kinase domain region. The nested PCR products undergo bidirectional dideoxynucleotide chain termination sequencing using a capillary electrophoresis instrument. The pathologist or other qualified health care professional evaluates the sequencing electropherograms for potential nucleotide sequence variants. The pathologist or other qualified health care professional compares this evaluation with possible variations suggested by computer software to ensure that all abnormalities are identified. The pathologist or other health care professional composes a report specifying the patient's ABL1 kinase domain mutation status. The report is edited and signed, and the results are communicated to appropriate caregivers.

 Clinical Example (81404)

A 30-year-old female who has relatives with head and neck paragangliomas presents to her physician complaining of an enlarging, otherwise asymptomatic right-sided neck mass. Imaging studies suggest a carotid body paraganglioma. The patient is referred to a surgeon, who suspects a hereditary paraganglioma-pheochromocytoma syndrome. An anticoagulated peripheral blood sample is submitted for SDHD gene sequencing.

Description of Procedure (81404)

High quality genomic DNA is isolated from whole blood and subjected to four individual PCR amplification reactions. The PCR products from each reaction undergo bidirectional dideoxynucleotide chain termination sequencing using a

⊘=Modifier 51 Exempt ⊙=Moderate Sedation ✚=Add-on Code 𝑵=FDA approval pending

capillary electrophoresis instrument. The pathologist or other qualified health care professional evaluates the sequencing electropherograms for potential nucleotide sequence variants, insertions, deletions, or other changes. The pathologist or other qualified health care professional compares this evaluation with possible variations suggested by computer software to ensure that all abnormalities are identified. The pathologist or other health care professional composes a report specifying the patient's mutation status. The report is edited and signed, and the results are communicated to appropriate caregivers.

 ### Clinical Example (81405)

A 30-year-old female with a family history that includes several relatives with chromaffin tumors presents to her physician complaining of episodic headaches, palpitations, sweating, and anxiety. Plasma metanephrines are elevated, and an MRI reveals a mass in the region of the organ of Zuckerkandl, that upon resection is confirmed to be a paraganglioma. A hereditary paraganglioma-pheochromocytoma syndrome is suspected, and an anticoagulated peripheral blood sample is submitted for SDHB gene sequencing.

Description of Procedure (81405)

High quality genomic DNA is isolated from whole blood and subjected to eight individual PCR amplification reactions. The PCR products from each reaction undergo bidirectional dideoxynucleotide chain termination sequencing using a capillary electrophoresis instrument. The pathologist or other qualified health care professional evaluates the sequencing electropherograms for potential nucleotide sequence variants, insertions, deletions, or other changes. The pathologist or other qualified health care professional compares this evaluation with possible variations suggested by computer software to ensure that all abnormalities are identified. The pathologist or other health care professional composes a report specifying the patient's SDHB mutation status. The report is edited and signed, and the results are communicated to appropriate caregivers.

 ### Clinical Example (81406)

A 10-month-old male of mixed Ashkenazi Jewish ancestry experiences progressive muscle weakness with a loss of motor skills, decreased attentiveness, and an increased startle response. His pediatrician suspects a diagnosis of Tay-Sachs disease, and the patient is tested for the common Ashkenazi Jewish HEXA gene variants. The patient is found to be heterozygous for the +TATC1278 variant, but no additional common mutations are detected. An anticoagulated peripheral blood sample is submitted for HEXA sequencing to assess the patient for the presence of a second HEXA mutation.

Description of Procedure (81406)

High quality genomic DNA is isolated from whole blood and subjected to 14 individual PCR amplification reactions. The PCR products from each reaction undergo bidirectional dideoxynucleotide chain termination sequencing using a capillary electrophoresis instrument. The pathologist or other qualified health care professional evaluates the sequencing electropherograms for potential nucleotide sequence variants, insertions, deletions, or other changes. The pathologist or other qualified health care professional compares this evaluation with possible variations suggested by computer software to ensure that all abnormalities are identified. The pathologist or other health care professional composes a report specifying the patient's HEXA mutation status. The report is edited and signed, and the results are communicated to appropriate caregivers.

Clinical Example (81407)

A 10-month-old female with a family history of epilepsy is taken to her pediatrician after experiencing a febrile seizure in association with a viral infection. An SCN1A-related seizure disorder is suspected. An anticoagulated peripheral blood sample is submitted for SCN1A sequencing to assess the patient for the presence of a SCN1A-related seizure disorder mutation.

Description of Procedure (81407)

High quality genomic DNA is isolated from whole blood and subjected to 30 individual PCR amplification reactions. The PCR products from each reaction undergo bidirectional dideoxynucleotide chain termination sequencing using a capillary electrophoresis instrument. The pathologist or other qualified health care professional evaluates the sequencing electropherograms for potential nucleotide sequence variants, insertions, deletions, or other changes. The pathologist or other qualified health care professional compares this evaluation with possible variations suggested by computer software to ensure that all abnormalities are identified. The pathologist or other health care professional composes a report specifying the patient's SCN1A mutation status. The report is edited and signed, and the results are communicated to appropriate caregivers.

Clinical Example (81408)

A 16-month-old female is found by her pediatrician to have mild axillary freckling and two large café-au-lait macules on routine physical examination. The history and physical examination is otherwise within normal limits. A diagnosis of neurofibromatosis is suspected. An anticoagulated peripheral blood sample is submitted for NF1 sequencing to assess the patient for the presence of a neurofibromatosis-related mutation.

Description of Procedure (81408)

High quality genomic DNA is isolated from whole blood and subjected to 58 individual PCR amplification reactions. The PCR products from each reaction undergo bidirectional dideoxynucleotide chain termination sequencing using a capillary electrophoresis instrument. The pathologist or other qualified health care professional evaluates the sequencing electropherograms for potential nucleotide sequence variants, insertions, deletions or other changes. The pathologist or other qualified health care professional compares this evaluation with possible variations suggested by computer software to ensure that all abnormalities are identified. The pathologist or other health care professional composes a report specifying the patient's NF1 mutation status. The report is edited and signed, and the results are communicated to appropriate caregivers.

86148   Anti-phosphatidylserine (phospholipid) antibody

(To report antiprothrombin [phospholipid cofactor] antibody, use Category III code 0030T)

▶(For cell enumeration using immunologic selection and identification in fluid specimen [eg, circulating tumor cells in blood], see 0279T, 0280T)◀

🔊 Rationale

In support of the addition of two new circulating tumor cell (CTC) enumeration Category III codes 0279T and 0280T, a cross-reference has been added following code 86148 directing users to these new codes. Please see the discussion of these new codes in the Category III section of this book.

86294   Immunoassay for tumor antigen, qualitative or semiquantitative (eg, bladder tumor antigen)

▶(For qualitative NMP22 protein, use 86386)◀

86300   Immunoassay for tumor antigen, quantitative; CA 15-3 (27.29)

86384   Nitroblue tetrazolium dye test (NTD)

●**86386**   Nuclear Matrix Protein 22 (NMP22), qualitative

(Ouchterlony diffusion, use 86331)

(Platelet antibodies, see 86022, 86023)

🔊 Rationale

Code 86386 has been established to report qualitative nuclear matrix protein 22 (NMP22) testing. This code was developed to allow for specific identification of the NMP22 protein. This assay was previously reported with code 86294, which does not identify the specific antigen tested. In conjunction with the addition of code 86386, a parenthetical note has been placed following code 86294 to direct users to the appropriate code for specifically reporting a qualitative NMP22 protein assay (86386).

86602   Antibody; actinomyces

▲**86703**   HIV-1 and HIV-2, single result

▶(For HIV-1 antigen(s) with HIV-1 and HIV-2 antibodies, single result, use 87389)◀

▶(When HIV immunoassay [HIV testing 86701-86703 or 87389] is performed using a kit or transportable instrument that wholly or in part consists of a single use, disposable analytical chamber, the service may be identified by adding modifier 92 to the usual code)◀

🔊 Rationale

In support of the establishment of HIV code 87389, code 86703 has been updated by replacing the term "assay" with the word "result." A cross-reference following code 86703 has been added to direct users to report code 87389 for HIV-1 antigen(s) with HIV-1 and HIV-2 antibodies, single result. The existing cross-reference following code 86703 has been updated to include code 87389 and delete reference to the word antibody.

Clinical Example (86386)
A 69-year-old female with a history of treated transitional cell carcinoma of the bladder presents for follow-up monitoring of disease status.

Description of Procedure (86386)
A urine specimen is collected and analyzed using a qualitative point of care test kit.

Tissue Typing

86812	HLA typing; A, B, or C (eg, A10, B7, B27), single antigen
86813	A, B, or C, multiple antigens
86816	DR/DQ, single antigen
86817	DR/DQ, multiple antigens
86821	lymphocyte culture, mixed (MLC)
86822	lymphocyte culture, primed (PLC)

▶(For HLA typing by molecular pathology techniques, see 81370-81383)◀

Rationale
An instructional note has been added following code 86822 to direct users to see codes 81730-81383 for HLA typing by molecular pathology techniques.

Microbiology

87301	Infectious agent antigen detection by enzyme immunoassay technique, qualitative or semiquantitative, multiple-step method; adenovirus enteric types 40/41
87385	Histoplasma capsulatum
●**87389**	HIV-1 antigen(s), with HIV-1 and HIV-2 antibodies, single result

Rationale
For CPT 2012, code 87389 has been established for reporting HIV-1 antigen(s), with HIV-1 and HIV-2 antibodies, single result. Currently codifiable procedures are those detecting only HIV antibodies, (CPT codes 86701, 86702, 86703) or separately tested antigen (CPT 87390). This procedure detects the presence of either the HIV-1 p24 antigen, the HIV-1 antibodies, or the HIV-2 antibodies by utilizing moderately complex enzyme immunoassay methodology with computer controlled

⊘=Modifier 51 Exempt   ⊙=Moderate Sedation   ✚=Add-on Code   ⊿=FDA approval pending

instrumentation. The presence of one or multiple analytes in the sample will be reported as "reactive." If none of the analytes are present, the result is "nonreactive." This procedure uniquely detects acute HIV infection approximately one to three weeks earlier than currently approved antibody-only tests.

In support of this change, code 86703 has been updated by replacing the term "assay" with the word "result." A cross-reference following code 86703 has been added to direct users to report code 87389 for HIV-1 antigen(s) with HIV-1 and HIV-2 antibodies, single result. The existing cross-reference following code 86703 has been updated to include code 87389 and delete reference to the word antibody.

In concert with these modifications, modifier 92, Alternative Laboratory Platform Testing, has been updated as well to include HIV code 87389.

Clinical Example (87389)

A 20-year-old male presented himself in the emergency room with a two-week history of headache and mild fever. Examination revealed no specific physical findings. He was discharged on aspirin with a diagnosis of possible influenza. One week later, he returned with similar symptoms at which time laboratory tests, including an HIV antibody test (because of newly-obtained history of homosexual activity), were all unremarkable. Antibiotics were prescribed. Because of additional complaints of fatigue and sore throat he presented at another facility two days later. There, he was offered an HIV Antigen/Antibody combination test.

Description of Procedure (87389)

A blood specimen was obtained in a routine fashion and serum free of red cells was used for testing. The technologist reviewed the positive and negative control specimens run earlier in the day, confirmed that the system was in control, and set the operating parameters of the computerized analyzer. A 150uL serum aliquot was accurately pipetted from the sample tube to initiate the multistep analysis for HIV infection. The result of the analysis as determined by the instrument computer software of the specimen was "reactive." As per testing protocol this presumptively reactive specimen had to be repeat tested in duplicate and both aliquots again tested with the result "reactive." The interpretation of the result by a qualified health care practitioner was that there is presumptive evidence of HIV p24 antigen and/or HIV-1/HIV-2 antibody presence. The recommendation for a supplementary confirmatory assay was made. Since the antibody test was negative two days earlier, this was likely to be a pre-seroconversion HIV antigenemia. This suspicion was confirmed by testing the sample for HIV RNA, which showed a viral load of 1 000 000 copies/mL.

Cytopathology

88104   Cytopathology, fluids, washings or brushings, except cervical or vaginal; smears with interpretation

88106   simple filter method with interpretation

▶(Do not report 88106 in conjunction with 88104)◀

►(88107 has been deleted. To report smears and simple filter preparation, see 88104, 88106)◄

(For nongynecological selective cellular enhancement including filter transfer techniques, use 88112)

✍🏻 Rationale

As part of the AMA/Specialty Society RVS Update Committee (RUC) analysis, the cytopathology code 88107 has been deleted, as this service is no longer in widespread clinical use. Therefore, in support of the deletion of code 88107, an exclusionary note has been added following code 88106 restricting the use of code 88106 in conjunction with code 88104. A cross-reference note was also added directing users to report codes 88104 and 88106 for smears and simple filter preparation services.

88187　Flow cytometry, interpretation; 2 to 8 markers

88188　　　9 to 15 markers

88189　　　16 or more markers

(Do not report 88187-88189 for interpretation of 86355, 86356, 86357, 86359, 86360, 86361, 86367)

►(For cell enumeration using immunologic selection and identification in fluid specimen [eg, circulating tumor cells in blood], see 0279T, 0280T)◄

✍🏻 Rationale

In support of the two new circulating tumor cell (CTC) enumeration Category III codes, a parenthetical note has been added following code 88189 directing users to these new codes. Please see the discussion of these new codes in the Category III section of this book.

Surgical Pathology

▲**88312**　Special stain including interpretation and report; Group I for microorganisms (eg, acid fast, methenamine silver)

►(Report one unit of 88312 for each special stain, on each surgical pathology block, cytologic specimen, or hematologic smear)◄

▲**88313**　　　Group II, all other (eg, iron, trichrome), except stain for microorganisms, stains for enzyme constituents, or immunocytochemistry and immunohistochemistry

►(Report one unit of 88313 for each special stain, on each surgical pathology block, cytologic specimen, or hematologic smear)◄

►(For immunocytochemistry and immunohistochemistry, use 88342)◄

+▲**88314**　　　histochemical stain on frozen tissue block (List separately in addition to code for primary procedure)

►(Use 88314 in conjunction with 17311-17315, 88302-88309, 88331, 88332)◄

　　⊘=Modifier 51 Exempt　⊙=Moderate Sedation　✚=Add-on Code　𝒩=FDA approval pending

►(Do not report 88314 with 17311-17315 for routine frozen section stain [eg, hematoxylin and eosin, toluidine blue], performed during Mohs surgery. When a nonroutine histochemical stain on frozen tissue during Mohs surgery is utilized, report 88314 with modifier 59)◄

►(Report one unit of 88314 for each special stain on each frozen surgical pathology block)◄

►(For a special stain performed on frozen tissue section material to identify enzyme constituents, use 88319)◄

►(88318 has been deleted)◄

►(For determinative histochemistry to identify chemical components, use 88313)◄

▲88319   Group III, for enzyme constituents

►(For each stain on each surgical pathology block, cytologic specimen, or hematologic smear, use one unit of 88319)◄

►(For detection of enzyme constituents by immunohistochemical or immunocytochemical technique, use 88342)◄

Rationale

The special stains codes have been revised to: (1) better define special stain codes 88312-88319; (2) eliminate confusion concerning special stains where procedures overlap two code definitions; (3) delete code 88318; and (4) revise existing and add new instructional and cross-reference parenthetical notes to create a defined hierarchy for codes 88314 and 88319.

Clinical Example (88312)

Microscopic examination of a Warthin Starry stain performed on stomach biopsy with gastritis obtained from a 70-year-old male.

Clinical Example (88313)

Microscopic examination of a Congo red stain performed on a bone marrow biopsy from a 75-year-old male with monoclonal gammopathy.

Clinical Example (88314)

Microscopic examination of an Oil Red O stain performed on a frozen skeletal muscle biopsy in a 30-year-old male with muscular dystrophy.

Clinical Example (88319)

Microscopic examination of a Nicotinamide adenosine dinucleotide-tetrazolium reductase (NADH-TR) stained slide performed on a skeletal muscle biopsy in a 30-year old-male with muscular dystrophy.

In Vivo (eg, Transcutaneous) Laboratory Procedures

(For all in vivo measurements not specifically listed, use 88749)

(For wavelength fluorescent spectroscopy of advanced glycation end products (skin), use 0233T)

▶(For transcutaneous oxyhemoglobin measurement in a lower extremity wound by near infrared spectroscopy, use 0286T)◄

88720 Bilirubin, total, transcutaneous

 Rationale

In support of the establishment of a Category III code for reporting transcutaneous oxyhemoglobin measurement in a lower extremity wound by near-infrared spectroscopy, a cross-reference note has been added to direct the user to report code 0286T.

⊘=Modifier 51 Exempt   ⊙=Moderate Sedation   ✚=Add-on Code   ⊿=FDA approval pending

Medicine

Numerous changes have been made to the Medicine section. A total of 18 codes have been added, 25 codes have been revised, and 17 codes have been deleted.

Code 90663 previously used for reporting the H1N1 vaccine has been deleted, as H1N1 vaccine is no longer offered.

A new code, 90869 and instructional notes have been added to the family of transcranial magnetic stimulation codes, and the existing codes, 90867 and 90868, have been revised to accommodate expansion of these services.

A new subsection has been added in the Medicine/Noninvasive Vascular Diagnostic Studies subsection, entitled Other Noninvasive Vascular Diagnostic Studies with a new code (93998) for reporting unlisted noninvasive vascular diagnostic studies.

The Pulmonary subsection incurred considerable changes. A number of codes used to identify pulmonary testing and the accompanying guidelines have been revised to combine a number of procedures that are commonly performed together for pulmonary testing procedures. This includes deletions of codes that were previously separately reported, the addition of new codes, a heading change that specifies the types of procedures included in the section, and inclusion of new guideline language that more appropriately reflects pulmonary testing procedures in the way that they are commonly performed.

The Neurology and Neuromuscular Procedures subsection now includes definitions to help clarify appropriate use of sleep medicine codes (95800-95811) following the revised subheading, now titled Sleep Medicine Testing.

Medicine

Immunization Administration for Vaccines/Toxoids

▶Report vaccine immunization administration codes 90460, 90461, 90471-90474 in addition to the vaccine and toxoid code(s) 90476-90749.◀

▶Report codes 90460 and 90461 only when the physician or qualified health care professional provides face-to-face counseling of the patient/family during the administration of a vaccine. For immunization administration of any vaccine that is not accompanied by face-to-face physician or qualified health care professional counseling to the patient/family or for administration of vaccines to patients over 18 years of age, report codes 90471-90474.◀

If a significant separately identifiable Evaluation and Management service (eg, office or other outpatient services, preventive medicine services) is performed, the appropriate E/M service code should be reported in addition to the vaccine and toxoid administration codes.

▶A component refers to all antigens in a vaccine that prevent disease(s) caused by one organism (90460 and 90461). Multi-valent antigens or multiple serotypes of antigens against a single organism are considered a single component of vaccines. Combination vaccines are those vaccines that contain multiple vaccine components. Conjugates or adjuvants contained in vaccines are not considered to be component parts of the vaccine as defined above.◀

▲90460   Immunization administration through 18 years of age via any route of administration, with counseling by physician or other qualified health care professional; first or only component of each vaccine or toxoid administered

+▲90461   each additional vaccine or toxoid component administered (List separately in addition to code for primary procedure)

▶(90470 has been deleted)◀

Rationale

An explanatory statement was added to the Immunization Administration for the Vaccines/Toxoids section guidelines to clarify that conjugates and adjuvants are not to be considered a component of a vaccine when reporting codes 90460 and 90461. Also, multivalent antigens or multiple serotypes of antigens against a single organism are considered a single component of a vaccine.

Further editorial revisions to the guidelines include the addition of the appropriate Immunization Administration code range, 90471-90474, to the first paragraph of the guidelines as codes that are reported in addition to the vaccine and toxoid code(s) 90476-90749.

Also, codes 90460 and 90461 were editorially revised to clarify that code 90460 can be reported only once per day of service.

Code 90470 for reporting the admininstration of the H1N1 vaccine product developed for the 2009 Swine Flu Pandemic has been deleted. The H1N1 vaccine is no longer offered. The seasonal vaccine developed for the 2010–2011 flu season incorporates H1N1 virus. The correct codes for the reformulated seasonal flu vaccines should be reported with the seasonal influenza vaccine codes (90655 et seq) and the immunization administration code(s) (90460 et seq). Information on reporting vaccines issued in the event of another pandemic flu outbreak with codes 90664-90668 are included in the AMA's CPT Category I Vaccine Codes under the fact sheet link, *http://www.ama-assn.org/resources/doc/cpt/ama-fact-sheet-report-cpt-codes-influenza.pdf.*

Vaccines, Toxoids

▲90581   Anthrax vaccine, for subcutaneous or intramuscular use

Rationale

The vaccine product code 90581 for anthrax vaccine, previously designated only for subcutaneous use, has been revised to accommodate the preferred intramuscular route of administration. The product has not changed, only the route and schedule of administration. Researchers found that fewer doses of intramuscularly injected anthrax vaccine results in similar levels of effectiveness and fewer adverse events. The subcutaneous route is still used when medically indicated (eg, vascular disorders).

✗▲90644   Meningococcal conjugate vaccine, serogroups C & Y and Hemophilus influenza B vaccine (Hib-MenCY), 4 dose schedule, when administered to children 2-15 months of age, for intramuscular use

Rationale

Code 90644 was revised to avoid misinterpreting this vaccine as a three-component vaccine when it is a two-component vaccine. With the establishment of the new immunization administration codes for CPT 2011 that consider the number of vaccine components, it was not clear how many components were included in the MenCY-Hib vaccine. The reference to the tetanus conjugate and its abbreviation in the code descriptor was being mistaken as an additional component. The elimination of the conjugate, tetanus toxoid, from the code descriptor clarifies that the vaccine is a two-component vaccine for Meningococcal and Hemophilus influenza B.

●90654   Influenza virus vaccine, split virus, preservative-free, for intradermal use

Rationale

A vaccine product code 90654 was established for the preservative-free vaccine for influenza virus intended for intradermal administration via a prefilled single dose disposable microinjection system consisting of a small needle for intradermal delivery. The vaccine consists of a lower antigen concentration than the influenza vaccines intended for intramuscular delivery reported with codes 90656 and 90658. A lower concentration is used due to efficiencies of dendrite cells accessed through the intradermal route of administration.

⊘=Modifier 51 Exempt   ⊙=Moderate Sedation   ✚=Add-on Code   ✗=FDA approval pending

Clinical Example (90654)

A 33-year-old male health care worker is required to obtain immunization against influenza to decrease the risk for transmitting influenza to his patients and to protect his own immunity. The health care worker is offered and accepts an intradermal administration as an alternative to an intramuscular injection.

Description of Procedure (90654)

Physician reviews patient's chart to determine if the patient meets the criteria to receive an influenza vaccine. Patient is counseled on the benefits of vaccination to prevent influenza disease. As with all vaccines, the physician discusses potential adverse reactions and answers any questions the patient might have. The patient is administered an intradermal injection of influenza vaccine through the epidermis into the upper layers of the dermis of the upper arm. As recommended for all vaccines, the patient is monitored for approximately 15 minutes for any adverse reaction. The patient's immunization record (and registry when applicable) is updated to reflect the vaccine administered.

90662   Influenza virus vaccine, split virus, preservative free, enhanced immunogenicity via increased antigen content, for intramuscular use

▶(90663 has been deleted)◀

Rationale

Code 90663 for reporting the H1N1 vaccine product developed for the 2009 Swine Flu Pandemic has been deleted. The H1N1 vaccine is no longer offered. The seasonal vaccine developed for the 2010–2011 flu season incorporates H1N1 virus. The correct codes for the reformulated seasonal flu vaccines should be reported with the seasonal influenza vaccine codes (90655 et seq) and the immunization administration code(s) (90460 et seq). Information on reporting vaccines issued in the event of another pandemic flu outbreak with codes 90664-90668 are included in the AMA's CPT Category I Vaccine Codes under the fact sheet link, *www.ama-assn.org/resources/doc/cpt/ama-fact-sheet-report-cpt-codes-influenza.pdf.*

Psychiatry

Psychiatric Therapeutic Procedures

OTHER PSYCHIATRIC SERVICES OR PROCEDURES

(For analysis/programming of neurostimulators used for vagus nerve stimulation therapy, see 95970, 95974, 95975)

90862   Pharmacologic management, including prescription, use, and review of medication with no more than minimal medical psychotherapy

90865   Narcosynthesis for psychiatric diagnostic and therapeutic purposes (eg, sodium amobarbital (Amytal) interview)

▲**90867**	Therapeutic repetitive transcranial magnetic stimulation (TMS) treatment; initial, including cortical mapping, motor threshold determination, delivery and management

(Report only once per course of treatment)

▶(Do not report 90867 in conjunction with 95928, 95929, 90868, 90869)◀

▲**90868**	subsequent delivery and management, per session
●**90869**	subsequent motor threshold re-determination with delivery and management

▶(Do not report 90869 in conjunction with 90867, 90868)◀

▶(If a significant, separately identifiable Evaluation and Management, medication management, psychotherapy or psychotherapy with evaluation and management service is performed, the appropriate E/M, psychotherapy, psychotherapy with E/M service or 90862 may be reported in addition to 90867-90869. Evaluation and management activities directly related to cortical mapping, motor threshold determination, delivery and management of TMS are not separately reported.)◀

✎ Rationale

For *CPT 2011*, codes 90867 and 90868 were added to describe therapeutic repetitive transcranial magnetic stimulation treatment planning, delivery, and management. In *CPT 2012*, this family of codes has been expanded to include 90869 and instructional notes. To accommodate expansion of these services, codes 90867 and 90868 have been revised.

Code 90869 has been established for reporting subsequent motor threshold re-determination with delivery and management. Codes 90867 and 90868 have been revised to report initial and subsequent transcranial magnetic stimulation delivery (TMS) and management. An exclusionary parenthetical note has been added following code 90867 to preclude reporting this code with codes 95928, 95929, 90868, 90869. Additionally, an exclusionary parenthetical note has been added following 90869 to preclude reporting this code with codes 90867 and 90868.

An instructional note has been added to this series to indicate that: (1) if a significant, separately identifiable Evaluation and Management, medication management, psychotherapy or psychotherapy with evaluation and management service is performed, the appropriate E/M, psychotherapy, psychotherapy with E/M service, or code 90862 may be reported in addition to codes 90867-90869; and (2) Evaluation and management activities directly related to cortical mapping, motor threshold determination, delivery and management of TMS are not separately reported.

Clinical Example (90867)

A 50-year-old female presents with a clinical diagnosis consistent with DSM-IV defined Major Depressive Disorder, severe, with a recurrent course of illness. She has a secondary diagnosis of generalized anxiety disorder, and has experienced a recurrent course of depressive illness, with at least prior episodes of major depression. Her history in the present episode is also significant for failure to receive benefit from treatment with three separate antidepressant medication trials, from two different chemical classes. She has also been treated with a combination of an

⃠=Modifier 51 Exempt ⊙=Moderate Sedation ✚=Add-on Code ⫫=FDA approval pending

antidepressant and an atypical antipsychotic medication, which she discontinued because of significant weight gain. The patient is to be treated with Transcranial Magnetic Stimulation (TMS) therapy.

Description of Procedure (90867)

The physician performs a brief focused interview to determine patient's mental status and ability to proceed with the procedure. Confirms with the patient: identity, current medications, and any significant clinical changes. Discusses the risks and benefits and alternate treatment options with the patient and obtains written consent. The physician responds to any patient questions.

Positioning the patient and in particular positioning the patient's head precisely by centering the head in the head positioner, using the laser attachment to identify the midline, placing the positioning tape to stabilize the head, and then locking the contralateral head support in place. The head positioner is adjusted along all 3 axes, and the parameters on each gauge are recorded.

Finding the thand muscle includes the following—Find the vertex and go laterally 5 cm. Place the coil in the estimated location and use single pulse TMS to search for the target hand muscle. Increase intensity slowly until a muscle twitch is obtained in the hand and use a grid approach to find the target muscle. Once the target muscle contraction is found, stimulate across the anterior-posterior plane to find the most anterior location and most posterior location that still produces a muscle twitch. Find the midpoint or area of maximal contraction and repeat this process along the medial-lateral plane. Find the cross point between these two planes and use this location to determine motor threshold.

Determining motor threshold (MT)—The MT value is defined as the lowest level of system output power that produces a visible movement in the targeted hand muscle. This is done using a computer program that calculates MT based on yes/no responses for stimulations at various intensities, or by using step-wise increases and decreases in intensity to identify at what intensity a contraction is seen in half of the stimulations.

Determining treatment site—Advance 5-6 cm anteriorly from the motor cortex site of the target hand muscle along the superior oblique plane or determine the treatment site using the EEG-F3 method.

Treatment and clinical monitoring—To initiate treatment the physician advances the treatment coil to the targeted treatment location and the prescribed treatment parameters are selected (frequency, intensity, number of stimuli, treatment train length, and inter-stimulus interval). The coil must remain in good contact with the patient's head for the duration of treatment. During the treatment session the patient must be closely monitored at all times to ensure good coil-to-head contact to optimize penetration of the electromagnetic pulses to the cortex. The clinician monitors the patient's clinical status for comfort and tolerability and, if necessary, adjusts coil position and customizes the stimulation parameters to mitigate discomfort. Although the risk of a seizure is low (<1%) it is a significant medical complication, thus patients must be monitored for any signs or symptoms that may indicate the emergence of an event, and the physician must be ready to respond if necessary. The physician leaves once it is determined that the treatment is proceeding appropriately.

 ## Clinical Example (90868)

A 50-year-old female presents with a clinical diagnosis consistent with DSM-IV defined Major Depressive Disorder, severe, with a recurrent course of illness. She has a secondary diagnosis of generalized anxiety disorder, and has experienced a recurrent course of depressive illness, with at least prior episodes of major depression. Her history in the present episode is also significant for failure to receive benefit from treatment with three separate antidepressant medication trials, from two different chemical classes. She has also been treated with a combination of an antidepressant and an atypical antipsychotic medication, which she discontinued because of significant weight gain. The patient is to be treated with Transcranial Magnetic Stimulation (TMS) therapy.

Description of Procedure (90868)

The physician performs a brief focused interview to determine patient's mental status and ability to proceed with the procedure. Confirms with the patient identity, current medications, and any significant clinical changes. The physician responds to any patient questions.

Treatment and clinical monitoring—The physician initiates treatment by advancing the treatment coil to the targeted treatment location and the prescribed treatment parameters are selected (frequency, intensity, number of stimuli, treatment train length, and inter-stimulus interval). The coil must remain in good contact with the patient's head for the duration of treatment. During the treatment session, the patient must be closely monitored at all times to ensure good coil-to-head contact to optimize penetration of the electromagnetic pulses to the cortex. The clinician monitors the patient's clinical status for comfort and tolerability and, if necessary, adjusts coil position and customizes the stimulation parameters to mitigate discomfort. Although the risk of a seizure is low (<1%), it is a significant medical complication, thus patients must be monitored for any signs or symptoms that may indicate the emergence of an event, and the physician must be ready to respond if necessary. The physician leaves once it is determined that the treatment is proceeding appropriately.

 ## Clinical Example (90869)

The patient is a 50-year-old female with a primary diagnosis consistent with DSM-IV defined Major Depressive Disorder, severe, with a recurrent course of illness, who presents for a routine daily TMS treatment. Since the last treatment, the patient's medication regimen has been revised to include clonazepam 1mg nightly, which is known to alter cortical excitability. This change makes it medically necessary for the physician to redetermine the motor threshold. The patient's motor threshold is redetermined after which the patient undergoes TMS treatment.

Description of Procedure (90869)

The physician performs a brief focused interview to determine patient's mental status and ability to proceed with the procedure. Confirms with the patient identity,

$\ominus$=Modifier 51 Exempt $\odot$=Moderate Sedation   ✚=Add-on Code   ✗=FDA approval pending

current medications, and any significant clinical changes. The physician responds to any patient questions.

Positioning the patient and in particular positioning the patient's head precisely by centering the head in the head positioner, using the laser attachment to identify the midline, placing the positioning tape to stabilize head, and then locking the contralateral head support in place. The head positioner is adjusted along all 3 axes, and the parameters on each gauge are recorded.

Finding the thand muscle includes the following—Place the coil in the previously estimated location and use single pulse TMS to search for the target hand muscle. Increase intensity slowly until a muscle twitch is obtained in the hand and use a grid approach to find the target muscle. Once the target muscle contraction is found, then stimulate across the anterior-posterior plane to find the most anterior location and most posterior location that still produces a muscle twitch. Find the midpoint or area of maximal contraction and repeat this process along the medial-lateral plane. Find the cross point between these two planes and use this location to determine motor threshold

Determining motor threshold (MT)—The MT value is defined as the lowest level of system output power that produces a visible movement in the targeted hand muscle. This is done using a computer program that calculates MT based on yes/no responses for stimulations at various intensities, or by using step-wise increases and decreases in intensity to identify at what intensity a contraction is seen in half of the stimulations.

Determining treatment site—Advance 5-6 cm anteriorly from the motor cortex site of the target hand muscle along the superior oblique plane or determine the treatment site using the EEG-F3 method.

Treatment and clinical monitoring—To initiate treatment the physician advances the treatment coil to the targeted treatment location and the prescribed treatment parameters are selected (frequency, intensity, number of stimuli, treatment train length, and inter-stimulus interval). The coil must remain in good contact with the patient's head for the duration of treatment. During the treatment session the patient must be closely monitored at all times to ensure good coil-to-head contact to optimize penetration of the electromagnetic pulses to the cortex. The clinician monitors the patient's clinical status for comfort and tolerability and, if necessary, adjusts coil position and customizes the stimulation parameters to mitigate discomfort. Although the risk of a seizure is low (<1%), it is a significant medical complication, thus patients must be monitored for any signs or symptoms that may indicate the emergence of an event, and the physician must be ready to respond if necessary. The physician leaves once it is determined that the treatment is proceeding appropriately.

▲**91010**   Esophageal motility (manometric study of the esophagus and/or gastroesophageal junction) study with interpretation and report;

▶(91011, 91012 have been deleted. To report esophageal motility studies with stimulant or perfusion, use 91013 in conjunction with 91010)◀

+▲**91013**   with stimulation or perfusion (eg, stimulant, acid or alkali perfusion) (List separately in addition to code for primary procedure)

(Use 91013 in conjunction with 91010)

(Do not report 91013 more than once per session)

▶(To report esophageal motility studies with high resolution esophageal pressure topography, use 0240T and with stimulant or perfusion, use 0241T)◀

Rationale

A revision was made to codes 91010 and 91013 in the Medicine section (as well as to codes 0240T and 0241T in the Category III section) to identify the intent for use of these codes to report two-dimensional or three-dimensional esophageal manometry studies performed *without* pressure topography. This included the removal of language that specified either two-dimensional or three-dimensional data within all of the codes (both in the Medicine and the Category III sections). Clarifications are also included via use of additions and revisions to parentheticals to note that: (1) code 91013 should be used ". . . in conjunction with code 91010" to report esophageal motility studies with stimulant or perfusion; and (2) the appropriate method of reporting esophageal motility studies with high resolution esophageal pressure topography by using code 0240T and additionally reporting code 0241T when stimulant or perfusion are used.

Clinical Example (91010)

A 48-year-old female has complaints of frequent heartburn. She has tried a number of pharmacologic agents without relief of symptoms. Esophagogastroduodenoscopy (EGD) was unremarkable. She is referred for evaluation.

Description of Procedure (91010)

The patient is positioned on the examination table and properly gowned. A swallow transducer is affixed to the neck with tape. The nares are inspected to determine which is most suitable for catheter insertion.

Topical anesthesia is administered to the nares. Under physician supervision, the esophageal pressure probe is passed transnasally into the esophagus to a depth of 60cm. Pressures are checked and the probe is positioned straddling the distal esophagus/proximal stomach based on interpretation of the measurements. After positioning is confirmed, the patient is instructed to perform 10 swallows of 5-ml liquid (typically water or saline) at no less than 30 second intervals. Pressure measurements are taken as the material moves through the esophagus into the stomach and the adequacy of the measurements is assessed. The probe is

⊘=Modifier 51 Exempt   ⊙=Moderate Sedation   ✚=Add-on Code   𝒩=FDA approval pending

withdrawn to the correct position in the esophageal body based on interpretation of the measurements, and additional pressure measurements are taken. At the conclusion of the procedure, the probe is withdrawn.

Clinical Example (91013)

A 49-year-old female has complaints of heartburn and chest pain. Cardiac evaluation and esophagogastroduodenoscopy (EGD) were unremarkable. She has tried a number of pharmacologic agents without relief of symptoms. She is referred for evaluation of esophageal function to assess symptoms in response to stimulation agents.

Description of Procedure (91013)

After a baseline esophageal motility study is performed, topical anesthesia is administered to the nares and a second small infusion catheter is placed through the contra-lateral nares into the esophagus to a distance of 30-35 cm from the nares. The motility probe is repositioned to straddle the distal esophagus, checking pressure measurements. The stimulant is infused through the infusion catheter. The patient is asked to perform a further series of swallows, and additional esophageal pressure measurements are taken. At the conclusion of this part of the procedure, the infusion catheter is removed. The recording is saved for subsequent interpretation.

Physician interpretation of the tracings includes the additional measurements obtained following administration of the provocative agent.

▶(For abdominal paracentesis, see 49082, 49083, 49084; with instillation of medication, see 96440, 96446)◀

(For peritoneoscopy, use 49320; with biopsy, use 49321)

(For peritoneoscopy and guided transhepatic cholangiography, use 47560; with biopsy, use 47561)

(For splenoportography, see 38200, 75810)

91110   Gastrointestinal tract imaging, intraluminal (eg, capsule endoscopy), esophagus through ileum, with physician interpretation and report

Rationale

In support of the establishment of codes 49082, 49083, and 49084, the cross-reference note preceding code 91110 has been updated.

Ophthalmology

Special Ophthalmological Services

▶(92070 has been deleted. To report, see 92071, 92072)◀

●92071   Fitting of contact lens for treatment of ocular surface disease

▶(Do not report 92071 in conjunction with 92072)◄

▶(Report supply of lens separately with 99070 or appropriate supply code)◄

●**92072**   Fitting of contact lens for management of keratoconus, initial fitting

▶(For subsequent fittings, report using Evaluation and Management services or General Ophthalmological services)◄

▶(Do not report 92072 in conjunction with 92071)◄

▶(Report supply of lens separately with 99070 or appropriate supply code)◄

Rationale

As part of the AMA/Specialty Society RVS Update Committee (RUC) analysis of codes, it was discovered that there were two distinct uses for code 92070, both involving substantially different levels of work. As a result of this review, code 92070 for contact lens fitting for treatment of ocular surface disease including supply of lens was deleted and two codes, 92071 and 92072, were established for reporting contact lens fitting for treatment of ocular surface disease (eg, corneal abrasion) and management of keratoconus. Additionally, parenthetical notes were added to: (1) instruct users to report E/M or the General Ophthalmological Services codes for subsequent fittings; (2) instruct users not to report the two new codes together; and (3) to report supply of the lens separately with code 99070 or the appropriate supply code.

Clinical Example (92071)

A 32-year-old male with eye pain, photophobia, and reduced vision after his eye was struck with a tree branch. He was found to have a corneal abrasion which requires a therapeutic contact lens to protect the corneal surface, reduce discomfort, and facilitate healing.

Description of Procedure (92071)

Topical anesthesia is administered. A therapeutic soft contact lens of the appropriate size and base curve is selected and applied to the cornea. A drop of topical antibiotic is administered. Fifteen minutes later the fit and centration of the lens is evaluated at the slit lamp.

Clinical Example (92072)

A 27-year-old female with keratoconus is unable to read or drive safely with glasses or conventional contact lenses. Her best corrected visual acuity is 20/60 OD and 20/200 OS due to irregular astigmatism from keratoconus. A custom contact lens fit and design is medically necessary for visual rehabilitation.

Description of Procedure (92072)

Results of diagnostic tests done prior to contact lens fitting to assess the corneal ectasia are used in concert with slit lamp examination to assess corneal shape and determine initial contact lens parameters (eg, diameter, base curve, and secondary curves). Lens designs can include corneal, scleral, hybrid, or piggyback systems. Keratometry, lid anatomy, tear film, and refraction are also performed/rechecked.

⊘=Modifier 51 Exempt   ⊙=Moderate Sedation   ✚=Add-on Code   𝑵=FDA approval pending

An initial diagnostic lens is selected for each eye and placed on the eyes. The patient is examined after adequate time for the lens to settle in order to evaluate the lens fit. Fluorescein dye is instilled in the eye to evaluate the posterior tear pattern, lens position, and corneal relationship. Based on the fit of the first diagnostic lens, the lens parameters are recalculated. This includes base curves, secondary curves, and lens design. This process is repeated until the lens is well-centered and comfortable. A typical fitting requires three different diagnostic lenses per eye. An over-refraction is performed to determine final contact lens power.

92100 Serial tonometry (separate procedure) with multiple measurements of intraocular pressure over an extended time period with interpretation and report, same day (eg, diurnal curve or medical treatment of acute elevation of intraocular pressure)

▶(92120, 92130 have been deleted)◀

▶(Ocular blood flow measurements are reported with 0198T. Single-episode tonometry is a component of general ophthalmological service or E/M service)◀

✍ Rationale

Codes 92120 and 92130 for tonography have been deleted due to extremely low use of these services. During the AMA/Specialty Society RVS Update Committee (RUC) surveying process, the involved specialty societies for ophthalmology discovered that an extremely low usage was associated with the services represented in codes 92120 and 92130. Thus, it was recommended that code 92120 should not be revised, but deleted along with code 92130. A cross-reference to direct the use of Category III code 0198T for ocular blood flow measurements has been added. This cross-reference also indicates that single-episode tonometry is a component of a general ophthalmological service or E/M service. A parenthetical note has also been added noting that codes 92120 and 92130 have been deleted.

OTHER SPECIALIZED SERVICES

▶For prescription, fitting, and/or medical supervision of ocular prosthetic (artificial eye) adaptation by a physician, see Evaluation and Management services including Office or Other Outpatient services (99201-99215), Office or Other Outpatient Consultations (99241-99245) or General Ophthalmological service codes 92002-92014.◀

92265 Needle oculoelectromyography, 1 or more extraocular muscles, 1 or both eyes, with interpretation and report

92270 Electro-oculography with interpretation and report

✍ Rationale

The parenthetical note following code 92326 in CPT 2011 has been relocated to the Special Ophthalmological Services, Other Specialized Services subsection in the Ophthalmology section. This parenthetical note has been revised to delineate the applicable Evaluation and Management (E/M) code ranges of office or other outpatient services (99201-99215) and office or other outpatient consultations (99241-99245). Additionally, the verbiage "artificial eye" was added in parenthesis following ocular prosthetic.

Contact Lens Services

The prescription of contact lens includes specification of optical and physical characteristics (such as power, size, curvature, flexibility, gas-permeability). It is NOT a part of the general ophthalmological services.

The fitting of contact lens includes instruction and training of the wearer and incidental revision of the lens during the training period.

Follow-up of successfully fitted extended wear lenses is reported as part of a general ophthalmological service (92012 et seq).

The supply of contact lenses may be reported as part of the service of fitting. It may also be reported separately by using the appropriate supply codes.

▶(For therapeutic or surgical use of contact lens, see 68340, 92071, 92072)◀

92310 Prescription of optical and physical characteristics of and fitting of contact lens, with medical supervision of adaptation; corneal lens, both eyes, except for aphakia

 Rationale

The cross-reference in the Contact Lens Services guidelines, which referenced codes for therapeutic or surgical use of contact lens has been updated to omit code 92070, and to include the new replacement codes 92071 for reporting contact lens fitting for treatment of ocular surface disease (eg, corneal abrasion) and 92072 for reporting management of keratoconus.

Special Otorhinolaryngologic Services

Audiologic Function Tests

92555 Speech audiometry threshold;

92556   with speech recognition

92557 Comprehensive audiometry threshold evaluation and speech recognition (92553 and 92556 combined)

(For hearing aid evaluation and selection, see 92590-92595)

(For automated audiometry, see 0208T-0212T)

▶**92558** Code is out of numerical sequence. See 92550-92597◀

92559 Audiometric testing of groups

#●**92558** Evoked otoacoustic emissions, screening (qualitative measurement of distortion product or transient evoked otoacoustic emissions), automated analysis

⃠=Modifier 51 Exempt   ⊙=Moderate Sedation   ✚=Add-on Code   ☏=FDA approval pending

▲**92587**   Distortion product evoked otoacoustic emissions; limited evaluation (to confirm the presence or absence of hearing disorder, 3-6 frequencies) or transient evoked otoacoustic emissions, with interpretation and report

▲**92588**   comprehensive diagnostic evaluation (quantitative analysis of outer hair cell function by cochlear mapping, minimum of 12 frequencies), with interpretation and report

(For central auditory function evaluation, see 92620, 92621)

✎ Rationale

Codes 92587 and 92588 have been revised and code 92558 added to identify changes made to evoked otoacoustic emissions studies.

Code 92587 has been revised deleting language that indicates ". . . *single stimulus level, either transient or distortion products . . . .*" and adding language that specifically notes ". . . *to confirm the presence or absence of hearing disorder, 3-6 frequencies or transient evoked otoacoustic emissions with interpretation and report.*" This language helps to confirm the intent of this code, ie, the use of a limited number of frequencies to determine if the patient has experienced hearing loss.

Code 92588 identifies a comprehensive analysis of cochlear function through establishing a functional map of the organ of hearing by using multiple frequencies per octave along multiple octaves. The descriptor for this code has been revised, eliminating generic language that notes ". . . *comparison of transient and/ or distortion product otoacoustic emissions at multiple levels and frequencies . . .*" and adding language that specifies ". . . *quantitative analysis of outer hair cell function by cochlear mapping, minimum of 12 frequencies . . .,*" with interpretation and report.

Code 92558 has been added for evoked otoacoustic emissions screening, automated analysis. Code 92558 appears with a number symbol (#) to indicate that this code is out of numerical sequence. A reference note has been added to instruct the user to the appropriate code range of 92550-92597 for the placement of code 92558.

🩺 Clinical Example (92558)

A 2-week-old female is being seen by her pediatrician because she did not pass a previous hearing screening at birth.

Description of Procedure (92558)

A qualified health care professional performs an otoscopic examination of each ear. An appropriately sized probe tip is selected and placed securely into each ear canal. An automated otoacoustic emission (OAE) screening protocol is initiated to stimulate the test and record the responses. The emissions are evaluated by the device in accordance with an automated algorithm. The qualified health care professional monitors the responses in accordance with automated algorithms. The algorithm determines the emissions to be present or not, yielding a result of pass or refer.

🩺 Clinical Example (92587)

A 2-year-old male is referred by his pediatrician for objective estimation of hearing sensitivity due to delays in speech and language development. Recent attempts to obtain behavioral hearing evaluation results yielded inconclusive information. Supplemental testing is needed to obtain additional information regarding hearing function.

Description of Procedure (92587)

The audiologist briefly affirms key elements of the history and presenting concerns, explains the purpose of the procedure to the patient's parents or guardian. The audiologist then informs the parent or guardian of what to expect when the test is under way and instructs the parent on the proper positioning of the child throughout the procedure. The audiologist performs an otoscopic examination of each ear, an appropriate-sized probe tip is selected, and the stimulus/recording probe assembly is inserted into the patient's ear canal. Once properly seated, the protocol is activated. Under the constant observation of the audiologist, the testing software performs a calibration to ensure proper probe placement and the absence of blockage. The test protocol continues with the evaluation of the first test frequency. Tonal pairs are presented to the patient's ear; after each presentation the OAE equipment waits approximately 2 to 6 milliseconds to record evidence of sensory cell movement in the cochlea. The process is repeated for approximately 500 samples in order to perform a signal-averaging algorithm to separate the anticipated otoacoustic emission from the noise floor from either the patient or the environment. Once the requisite number of samples is collected for the first frequency pair, the OAE equipment changes frequency pairs according to the selected protocol and repeats the procedure. This algorithm is repeated until data for three to six frequency pairs are collected. Results are then displayed on the OAE equipment screen by frequency for the otoacoustic emission amplitude and the level of the noise floor in decibels. When the first ear is completed, the process is repeated for the second ear. The audiologist evaluates the data to determine whether a biologic (in contrast to artifactual) response was obtained at each frequency. Results are printed for placement in the patient's medical chart. The audiologist prepares a report describing the measurements, outcomes, and recommendations.

 ### Clinical Example (92588)

A 56-year-old female with a diagnosis of cancer is referred by her oncologist for a baseline assessment of cochlear hair cell function prior to the initiation of a potentially ototoxic regimen of chemotherapy.

Description of Procedure (92588)

The audiologist performs an otoscopic examination of each ear. Once the appropriate-sized probe tip is selected and placed on the acoustic probe assembly, it is inserted directly into each ear canal. During the test administration the audiologist continually assesses the collected data to determine if changes to the test protocol are warranted. The measurement of distortion product otoacoustic emissions is repeated for multiple frequencies per octave across multiple octaves. The responses are then replicated to establish validity and reliability of the distortion products. The amplitudes of the distortion product otoacoustic emissions relative to the noise floor are evaluated for distinct response patterns signifying frequency regions of good cochlear function, frequency regions where function is compromised but not eliminated, and frequency regions where there is no residual function. The audiologist performs a detailed analysis of the graphic display of these collective responses which constitutes a frequency map of the cochlea consistent with the status of the cochlear outer hair cells. After the protocol has been completed on the first ear, the procedure is repeated for the second ear. When the test protocol has been completed for both ears, the audiologist interprets the test results by comparing the response amplitudes to normative data and/or previous test results. The audiologist then prepares a report for the referring physician.

Evaluative and Therapeutic Services

▲92605   Evaluation for prescription of non-speech-generating augmentative and alternative communication device, face-to-face with the patient; first hour

#+●92618   each additional 30 minutes (List separately in addition to code for primary procedure)

►(Use 92618 in conjunction with 92605)◄

►92618   Code 92618 is out of numerical sequence. See 92601-92633◄

Rationale

Code 92605 has been revised to include time by adding the phrase "face-to-face with the patient, first hour" in the descriptor. In addition, an add-on code (92618) has been added for reporting each additional 30 minutes of time provided. Following code 92618 a parenthetical note has been added to instruct the user to report code 92618 in conjunction with code 92605.

A reference note has been added to instruct the user to the appropriate code range of 92601-92633 for placement of code 92618.

Clinical Example (92605)

A 4-year-old male with cerebral palsy, severely unintelligible speech, and severe motoric impairment is referred for a non-speech-generating augmentative and alternative communication device evaluation.

Description of Procedure (92605)

Conduct observations, interactions, and evaluations to gather information about functional vision, hearing, motor, cognition, communication, and language skills that will be utilized in a communication system.

Determine optimal access method, level of symbolic representation, symbol size, display layout, vocabulary, message formulation methods, and accessories needed to carry or mount communication displays/boards.

Identify techniques that will maximize effective communication between the patient and his/her communication partners.

Interact with patient and caregiver to appropriately interpret feedback/communication for the patient and counsel caregiver throughout evaluation, including discussion of recommendations.

Clinical Example (92618)
A 4-year-old male with cerebral palsy, severely unintelligible speech, and severe motoric impairment is referred for a non-speech-generating augmentative and alternative communication device evaluation.

Description of Procedure (92618)
Conduct observations, interactions, and evaluations to gather information about functional vision, hearing, motor, cognition, communication, and language skills that will be utilized in a communication system.

Determine optimal access method, level of symbolic representation, symbol size, display layout, vocabulary, message formulation methods, and accessories needed to carry or mount communication displays/boards.

Identify techniques that will maximize effective communication between the patient and his/her communication partners.

Interact with patient and caregiver to appropriately interpret feedback/communication for the patient and counsel caregiver throughout evaluation including discussion of recommendations.

92620　　Evaluation of central auditory function, with report; initial 60 minutes

+▲92621　　　each additional 15 minutes (List separately in addition to code for primary procedure)

▶(Use 92621 in conjunction with 92620)◀

 Rationale
Code 92621 was editorially revised to reflect the status of this code as an add-on code with addition of standard add-on code language to the descriptor and an add-on symbol. A parenthetical note has been added instructing the use of code 92621 with code 92620.

Cardiovascular

Echocardiography

Echocardiography includes obtaining . . .

A complete transthoracic echocardiogram . . .

A complete transthoracic echocardiogram . . .

A follow-up or limited echocardiographic . . .

In stress echocardiography . . .

▶When a stress echocardiogram is performed with a complete cardiovascular stress test (continuous electrocardiographic monitoring, physician supervision, interpretation and report), use 93351. When only the professional components of a complete stress test and a stress echocardiogram are provided (eg, in a facility setting) by the same physician, use 93351 with modifier 26. When

　　　⊘=Modifier 51 Exempt　⊙=Moderate Sedation　✚=Add-on Code　𝒩=FDA approval pending

all professional services of a stress test are not performed by the same physician performing the stress echocardiogram, use 93350 in conjunction with the appropriate codes (93016-93018) for the components of the cardiovascular stress test that are provided.◄

When left ventricular endocardial borders . . .

Report of an echocardiographic study . . .

Use of an ultrasound . . .

93350   Echocardiography, transthoracic, real-time with image documentation (2D), includes M-mode recording, when performed, during rest and cardiovascular stress test using treadmill, bicycle exercise and/or pharmacologically induced stress, with interpretation and report;

(Stress testing codes 93016-93018 should be reported, when appropriate, in conjunction with 93350 to capture the cardiovascular stress portion of the study)

(Do not report 93350 in conjunction with 93015)

93351   including performance of continuous electrocardiographic monitoring, with physician supervision

►(Do not report 93351 in conjunction with 93015-93018, 93350. Do not report 93351-26 in conjunction with 93016, 93018, 93350-26)◄

✍️ Rationale

In CPT 2009, code 93351 was established to report a complete stress test and stress echocardiogram when performed together. The introductory language in the Medicine/Cardiovascular/Echocardiography section has been revised in 2012 to clarify how to report the professional components of these services.

When only the professional components of a complete stress test and a stress echocardiogram are provided by the same physician, code 93351 should be reported with modifier 26 appended. In the instance when all the professional services of a stress test are not performed by the same physician who is performing the stress echocardiogram, code 93350 should be reported with the appropriate code(s) from the 93016-93018 series for the components of the stress test that are provided. The parenthetical note following code 93351 has also been revised to reflect these revisions.

Cardiac Catheterization

When cardiac catheterization is combined . . .

Contrast injection to image the access . . .

Modifier 51 should not be appended . . .

►Please see the cardiac catheterization table located following 93572.◄

⊙⊘**93451**   Right heart catheterization including measurement(s) of oxygen saturation and cardiac output, when performed

(Do not report 93451 in conjunction with 93453, 93456, 93457, 93460, 93461)

Rationale

An instructional note been added following the Cardiac Catheterization guidelines to see the Cardiac Catheterization table to assist users in proper code selection based on the type of catheter placement and services performed during the catheterization procedure.

INJECTION PROCEDURES

⊙▲**93561**   Indicator dilution studies such as dye or thermodilution, including arterial and/or venous catheterization; with cardiac output measurement (separate procedure)

⊙▲**93562**   subsequent measurement of cardiac output

▶(Do not report 93561, 93562 in conjunction with 93451-93462)◀

(For radioisotope method of cardiac output, see 78472, 78473, or 78481)

 Rationale

Codes 93561 and 93562 have been revised by changing the term "thermal dilution" to "thermodilution" to better reflect current terminology. In addition, the exclusionary parenthetical note following code 93562 was revised by removing the language "are not to be used with cardiac catheterization codes" and replacing it with the applicable cardiac catheterization code range of 93451-93462 and the standard exclusionary note language "Do not report in conjunction with."

Noninvasive Physiologic Studies and Procedures

93701   Bioimpedance-derived physiologic cardiovascular analysis

(For left ventricular filling pressure indirect measurement by computerized calibration of the arterial waveform response to Valsalva, use 93799)

▶(93720-93722 have been deleted. To report, use 94726)◀

✍ **Rationale**

The codes previously used to identify plethysmography procedures (93720-93722) have been deleted and replaced by code 94726, which is now used to identify all services related to plethysmography testing. This includes all lung volume determinations and airway resistance determinations, when performed. A deletion parenthetical note has been included for these codes to direct users to the appropriate code for reporting plethysmography procedures.

Noninvasive Vascular Diagnostic Studies

Vascular studies include patient . . .

The use of a simple hand-held . . .

⊘=Modifier 51 Exempt   ⊙=Moderate Sedation   ✚=Add-on Code   ✔=FDA approval pending

Duplex scan (eg, 93880, 93882) describes . . .

▶***Physiologic studies*** Noninvasive physiologic studies are performed using equipment separate and distinct from the duplex ultrasound imager. Codes 93922, 93923, 93924, and 93965 describe the evaluation of non-imaging physiologic recordings of pressures with Doppler analysis of bi-directional blood flow, plethysmography, and/or oxygen tension measurements appropriate for the anatomic area studied.◀

Cerebrovascular Arterial Studies

A complete transcranial Doppler (TCD) study (93886) includes ultrasound evaluation of the right and left anterior circulation territories and the posterior circulation territory (to include vertebral arteries and basilar artery). In a limited TCD study (93888) there is ultrasound evaluation of two or fewer of these territories. For TCD, ultrasound evaluation is a reasonable and concerted attempt to identify arterial signals through an acoustic window.

▶(93875 has been deleted)◀

93880   Duplex scan of extracranial arteries; complete bilateral study

Rationale

As part of the AMA/Specialty Society RVS Update Committee (RUC) analysis, the noninvasive physiologic studies code 93875 was deleted due to the evidence that these services are no longer being performed. It was determined that this service is considered obsolete and did not warrant referencing an unlisted code. Due to the deletion of code 93875, the Noninvasive Vascular Diagnostic Studies guidelines have been revised to remove reference to deleted code 93875.

Extremity Arterial Studies (Including Digits)

93922   Limited bilateral noninvasive physiologic studies of upper or lower extremity arteries, (eg, for lower extremity: ankle/brachial indices at distal posterior tibial and anterior tibial/dorsalis pedis arteries plus bidirectional, Doppler waveform recording and analysis at 1-2 levels, or ankle/brachial indices at distal posterior tibial and anterior tibial/dorsalis pedis arteries plus volume plethysmography at 1-2 levels, or ankle/brachial indices at distal posterior tibial and anterior tibial/dorsalis pedis arteries with, transcutaneous oxygen tension measurement at 1-2 levels)

(When only 1 arm or . . .

(Report 93922 only once . . .

▶(For transcutaneous oxyhemoglobin measurement in a lower extremity wound by near infrared spectroscopy, use 0286T)◀

93923   Complete bilateral noninvasive physiologic studies of upper or lower extremity arteries, 3 or more levels (eg, for lower extremity: ankle/brachial indices at distal posterior tibial and anterior tibial/dorsalis pedis arteries plus segmental blood pressure measurements with bidirectional Doppler waveform recording and analysis, at 3 or more levels, or ankle/brachial indices at distal posterior tibial and anterior tibial/dorsalis pedis arteries plus segmental volume plethysmography at 3 or more levels, or ankle/brachial indices at distal posterior tibial and anterior tibial/dorsalis pedis arteries plus segmental transcutaneous oxygen tension measurements at 3 or more levels), or single level study with provocative functional maneuvers (eg, measurements with postural provocative tests, or measurements with reactive hyperemia)

(When only 1 arm or . . .

(Report 93923 only once in the upper extremity(s) and/or once in the lower extremity(s). When both the upper and lower extremities are evaluated in the same setting, 93923 may be reported twice by adding modifier 59 to the second procedure)

▶(For transcutaneous oxyhemoglobin measurement in a lower extremity wound by near infrared spectroscopy, use 0286T)◀

▶Other Noninvasive Vascular Diagnostic Studies◀

●93998   Unlisted noninvasive vascular diagnostic study

 Rationale

In support of the addition of a new Category III code (0286T) for reporting near-infrared spectroscopy studies of lower extremity wounds, a new subsection has been added in the Medicine/Noninvasive Vascular Diagnostic Studies subsection entitled "Other Noninvasive Vascular Diagnostic Studies." Also, a Category I code for reporting unlisted noninvasive vascular diagnostic studies (93998) has been created.

Finally, cross-reference notes following codes 93922 and 93923 have been added instructing users to report code 0286T for transcutaneous oxyhemoglobin measurement in a lower extremity wound by near-infrared spectroscopy.

Pulmonary

▶Pulmonary Diagnostic Testing and Therapies◀

▶Codes 94010-94799 include laboratory procedure(s) and interpretation of test results. If a separate identifiable Evaluation and Management service is performed, the appropriate E/M service code may be reported in addition to 94010-94799.

Spirometry (94010) measures expiratory airflow and volumes and forms the basis of most pulmonary function testing. When spirometry is performed before and after administration of a bronchodilator, report 94060. Measurement of vital capacity (94150) is a component of spirometry and is only reported when performed alone. The flow-volume loop (94375) is used to identify patterns of inspiratory and/or expiratory obstruction in central or peripheral airways. Spirometry (94010, 94060) includes maximal breathing capacity (94200) and flow-volume loop (94375), when performed.

Measurement of lung volumes may be performed using plethysmography, helium dilution or nitrogen washout. Plethysmography (94726) is utilized to determine total lung capacity, residual volume, functional residual capacity, and airway resistance. Nitrogen washout or helium dilution (94727) may

⊘=Modifier 51 Exempt   ⊙=Moderate Sedation   ✛=Add-on Code   𝑁=FDA approval pending be used to measure lung volumes, distribution of ventilation and closing volume. Impulse oscillometry (94728) assesses airway resistance and may be reported in addition to gas dilution techniques. Spirometry (94010, 94060) and bronchial provocation (94070) are not included in 94726 and 94727 and may be reported separately.

Diffusing capacity (94729) is most commonly performed in conjunction with lung volumes or spirometry and is an add-on code to 94726-94728, 94010, 94060, 94070, and 94375.

Pulmonary function tests (94011-94013) are reported for measurements in infants and young children through 2 years of age.

Pulmonary function testing measurements are reported as actual values and as a percent of predicted values by age, gender, height, and race.◄

94010　Spirometry, including graphic record, total and timed vital capacity, expiratory flow rate measurement(s), with or without maximal voluntary ventilation

►(Do not report 94010 in conjunction with 94150, 94200, 94375, 94728)◄

94060　Bronchodilation responsiveness, spirometry as in 94010, pre- and post-bronchodilator administration

►(Do not report 94060 in conjunction with 94150, 94200, 94375, 94728)◄

94150　Vital capacity, total (separate procedure)

►(Do not report 94150 in conjunction with 94010, 94060, 94728. To report thoracic gas volumes, see 94726, 94727)◄

94200　Maximum breathing capacity, maximal voluntary ventilation

►(Do not report 94200 in conjunction with 94010, 94060)◄

►(94240 has been deleted. To report thoracic gas volumes, see 94726, 94727)◄

94250　Expired gas collection, quantitative, single procedure (separate procedure)

►(94260 has been deleted. To report thoracic gas volumes, see 94726, 94727)◄

►(94350 has been deleted. To report, see 94726, 94727)◄

►(94360 has been deleted. To report, see 94726, 94728)◄

►(94370 has been deleted. To report, see 94726, 94727)◄

94375　Respiratory flow volume loop

►(Do not report 94375 in conjunction with 94010, 94060, 94728)◄

►(94720, 94725 have been deleted. To report, see 94729)◄

●**94726**　Plethysmography for determination of lung volumes and, when performed, airway resistance

►(Do not report 94726 in conjunction with 94727, 94728)◄

●**94727**　Gas dilution or washout for determination of lung volumes and, when performed, distribution of ventilation and closing volumes

►(Do not report 94727 in conjunction with 94726)◄

●**94728**　Airway resistance by impulse oscillometry

▶(Do not report 94728 in conjunction with 94010, 94060, 94070, 94375, 94726)◀

+●94729   Diffusing capacity (eg, carbon monoxide, membrane) (List separately in addition to code for primary procedure)

▶(Report 94729 in conjunction with 94010, 94060, 94070, 94375, 94726-94728)◀

 Rationale

A number of codes used to identify pulmonary testing and the accompanying guidelines have been revised to combine a number of procedures that are commonly performed together for pulmonary testing procedures. This includes deletions of codes that were previously separately reported, the addition of new codes, a heading change that specifies the types of procedures included in the section, and inclusion of new guideline language that more appropriately reflects pulmonary testing procedures in the way that they are commonly performed.

The subheading for pulmonary testing procedure and therapies has been revised to more accurately describe the services that are included in this section. The previous generic heading, "Other Procedures," has now been replaced by the subheading "Pulmonary Diagnostic Testing and Therapies" to provide users with a quick reference that notes the types of codes that are included within this section.

The codes previously used to identify plethysmography procedures (93720-93722) have been deleted and replaced by code 94726, which is now used to identify all services related to plethysmography testing. This includes all lung volume determinations and airway resistance determinations, when performed.

New guidelines have been included in this section to identify services that are included when reporting spirometry and plethysmography procedures. The guidelines provide users with a definition of spirometry, noting that this service measures expiratory airflow and volumes and forms the basis of most pulmonary function testing. They also note that spirometry performed before and after administration of a bronchodilator is reported using code 94060. The guidelines also note services that are commonly performed with spirometry (vital capacity [94150], maximal breathing capacity [94200], and flow volume loop [94375]), which are therefore inherently included when code 94010 is reported.

New guidelines have also been added to identify measurement of lung volumes by use of plethysmography (94726) and by helium dilution or nitrogen washout procedures (94727). This includes determination of the total lung capacity and all contributory lung volume determinations (residual volume and the functional residual capacity). The guidelines also note that plethysmography (94726) includes airway resistance testing. The new guidelines additionally provide a definition for impulse oscillometry (94728) and note that impulse oscillometry (94728) is a separately reportable procedure from gas dilution techniques. Spirometry services (94010, 94060) and bronchial provocation (94070) are not included in 94726 and 94727, and is therefore separately reported.

New guidelines have also been added to direct users to the appropriate method to report diffusing capacity (94729) and pulmonary function testing. Diffusing capacity testing has been included as an add-on procedure. In addition, guidelines have

⊘=Modifier 51 Exempt   ⊙=Moderate Sedation   ✚=Add-on Code   𝑵=FDA approval pending

been included in the CPT codebook to identify pulmonary function testing for infants and young children (94011-94013). The guideline language included for pulmonary function testing also includes information noting how these services are usually reported (percent of predicted values by age, gender, height, and race).

In conjunction with the new guidelines, new exclusionary parentheticals have been included following codes 94010 and 94060 that restrict use of these codes when provided with infusion oscillometry (94728), total capacity (94150), maximal breathing capacity (94200), and use of a flow volume loop (94375).

Other exclusionary parentheticals and code deletions have been provided to direct users to the appropriate codes to report various other services. This includes: (1) use of an exclusionary parenthetical for reporting vital capacity (94150) when provided in conjunction with infusion oscillometry (94728), spirometry (94010), and spirometry with bronchodilation (94060) (with directions to report code 94726 or 94727 for report of thoracic gas volume determinations); (2) addition of an exclusion parenthetical following code 94200 that restricts use of this code with bronchodilation procedures (94010, 94060); (3) deletion of codes 94240 (previously used to identify functional residual capacity/residual volume measurement), 94260 (previously used to identify thoracic gas volume measurement), 94350 (previously used for determination of maldistribution of inspired gas), 94360 (previously used for determination of resistance to airflow), and 94370 (previously used for determination of airway closing volume) with replacement by deletion parentheticals that direct users to report of codes 94726, 94727, or 94728 for thoracic gas volume or impulse oscillometry determinations; and (4) deletion of codes 94720 (carbon monoxide diffusing capacity) and 94725 (membrane diffusion capacity) with replacement by a deletion parenthetical that directs users to add-on code 94729 for diffusion capacity testing.

As noted in the guidelines, exclusion parentheticals have also been placed following new codes 94726-94729 to restrict use of these codes when combined service codes are available for report.

Clinical Example (94726)

A 65-year-old male complains of respiratory symptoms. Pulmonary function tests using body plethysmography are performed.

Description of Procedure (94726)

Verify that predicted values are correct for the patient tested. Review pressure volumes' curves from plethysmography. Review pressure/flow results from airway resistance. Check results for errors in the three to eight maneuvers as noted by the RN/RT. Interpret the test results. Record interpretation and findings in the patient record.

Clinical Example (94727)

A 65-year-old male complains of respiratory symptoms. Pulmonary function tests assessed by gas dilution are performed.

Description of Procedure (94727)

Verify that predicted values are correct for the patient tested. Review nitrogen wash-out or helium wash-in curves. Interpret the test results. Record interpretation and findings in the patient record.

 Clinical Example (94728)

A 4-year-old male presents with respiratory symptoms. Diagnostic pulmonary function tests by impulse oscillometry are performed.

Description of Procedure (94728)

Verify that predicted values are correct for the patient tested. Review resistance and reactance distribution over different phases of tidal breathing. Checking results for errors in the three to eight maneuvers before and after the administration of the bronchodilator as noted by the RN/RT. Interpret the test results. Record interpretation and findings in the patient record.

 Clinical Example (94729)

A 65-year-old male complains of shortness of breath. In addition to other pulmonary function tests, diffusing capacity is performed to assess for emphysema or interstitial lung disease.

Description of Procedure (94729)

Verify that predicted values are correct for the patient tested. Check results for errors in the two to three maneuvers as noted by the RN/RT. Check inspired vital capacity values for comparison to vital capacity. Check breath hold times. Interpret the test results. Record interpretation and findings in the patient record.

●94780   Car seat/bed testing for airway integrity, neonate, with continual nursing observation and continuous recording of pulse oximetry, heart rate and respiratory rate, with interpretation and report; 60 minutes

    ▶(Do not report 94780 for less than 60 minutes)◀

    ▶(Do not report 94780 in conjunction with 93040-93042, 94760, 94761, 99468-99472, 99477-99480)◀

+●94781   each additional full 30 minutes (List separately in addition to code for primary procedure)

    ▶(Use 94781 in conjunction with 94780)◀

 Rationale

A set of codes were established based on time increments of 60 minutes (94780) and each additional 30 minutes (94781) of testing of the cardio/respiratory responses of preterm or high-risk infants in the car seat/bed that will be used to transport them. Car seat testing is performed before discharge of a premature or other high-risk infant from the hospital to determine whether the infant can be safely transported using a standard car seat or if a car bed is necessary. Preterm infants and high-risk infants (eg, infants with craniofacial anomalies, presence of neuromuscular diseases) are at increased risk of adverse cardiorespiratory events when placed in a semi-upright position typical in an infant car seat.

Clinical Example (94780)

An infant born at 35 weeks' gestation requires and fails a car seat/bed test before discharge from the hospital and is sent home in a car bed. The parent brings the child to the physician's office for retesting to determine whether the infant is medically stable to transition to a car seat.

Description of Procedure (94780)

The physician reviews the results, interprets them, and documents his/her recommendation in the medical record.

Clinical Example (94781)

An infant born at 35 weeks' gestation requires and fails a car seat/bed test before discharge from the hospital and is sent home in a car bed. The parent brings the child to the physician's office for retesting to determine whether the infant is medically stable to transition to a car seat.

Description of Procedure (94781)

The physician reviews the results, interprets them, and documents his/her recommendation in the medical record.

Neurology and Neuromuscular Procedures

►Sleep Medicine Testing◄

►Sleep medicine services include procedures that evaluate adult and pediatric patients for a variety of sleep disorders. Sleep medicine testing services are diagnostic procedures using in-laboratory and portable technology to assess physiologic data and therapy.

All sleep services (95800-95811) include recording, interpretation and report. (Report with modifier 52 if less than 6 hours of recording for 95800, 95801 and 95806-95811, and if less than four nap opportunities are recorded for 95805).

Definitions

For purposes of CPT reporting of sleep medicine testing services, the following definitions apply:

Actigraphy: the use of a portable, non-invasive, device that continuously records gross motor movement over an extended period of time. The periods of activity and rest are indirect parameters for estimates of the periods of wakefulness and sleep of an individual.

Attended: a technologist or qualified health care professional is physically present (ie, sufficient proximity such that the qualified health care professional can physically respond to emergencies, to other appropriate patient needs or to technical problems at the bedside) throughout the recording session.

Electrooculogram (EOG): a recording of electrical activity indicative of eye movement.

Maintenance of wakefulness test (MWT): a standardized objective test used to determine a person's ability to stay awake. MWT requires sleep staging of the trials that are performed at defined intervals and is attended by a qualified health care professional.

Multiple sleep latency test (MSLT): a standardized objective test of the tendency to fall asleep. MSLT requires sleep staging of the nap opportunities that are performed at defined intervals and is attended by a technologist or qualified health care professional.

Peripheral arterial tonometry (PAT): a plethysmography technique that continuously measures pulsatile volume changes in a digit. This reflects the relative change of blood volume as an indirect measure of sympathetic nervous system activity which is used in respiratory analysis.

Physiological measurements of sleep as used in 95805: the parameters measured are a frontal, central and occipital lead of EEG (3 leads), submental EMG lead and a left and right EOG. These parameters are used together for staging sleep.

Polysomnography: a sleep test involving the continuous, simultaneous, recording of physiological parameters for a period of at least 6 hours that is performed in a sleep laboratory and attended by a technologist or qualified health care professional. The parameters measured are a frontal, central and occipital lead of EEG (3 leads), submental EMG lead and a left and right EOG, (from which sleep is staged), plus four or more additional parameters. The additional parameters typically required in polysomnography are listed below:

A. Electrocardiogram (ECG)

B. Nasal and/or oral airflow

C. Respiratory effort

D. Oxyhemoglobin saturation, SpO2

E. Bilateral anterior tibialis EMG

Positive airway pressure (PAP): a device used to treat sleep-related breathing disorders with the use of non-invasive delivery of positive pressure to the airway. Examples include but are not limited to: CPAP (continuous positive airway pressure), bilevel PAP, AutoPAP (autotitrating or adjusting PAP), ASV (adaptive-servo ventilation).

Remote: the site of service is distant from the monitoring center. Neither a technologist nor a qualified health care professional is physically present at the testing site.

Respiratory airflow (ventilation): the movement of air during inhaled and exhaled breaths. This is typically assessed using thermistor and nasal pressure sensors.

Respiratory analysis: generation of derived parameters that describe components of respiration obtained by using direct or indirect parameters, eg, by airflow or peripheral arterial tone.

Respiratory effort: contraction of the diaphragmatic and/or intercostal muscles to cause (or attempt to cause) respiratory airflow. This is typically measured using transducers that estimate motion of the thorax and abdomen such as respiratory inductive plethysmography, transducers that estimate pressures generated by breathing muscles such as esophageal monometry, or by contraction of breathing muscles, such as diaphragmatic/intercostal EMG.

Respiratory (thoracoabdominal) movement: movement of the chest and abdomen during respiratory effort.

Sleep latency: the length of time it takes to transition from wakefulness to sleep. In the sleep laboratory it is the time from "lights out" to the first epoch scored as any stage of sleep.

Sleep staging: the delineation of the distinct sleep levels through the simultaneous evaluation of physiologic measures including a frontal, central and occipital lead of EEG (3 leads), submental EMG lead and a left and right EOG.

Sleep testing (or sleep study): the continuous, simultaneous monitoring of physiological parameters during sleep (eg, polysomnography, EEG).

Total sleep time: a derived parameter obtained by sleep staging or may be estimated indirectly using actigraphy or other methods.

Unattended: a technologist or qualified health care professional is not physically present with the patient during the recording session.◄

🖎 Rationale

For *CPT 2011*, two sleep study codes were added (95800-95801) for reporting unattended sleep study testing services. For *CPT 2012*, this subsection has been updated and expanded to reflect current practice of sleep medicine testing. The heading has been revised by adding the word, "Medicine." In addition, definitions have been added to help clarify appropriate use of sleep medicine codes (95800-95811).

Electromyography

▶Needle electromyographic (EMG) procedures include the interpretation of electrical waveforms measured by equipment that produces both visible and audible components of electrical signals recorded from the muscle(s) studied by the needle electrode.

Use 95870 or 95885 when four or fewer muscles are tested in an extremity. Use 95860-95864 or 95886 when five or more muscles are tested in an extremity.

Use EMG codes (95860-95864 and 95867-95870) when no nerve conduction studies (95900-95904) are performed on that day. Use 95885, 95886 and 95887 for EMG services when nerve conduction studies (95900-95904) are performed in conjunction with EMG on the same day.

Report either 95885 or 95886 once per extremity. Codes 95885 and 95886 can be reported together up to a combined total of four units of service per patient when all four extremities are tested.◄

95872	Needle electromyography using single fiber electrode, with quantitative measurement of jitter, blocking and/or fiber density, any/all sites of each muscle studied
#✚●95885	Needle electromyography, each extremity, with related paraspinal areas, when performed, done with nerve conduction, amplitude and latency/velocity study; limited (List separately in addition to code for primary procedure)
#✚●95886	complete, five or more muscles studied, innervated by three or more nerves or four or more spinal levels (List separately in addition to code for primary procedure)

▶(Use 95885, 95886 in conjunction with 95900-95904)◄

▶(Do not report 95885, 95886 in conjunction with 95860-95864, 95870, 95905)◄

#+●95887 Needle electromyography, non-extremity (cranial nerve supplied or axial) muscle(s) done with nerve conduction, amplitude and latency/velocity study (List separately in addition to code for primary procedure)

▶(Use 95887 in conjunction with 95900-95904)◀

▶(Do not report 95887 in conjunction with 95867-95870, 95905)◀

Ischemic Muscle Testing

95873 Electrical stimulation for guidance in conjunction with chemodenervation (List separately in addition to code for primary procedure)

95874 Needle electromyography for guidance in conjunction with chemodenervation (List separately in addition to code for primary procedure)

(Use 95873, 95874 in conjunction with 64612-64614)

(Do not report 95874 in conjunction with 95873)

(Do not report 95873, 95874 in conjunction with 95860-95870)

95875 Ischemic limb exercise test with serial specimen(s) acquisition for muscle(s) metabolite(s)

(For listing of nerves considered for separate study, see Appendix J)

95885 Code is out of numerical sequence. See 95860-95887

95886 Code is out of numerical sequence. See 95860-95887

95887 Code is out of numerical sequence. See 95860-95887

🖉 Rationale

To address the concerns of the AMA/Specialty Society RVS Update Committee (RUC) related to the screening of codes that are performed together more than 75% of the time, three add-on codes and introductory language for needle electromyography (EMG) performed in conjunction with nerve conduction study(s) have been established. Code 95885 has been established for reporting a limited needle EMG study per extremity when performed with a nerve conduction study(s). Code 95886 is for reporting a complete study, per extremity, performed with a nerve conduction study(s). Codes 95885 and 95886 can be reported together up to a combined total of four units of service per patient when all four extremities are tested.

Code 95887 has been established for reporting needle EMG procedures performed on a nonextremity muscle(s) (cranial nerve supplied or axial) performed in conjuction with a nerve conduction study(ies).

Codes 95885, 95886, and 95887 appear with a number symbol (#) to indicate that these codes appear out of numerical sequence. Reference notes have been added (where these codes would have been found numerically) to direct users to the appropriate code range 95860-95887. These new needle EMG add-on codes

⊘=Modifier 51 Exempt ⊙=Moderate Sedation ✚=Add-on Code ✗=FDA approval pending

are reported in addition to the nerve conduction codes 95900-95904 when nerve conduction studies are performed in conjunction with EMG on the same day.

As indicated in the instructional parenthetical note, codes 95885, 95886, and 95887 are excluded from use in conjunction with needle electromyography codes 95860-95864, 95867-95870, and 95905.

Clinical Example (95885)

A 45-year-old female has a 5-month history of frequent awakening at night due to right hand and arm pain. Prolonged typing also causes distal right upper extremity numbness, tingling, and pain and she sometimes drops things out of the right hand. Physical examination reveals numbness of the palmar aspects of the right index and middle fingers; and a questionable Tinel's sign over the right median nerve at the carpal tunnel. Three motor and four sensory nerve conduction studies were performed. Right median sensory nerve conduction is slowed across the carpal tunnel. Needle electromyography examination of a thenar muscle innervated by the median nerve of the symptomatic limb is indicated, along with an ulnar and radial-innervated muscle to confirm the diagnosis of median neuropathy at the wrist, evaluate severity, and rule out more widespread pathology.

Description of Procedure (95885)

Intraservice work includes physician participation in patient preparation, focusing on discussing the needle EMG test with the patient and answering questions regarding the pain associated with the procedure. The physician must specifically assess the risk of the procedure (eg, bleeding, infection) by reviewing the patient's medical history and medications. The physician places the ground surface electrode, cleans the skin overlying anticipated muscle puncture sites, and dons gloves prior to the examination. Prior to inserting the needle electrode into each muscle to be examined, the electromyographer must perform a focused physical examination to determine surface anatomic landmarks, and identify structures to avoid during the needle insertion. Under minimal voluntary contraction of the muscle at least 20 voluntary motor unit potentials are analyzed along multiple passes through the muscle, noting duration, amplitude, configuration, and other diagnostic variables both visually and by sound that allow the waveform to be classified as normal or abnormal. The patient is examined after the needle is withdrawn from each puncture site to insure hemostasis and to apply any needed manual pressure or bandage where minor bleeding may be observed. Four or fewer muscles are examined individually using the steps outlined above. The muscles are located in an upper or lower extremity and its related cervical or lumbar paraspinal areas.

Clinical Example (95886)

A 55-year-old diabetic male has a 2-month history of pain, numbness, and tingling of the left upper extremity. There was no preceding injury and there are no clear cut provocative or palliative factors. Physical examination reveals no definite motor, sensory, or reflex abnormalities. Three motor and four sensory nerve conduction studies were performed. No abnormalities are noted on these studies. Needle electromyography examination of at least one muscle innervated by the C5, C6, C7, C8, and T1 spinal roots in the symptomatic limb, and cervical paraspinal muscles at one or more levels, is indicated to evaluate for mononeuropathy, peripheral neuropathy, brachial plexopathy, or cervical radiculopathy as a cause for these symptoms.

Description of Procedure (95886)

Intraservice work includes physician participation in patient preparation, focusing on discussing the needle EMG test with the patient and answering questions regarding the pain associated with the procedure. The physician must specifically assess the risk of the procedure (eg, bleeding, infection) by reviewing the patient's medical history and medications. The physician places the ground surface electrode, cleans the skin overlying anticipated muscle puncture sites, and dons gloves prior to the examination. Prior to inserting the needle electrode into each muscle to be examined, the electromyographer must perform a focused physical examination to determine surface anatomic landmarks, and identify structures to avoid during the needle insertion. Under minimal voluntary contraction of the muscle at least 20 voluntary motor unit potentials are analyzed along multiple passes through the muscle, noting duration, amplitude, configuration, and other diagnostic variables both visually and by sound that allow the waveform to be classified as normal or abnormal. The patient is examined after the needle is withdrawn from each puncture site to insure hemostasis and to apply any needed manual pressure or bandage where minor bleeding may be observed. Five or more muscles are examined individually using the steps outlined above. The muscles are located in an upper or lower extremity and its related cervical or lumbar paraspinal areas, and are innervated by three or more nerves or four or more spinal levels.

 Clinical Example (95887)

A 65-year-old female has a 2-month history of right facial weakness involving the forehead, eyelid, and mouth. Initially she was treated with steroids for a presumptive diagnosis of Bell's palsy, but her deficits persisted. Physical examination demonstrates a peripheral distribution right facial palsy. Right facial motor nerve conduction study was abnormal due to prolonged distal motor latency and low compound muscle action potential amplitude. Needle electromyography of right cranial nerve innervated muscles (V, VII, XI, XII) is indicated to confirm the diagnosis, help establish the prognosis, and determine the need for facial nerve decompression.

Description of Procedure (95887)

Intraservice work includes physician participation in patient preparation, focusing on discussing the needle EMG test with the patient, and answering questions regarding the pain associated with the procedure. The physician must specifically assess the risk of the procedure (eg, bleeding, infection) by reviewing the patient's medical history and medications. The physician places the ground surface electrode, cleans the skin overlying anticipated muscle puncture sites, and dons gloves prior to the examination. Prior to inserting the needle electrode into each muscle to be examined, the electromyographer must perform a focused physical examination to determine surface anatomic landmarks, and identify structures to avoid during the needle insertion. Under minimal voluntary contraction of the muscle at least 20 voluntary motor unit potentials are analyzed along multiple passes through the muscle, noting duration, amplitude, configuration and other diagnostic variables both visually and by sound that allow the waveform to be classified as normal or abnormal. The patient is examined after the needle is withdrawn from each puncture site to insure hemostasis and to apply any needed manual pressure or bandage where minor bleeding may be observed. Cranial nerve innervated muscles (eg, face or tongue muscles) or axial muscles (eg, serratus anterior or thoracic paraspinal muscles) on one side of the body are examined individually using the steps outlined above. Special care must be taken during the study since many muscles are thin and located adjacent to critical structures (eg, eye or lung).

Nerve Conduction Tests

The following applies to nerve conduction tests . . .

Code 95905 describes nerve conduction tests when . . .

⊘ **95900**   Nerve conduction, amplitude and latency/velocity study, each nerve; motor, without F-wave study

⊘**95903**   motor, with F-wave study

⊘**95904**   sensory

(Report 95900, 95903, and/or 95904 only once when multiple sites on the same nerve are stimulated or recorded)

▶(Use 95885-95887 in conjunction with 95900-95904 when performing electromyography with nerve conduction studies)◀

⊘ **95905**   Motor and/or sensory nerve conduction, using preconfigured electrode array(s), amplitude and latency/velocity study, each limb, includes F-wave study when performed, with interpretation and report

(Report 95905 only once per limb studied)

▶(Do not report 95905 in conjunction with 95885, 95886, 95900-95904, 95934-95936)◀

✎ Rationale

In support of the establishment of the three add-on codes 95885-95887 for needle electromyography (EMG) performed in conjunction with nerve conduction study(s), a parenthetical note has been added following code 95904 instructing the appropriate use with the new codes. An exclusionary parenthetical note has also been added following code 95905 precluding its use with 95885, 95886, 95900-95904, 95934-95936.

Evoked Potentials and Reflex Tests

95925   Short-latency somatosensory evoked potential study, stimulation of any/all peripheral nerves or skin sites, recording from the central nervous system; in upper limbs

▶(Do not report 95925 in conjunction with 95926)◀

95926   in lower limbs

▶(Do not report 95926 in conjunction with 95925)◀

#●95938   in upper and lower limbs

▶(Do not report 95938 in conjunction with 95925, 95926)◀

95927   in the trunk or head

(To report a unilateral study, use modifier 52)

(For auditory evoked potentials, use 92585)

95928   Central motor evoked potential study (transcranial motor stimulation); upper limbs

▶(Do not report 95928 in conjunction with 95929)◀

95929   lower limbs

▶(Do not report 95929 in conjunction with 95928)◀

#●95939   in upper and lower limbs

▶(Do not report 95939 in conjunction with 95928, 95929)◀

95930   Visual evoked potential (VEP) testing central nervous system, checkerboard or flash

95933   Orbicularis oculi (blink) reflex, by electrodiagnostic testing

95934   H-reflex, amplitude and latency study; record gastrocnemius/soleus muscle

95936   record muscle other than gastrocnemius/soleus muscle

(To report a bilateral study, use modifier 50)

95937   Neuromuscular junction testing (repetitive stimulation, paired stimuli), each nerve, any 1 method

▶95938   Code is out of numerical sequence. See 95925-95939◀

▶95939   Code is out of numerical sequence. See 95925-95939◀

✍ Rationale

Codes combining both upper and lower limbs into a single code have been added to the evoked potentials and reflex tests series of codes. Code 95938 combines both upper and lower limbs into a code when performing short-latency somatosensory evoked potential studies. Code 95939 combines both upper and lower limbs into a single code when performing central motor evoked potential studies. In support of the establishment of these combination codes, several exclusionary parenthetical notes have been added following: (1) 95925 to preclude the use of 95925 with 95926; (2) 95926 to preclude its use with 95925; (3) 95938 precluding its use with 95925 and 95926; (4) 95928 precluding its use with 95929; (5) 95929 to preclude its use with 95928; and (6) 95939 precluding its use with 95928 and 95929. Codes 95938 and 95939 appear with a number symbol (#) to indicate that these codes appear out of numerical sequence. Reference notes have been added (where these codes would have been found numerically) to direct users to the appropriate code range 95925-95939 for placement of codes 95938 and 95939.

⊘=Modifier 51 Exempt   ⊙=Moderate Sedation   ✚=Add-on Code   ✗=FDA approval pending

Clinical Example (95938)

A 45-year-old female complains of 1 month of numbness in her left leg. Three years ago she had an episode of visual blurriness lasting one month, which was not medically evaluated. A somatosensory evoked potential study (SEP) test was ordered to assess for and localize central conduction impairment, and to separate a central from a peripheral nervous system cause of sensory impairment.

Description of Procedure (95938)

Intraservice work includes physician supervision of patient preparation, placement of ground, stimulating and recording surface electrodes, stimulation of nerves and/or dermatomes and recording the resulting evoked potentials at several sites from periphery to cerebral cortex. Many hundreds of trials are averaged since the signals are very small, and each of the 4 limbs is studied successively. Test design changes may occur during the course of the study in response to the information obtained.

Clinical Example (95939)

A 65-year-old male has 3 months of progressive, bilateral lower limb weakness and stiffness. MRI showed severe cervical stenosis with impingement of cervical cord. An anterior and posterior cervical decompression and fusion was planned. A transcranial electrical MEP with 4-limb, 12-muscle recording was performed preoperatively to establish a baseline for use in surgical monitoring.

Description of Procedure (95939)

Insert needle electrodes into left and right biceps, triceps, abductor pollicis brevis, and abductor digiti minimi, medial gastrocnemius, tibialis anterior, and abductor hallucis muscles. Secure electrodes in place. Assure a bite block is comfortably in place. Place 10 scalp recording electrodes at sites measured using the 10-20 electrode placement system. Check impedances, and replace or move electrodes as needed. Prior to performing transcranial brain electrical stimulation, perform routine motor nerve conduction studies of the and/or median nerves to establish baseline compound muscle action potentials (CMAP). Stimulate at point and distal nerve segments. Identify evidence of peripheral neuropathy or other pathology interfering with peripheral conduction, and adjust muscles tested to accommodate for those pre-existing disorders. Throughout the brain electrical stimulation procedure, monitor scalp EEG to assess for any epileptic spikes, seizures, or after-discharges that were caused by the electrical brain stimulation. Be prepared abruptly to stop stimulation if it provokes an epileptic seizure, and to care for the patient during any seizure that occurs. Determine the initial scalp location for stimulating electrodes by carefully measuring the head. Stimulate at each of several scalp sites and measure latency and amplitudes of responses at the muscle. Vary the stimulus location to identify better stimulation locations for this patient. Vary the stimulus voltage intensity at each location in 10% increments to find locations and voltages that produce adequate responses for that muscle. Limit the brain stimulation to 500 volts maximum except in unusual cases. After determining the threshold, measure the transcranial MEP amplitude and initial peak latency to establish baseline studies. Adjust the stimulus pulse duration, number of stimuli in a train, and interstimulus interval to identify the best motor responses, while adjusting the voltage as needed. Mark the stimulation sites, and note the voltages, pulse width, train length, and interstimulus intervals needed to obtain optimal responses for that muscle. Replicate data. Store the signals for later review and analysis. Repeat this procedure for three to four selected muscles on the same limb. Repeat this procedure on the other upper extremity. Repeat this procedure in the lower extremities. Repeat as needed to obtain adequate data. Chart the latency and amplitude findings, measuring latency to the nearest 100 microseconds, and amplitude in microvolt units. Compare the patient's results to normative data adjusted for the patient's individual age, height, and gender. Account for limb temperature. Interpret the pattern of changes, identifying confirmed or suspected sites of pathway disruption due to pathology, and providing a diagnostic interpretation for the results that takes into account the patient's findings, history, exam, and prior test and imaging results.

Neurostimulators, Analysis-Programming

▶Simple intraoperative or subsequent programming of the neurostimulator pulse generator/transmitter (95971) includes changes to three or fewer of the following parameters: rate, pulse amplitude, pulse duration, pulse frequency, eight or more electrode contacts, cycling, stimulation train duration, train spacing, number of programs, number of channels, alternating electrode polarities, dose time (stimulation parameters changing in time periods of minutes including dose lockout times), more than one clinical feature (eg, rigidity, dyskinesia, tremor). Complex intraoperative or subsequent programming (95972-95979) includes changes to more than three of the above.◀

Code 95970 describes subsequent . . .

Code 95980 describes intraoperative . . .

▶For 95972, 95974 and 95978, use modifier 52 if less than 31 minutes in duration.◀

▶(For electronic analysis and reprogramming of a peripheral subcutaneous field stimulation pulse generator, use 0285T)◀

(For insertion of neurostimulator pulse generator, see 61885, 63685, 64590)

(For revision or removal of neurostimulator pulse generator or receiver, see 61888, 63688, 64595)

▶(For implantation of neurostimulator electrodes, see 43647, 43881, 61850-61875, 63650-63655, 64553-64580. For revision or removal of neurostimulator electrodes, see 43648, 43882, 61880, 63661-63664, 64585)◀

▲95970   Electronic analysis of implanted neurostimulator pulse generator system (eg, rate, pulse amplitude, pulse duration, configuration of wave form, battery status, electrode selectability, output modulation, cycling, impedance and patient compliance measurements); simple or complex brain, spinal cord, or peripheral (ie, cranial nerve, peripheral nerve, sacral nerve, neuromuscular) neurostimulator pulse generator/transmitter, without reprogramming

▲95971   simple spinal cord, or peripheral (ie, peripheral nerve, sacral nerve, neuromuscular) neurostimulator pulse generator/transmitter, with intraoperative or subsequent programming

▲95972   complex spinal cord, or peripheral (ie, peripheral nerve, sacral nerve, neuromuscular) (except cranial nerve) neurostimulator pulse generator/transmitter, with intraoperative or subsequent programming, first hour

+▲95973   complex spinal cord, or peripheral (ie, peripheral nerve, sacral nerve, neuromuscular) (except cranial nerve) neurostimulator pulse generator/transmitter, with intraoperative or subsequent programming, each additional 30 minutes after first hour (List separately in addition to code for primary procedure)

    (Use 95973 in conjunction with 95972)

▲95974   complex cranial nerve neurostimulator pulse generator/transmitter, with intraoperative or subsequent programming, with or without nerve interface testing, first hour

+▲95975   complex cranial nerve neurostimulator pulse generator/transmitter, with intraoperative or subsequent programming, additional 30 minutes after first hour (List separately in addition to code for primary procedure)

🖎 Rationale

In support of [ ] codes 0282T-0285T, a parenthetical not [ ] eurology and Neuromuscular Procedures [ ] ming section directing users to code 0285 [ ] ogramming of a peripheral subcutaneous field stimulation [ ] ease see the discussion of codes 0282T-0285T in the Category III section [ ] his book.

Changes have also been made to the neurostimulation codes throughout the CPT codebook to provide parallel language for these procedures as well as to more clearly portray the intended use for these procedures. This includes clarifications for guidelines to differentiate "simple" versus "complex" programming procedures, identifying three or fewer parameters for simple versus four or more for complex procedures. There have also been changes to instruct users to append modifier 52 to services for sessions lasting less than 31 minutes in duration.

Codes 95970, 95971, and 95972 have also been revised to remove the language, autonomic nerve. For codes 95970-95972, "sacral nerve" was added to provide more specific language regarding the nerves being tested.

Other Procedures

▲95990   Refilling and maintenance of implantable pump or reservoir for drug delivery, spinal (intrathecal, epidural) or brain (intraventricular), includes electronic analysis of pump, when performed;

▲95991   requiring physician's skill

    ▶(Do not report 95990, 95991 in conjunction with 62367-62370. For analysis and/or reprogramming of implantable infusion pump, see 62367-62370)◀

    ▶(For refill and maintenance of implanted infusion pump or reservoir for systemic drug therapy [eg, chemotherapy], use 96522)◀

Rationale

The AMA/Specialty Society RVS Update Committee (RUC) identified codes 62367, 62368, 95990, and 95991 in the "Codes Reported Together 75% or More" screen. As a result, the services described by these codes have been combined as appropriate by revising code 62367, adding two new codes to this code family and revising codes 95990 and 95991. See the Surgery/Nervous System/Spine and Spinal Cord/Reservoir/Pump Implantation section of this book for an explanation of revised code 62367 and new codes 62369 and 62370.

Codes 95990 and 95991 were revised to include electronic analysis of a pump for intrathecal, epidural, or intraventricular drug delivery when performed in conjunction with refilling and maintenance of the pump. Code 95991 has been further revised to clarify that physician's skill is required by changing the language from "administered by physician" to "requiring physician's skill."

The parenthetical note following code 95990 directing users to codes 62367 and 62368 for analysis and/or reprogramming of implantable infusion pump has been deleted. The parenthetical note following code 95990 directing users to code 96522 for refill and maintenance of implanted infusion pump or reservoir for systemic drug therapy has also been deleted. Two parenthetical notes have been added following code 95991. The first note instructs users not to report codes 95990 and 95991 in conjunction with codes 62367-62370 and to report codes 62367-62370 for analysis and/or reprogramming of implantable infusion pump. The second note is a cross-reference directing users to report code 96522 for refill and maintenance of an implanted infusion pump or reservoir for systemic drug therapy (eg, chemotherapy).

Central Nervous System Assessments/Tests (eg, Neuro-Cognitive, Mental Status, Speech Testing)

▲96110   Developmental screening, with interpretation and report, per standardized instrument form

▲96111   Developmental testing, (includes assessment of motor, language, social, adaptive, and/or cognitive functioning by standardized developmental instruments) with interpretation and report

Rationale

Codes 96110 and 96111 have been editorially revised to reflect current practice and to avoid use of inaccurate terms associated with these codes. Code 96110, previously described as developmental testing, was inaccurate and was changed to the term developmental screening. Code 96111 is still intended for developmental testing, but it is now a stand-alone code. Testing is a face-to-face objective service in which the physician directly observes the child performing tasks on a standardized test. Screening, on the other hand, asks a child's observer to provide his or her observations of the child's skills, and these are recorded on a standardized and validated screening instrument. Screening is subjective. Testing actually measures what the patient is able to do on a standardized psychometric instrument at that

⃠=Modifier 51 Exempt   ⊙=Moderate Sedation   ✚=Add-on Code   𝒩=FDA approval pending

time while screening only reports the assessment of the patient's skills through the observation of the informal observer.

The terms "limited" and "extended" were deleted from codes 96110 and 96111. Also, the parenthetical note following code 96110 with names of specific tests (eg, Developmental Screening Test II, Early Language Milestone Screen) was deleted to avoid reference to tests that have become obsolete or may be replaced by newer tests. To replace the omission of the explanatory parenthetical note, the term "per standardized instrument form" was added to code 96110.

Hydration, Therapeutic, Prophylactic, Diagnostic Injections and Infusions, and Chemotherapy and Other Highly Complex Drug or Highly Complex Biologic Agent Administration

Physician work related to hydration, injection, and infusion services predominantly involves affirmation of treatment plan and direct supervision of staff.

►Codes 96360-96379, 96401, 96402, 96409-96425, 96521-96523 are not intended to be reported by the physician in the facility setting. If a significant, separately identifiable office or other outpatient Evaluation and Management service is performed, the appropriate E/M service (99201-99215, 99241-99245, 99354-99355) should be reported using modifier 25 in addition to 96360-96549. For same day E/M service, a different diagnosis is not required.◄

If performed to facilitate the infusion or injection, the following services are included and are not reported separately:

a. Use of local anesthesia

b. IV start

c. Access to indwelling IV, subcutaneous catheter or port

d. Flush at conclusion of infusion

e. Standard tubing, syringes, and supplies

(For declotting a catheter or port, use 36593)

When multiple drugs are administered, report the service(s) and the specific materials or drugs for each.

►When administering multiple infusions, injections or combinations, only one "initial" service code should be reported for a given date, unless protocol requires that two separate IV sites must be used. Do not report a second initial service on the same date due to an intravenous line requiring a re-start, an IV rate not being able to be reached without two lines, or for accessing a port of a multi-lumen catheter. If an injection or infusion is of a subsequent or concurrent nature, even if it is the first such service within that group of services, then a subsequent or concurrent code from the appropriate section should be reported (eg, the first IV push given subsequent to an initial one-hour infusion is reported using a subsequent IV push code).

Initial infusion: For physician reporting, an initial infusion is the *key or primary reason for the encounter* reported irrespective of the temporal order in which the infusion(s) or injection(s) are administered. For facility reporting, an initial infusion is based using the hierarchy. For both physician and facility reporting, only one *initial* service code (eg, 96365) should be reported unless the protocol or patient condition requires that two separate IV sites must be utilized. The difference in time and effort in providing this second IV site access is also reported using the *initial* service code with modifier 59 appended (eg, 96365, 96365-59).

Sequential infusion: A sequential infusion is an infusion or IV push of a new substance or drug following a primary or initial service. All sequential services require that there be a new substance or drug, except that facilities may report a sequential intravenous push of the same drug using 96376.

Concurrent infusion: A concurrent infusion is an infusion of a new substance or drug infused at the same time as another substance or drug. A concurrent infusion service is not time based and is only reported once per day regardless of whether an additional new drug or substance is administered concurrently. Hydration may not be reported concurrently with any other service. A separate subsequent concurrent administration of another new drug or substance (the third substance or drug) is not reported.◄

In order to determine which service . . .

When these codes are reported . . .

►When reporting multiple infusions of the same drug/substance on the same date of service, the initial code should be selected. The second and subsequent infusion(s) should be reported based on the individual time(s) of each additional infusion(s) of the same drug/substance using the appropriate add-on code.

Example: In the outpatient observation setting, a patient receives one-hour intravenous infusions of the same antibiotic every 8 hours on the same date of service through the same IV access. The hierarchy for facility reporting permits the reporting of code 96365 for the first one-hour dose administered. Add-on 96366 would be reported twice (once for the second and third one-hour infusions of the same drug).

When reporting codes for which infusion time is a factor, use the actual time over which the infusion is administered. Intravenous or intra-arterial push is defined as: (a) an injection in which the health care professional who administers the drug/substance is continuously present to administer the injection and observe the patient, or (b) an infusion of 15 minutes or less. If intravenous hydration (96360, 96361) is given from 11 PM to 2 AM, 96360 would be reported once and 96361 twice. However, if instead of a continuous infusion, a medication was given by intravenous push at 10 PM and 2 AM, as the service was not continuous, both administrations would be reported as an initial service (96374). For continuous services that last beyond midnight, use the date in which the service began and report the total units of time provided continuously. A "keep open" infusion of any type is not separately reported.◄

Hydration

Codes 96360-96361 are intended . . .

►Some chemotherapeutic agents and other therapeutic agents require pre- and/or post-hydration to be given in order to avoid specific toxicities. A minimum time duration of 31 minutes of hydration infusion is required to report the service. However, the hydration codes 96360 or 96361 are not used when the purpose of the intravenous fluid is to "keep open" an IV line prior or subsequent to a therapeutic infusion, or as a free-flowing IV during chemotherapy or other therapeutic infusion.◄

96360   Intravenous infusion, hydration; initial, 31 minutes to 1 hour

(Do not report 96360 if performed as a concurrent infusion service)

(Do not report intravenous infusion for hydration of 30 minutes or less)

+ 96361   each additional hour (List separately in addition to code for primary procedure)

Therapeutic, Prophylactic, and Diagnostic Injections and Infusions (Excludes Chemotherapy and Other Highly Complex Drug or Highly Complex Biologic Agent Administration)

A therapeutic, prophylactic, or diagnostic IV . . .

See codes 96401-96549 for the administration . . .

(Do not report 96365-96379 with codes for which IV push or infusion is an inherent part of the procedure [eg, administration of contrast material for a diagnostic imaging study])

96365   Intravenous infusion, for therapy, prophylaxis, or diagnosis (specify substance or drug); initial, up to 1 hour

+ 96366   each additional hour (List separately in addition to code for primary procedure)

(Report 96366 in conjunction with 96365, 96367)

(Report 96366 for additional hour[s] of sequential infusion)

(Report 96366 for infusion intervals of greater than 30 minutes beyond 1 hour increments)

►(Report 96366 in conjunction with 96365 to identify each second and subsequent infusions of the same drug/substance)◄

+▲ 96367   additional sequential infusion of a new drug/substance, up to 1 hour (List separately in addition to code for primary procedure)

►(Report 96367 in conjunction with 96365, 96374, 96409, 96413 to identify the infusion of a new drug/substance provided as a secondary or subsequent service after a different initial service is administered through the same IV access. Report 96367 only once per sequential infusion of same infusate mix)◄

+ 96368   concurrent infusion (List separately in addition to code for primary procedure)

►(Report 96368 only once per date of service)◄

(Report 96368 in conjunction with 96365, 96366, 96413, 96415, 96416)

+ 96376   each additional sequential intravenous push of the same substance/drug provided in a facility (List separately in addition to code for primary procedure)

(Do not report 96376 for a push performed within 30 minutes of a reported push of the same substance or drug)

(96376 may be reported by facilities only)

▶(Report 96376 in conjunction with 96365, 96374, 96409, 96413)◀

96379   Unlisted therapeutic, prophylactic, or diagnostic intravenous or intra-arterial injection or infusion

🖎 Rationale

Following the structural algorithm of the hierarchy created for facility reporting, additional instruction and specific definitions have been added to the chemotherapy, therapeutic, prophylactic, diagnostic infusion/injection, and hydration services guidelines. The instruction represents the intent and use of codes 96360-96379 based on the principles of the entire set of infusion codes with particular attention to the reporting of these service(s) in 24-hour hospital outpatient settings (eg, emergency department, outpatient observation).

A specific code listing reiterates that codes 96360-96379, 96401, 96402, 96409-96425, and 96521-96523 are not intended to be reported by the physician in the facility setting. Also explicitly stated are the Evaluation and Management Services codes (99201-99215, 99241-99245, 99354-99355) that should be additionally reported in the event a separately identifiable office or other outpatient Evaluation and Management service is performed.

The reporting of more than one "initial" service code is reiterated when drug/substance administration protocol or the patient's condition requires two distinctly separate IV site accesses. The difference in time and effort in providing this second IV site access is also reported using the initial service code with the modifier 59, Distinct Procedural Service, appended (eg, 96365, 96365 59). However, providers are reminded that it is not appropriate to report a second initial service on the same date due to an intravenous line requiring a restart, an IV rate not being able to be reached without two lines, or for accessing a port of a multilumen catheter.

The Hydration guidelines offer further definition of "hydration," chemotherapeutic and other therapeutic agent pre-and/or posthydration. Also included is the reminder that Hydration codes 96360 or 96361 are not used when the purpose of the intravenous fluid is to "keep open" an IV line prior or subsequent to a therapeutic infusion, or as a free-flowing IV during chemotherapy or other therapeutic infusion.

Definitions have been added to delineate that which comprises an "initial", "sequential," and "concurrent" infusion as it pertains to either physician or facility reporting.

Reporting of multiple infusions of the same or different drugs/substances on the same calendar date is based on the individual time(s) of each additional infusion(s) using the appropriate add-on code. An example has been added depicting a one-hour infusion of the same drug every eight hours on the same date of service. Using the facility reporting hierarchy, code 96365 is reported for the first one-hour dose administered. Add-on code 96366 would be reported twice (once for the second and third one-hour infusions of the same drug). A parenthetical instruction follows add-on code 96366 instructing the use of 96366 in conjunction with 96365 to identify each second and subsequent infusions of the same drug/substance.

⊘=Modifier 51 Exempt   ⊙=Moderate Sedation   ✚=Add-on Code   ✗=FDA approval pending

To differentiate usage, the descriptor of add-on code 96367 was revised to reflect the additional sequential infusion of a new drug/substance. The parenthetical note following add-on code 96367 was revised to correspond with the descriptor revision, ie, code 96367 is reported with "initial" codes 96365, 96374, 96409, and 96413 to identify the infusion of a new drug/substance. Code 96367 continues to represent a secondary or subsequent service after a different initial service is administered through the same IV access and is reported only once per sequential infusion of the same infusate mix.

The parenthetical note following the sequential intravenous push code 96376 (only for facility reporting) designates its usage with "initial" codes 96365, 96374, 96409, 96413.

Consistent with the Time instruction in the Introduction of the CPT code set, code choice continues to be based on the actual time over which the infusion is administered (ie, start and stop time). An example has been added outlining the circumstance wherein an infusion was started prior to midnight on one calendar date extends beyond midnight of the next calendar date. For continuous services that last beyond midnight, providers are instructed to use the date in which the services began and report the total units of time provided continuously.

The parenthetical note following concurrent infusion add-on code 96368 was revised to reflect the reporting of code 96368 only once per date of service.

Special Dermatological Procedures

96900   Actinotherapy (ultraviolet light)

▶(For rhinophototherapy, intranasal application of ultraviolet and visible light, use 30999)◀

🖎 Rationale

In support of the deletion of Category III code 0168T, a cross-reference note has been added to direct the users to report code 30999.

Physical Medicine and Rehabilitation

Modalities

CONSTANT ATTENDANCE

The application of a modality that requires direct (one-on-one) patient contact by the provider.

97032   Application of a modality to 1 or more areas; electrical stimulation (manual), each 15 minutes

▶(For transcutaneous electrical modulation pain reprocessing [TEMPR/scrambler therapy], use 0278T)◀

A parenthetical note has been placed following code 97032 to direct users to the appropriate code to use to identify transcutaneous electrical modulation pain reprocessing (TEMPR/scrambler therapy). For more information regarding reporting for this type of service, see the rationale following code 0278T.

Therapeutic Procedures

97140 Manual therapy techniques (eg, mobilization/ manipulation, manual lymphatic drainage, manual traction), 1 or more regions, each 15 minutes

▶(Do not report 97140 in conjunction with 29581-29584)◀

 Rationale

In support of the addition of new multi-layer compression procedures, an exclusionary parenthetical note has been added following 97140 precluding the reporting of manual therapeutic techniques code 97140 in conjunction with the application of multilayer compression procedures 29581, 29582, 29583, or 29584.

Special Services, Procedures and Reports

The procedures with code numbers . . .

Code 99091 should be reported no . . .

If the services described by 99091 . . .

Do not report 99091 if it occurs within . . .

▶Codes 99050-99060 are reported in addition to an associated basic service. Do not append modifier 51 to 99050-99060. Typically only a single adjunct code from among 99050-99060 would be reported per patient encounter. However, there may be circumstances in which reporting multiple adjunct codes per patient encounter may be appropriate.◀

Rationale

The Special Services, Procedures and Reports introductory guidelines have been revised to note that modifier 51 should not be appended to the adjunct to basic services codes 99050-99060.

MISCELLANEOUS SERVICES

99000 Handling and/or conveyance of specimen for transfer from the physician's office to a laboratory

99090 Analysis of clinical data stored in computers (eg, ECGs, blood pressures, hematologic data);

▶(For physician/qualified health care professional collection and interpretation of physiologic data stored/transmitted by patient/caregiver, see 99091)◀

⊘=Modifier 51 Exempt ⊙=Moderate Sedation ✚=Add-on Code 𝗡=FDA approval pending

►(Do not report 99090 if other more specific CPT codes exist, eg, 93227, 93272, 0206T for cardiographic services; 95250 for continuous glucose monitoring; 97750 for musculoskeletal function testing)◄

✍ Rationale

The two parenthetical notes following code 99090 have been revised. For consistency with the language in the "Instructions for Use" of the CPT codebook, the first note has been updated to include the term, "qualified." The second parenthetical note following code 99090 was revised to include codes 93272 and 0206T as examples of more specific codes for reporting cardiographic services.

Category II Codes

This section of the CPT codebook has continued its expansion with the addition of 59 new codes, 3 revised codes, and new and revised clinical conditions.

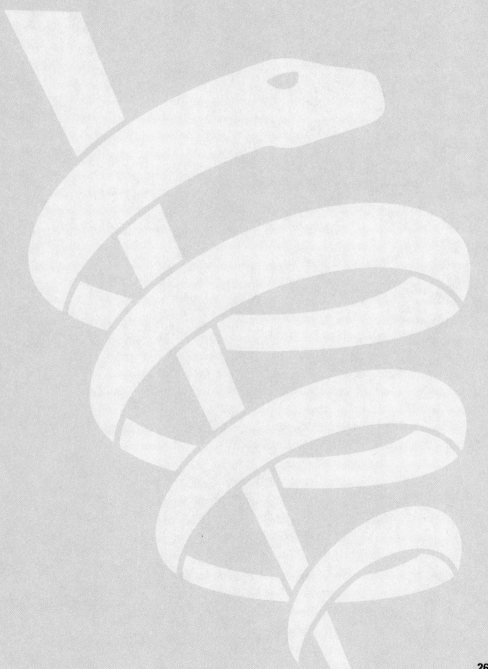

Category II Codes

FOOTNOTES

1. Physician Consortium for Performance Improvement® (PCPI), www.physicianconsortium.org.

2. National Committee on Quality Assurance (NCQA), Health Employer Data Information Set (HEDIS®), www.ncqa.org.

3. Joint Commission on Accreditation of Healthcare Organizations (JCAHO), ORYX Initiative Performance Measures, www.jcaho.org/pms.

4. National Diabetes Quality Improvement Alliance (NDQIA), www.nationaldiabetesalliance.org

5. Joint measure from The Physician Consortium for Performance Improvement, www.physician consortium.org and National Committee on Quality Assurance (NCQA), www.ncqa.org.

6. The Society of Thoracic Surgeons at www.sts.org and National Quality Forum, www.qualityforum.org.

7. Ingenix, www.ingenix.com.

8. American Academy of Neurology, www.aan.com/go/practice/quality/measurements or quality@aan.com.

▶9. College of American Pathologists (CAP), www.cap.org/apps/docs/advocacy/pathology performance measurement.pdf◀

 Rationale

A new measure developer has been included within the footnotes. The College of American Pathologists (CAP) has been added to the listing with appropriate Web information to allow users the ability to locate the actual measures from the developers. In addition, codes that are used within CAP-developed measures include a "9" reference to assist users in locating the full measure information from the CAP Web site.

Composite Codes

0001F   Heart failure assessed (includes assessment of all the following components) (CAD)[1]:

Blood pressure measured (2000F)[1]

Level of activity assessed (1003F)[1]

Clinical symptoms of volume overload (excess) assessed (1004F)[1]

Weight, recorded (2001F)[1]

Clinical signs of volume overload (excess) assessed (2002F)[1]

Rationale

The previous Heart Failure measures listed within the Heart Failure measure set have been replaced with new measures. As a result, code 0001F is no longer used for reporting for the Heart Failure measure set and the "HF" suffix has been removed from the 0001F composite code.

Patient Management

●**0550F**   Cytopathology report on routine nongynecologic specimen finalized within two working days of accession date (PATH)[9]

●**0551F**   Cytopathology report on nongynecologic specimen with documentation that the specimen was non-routine (PATH)[9]

Rationale

Codes 0550F and 0551F are used to report services within the Pathology measure set. Specifically, they are used to identify services for the Turn-Around Time (TAT) for Routine Non-Gynecologic Cytopathology Specimens[9] measure. The measure notes whether a cytopathology report on a routine nongynecologic specimen was finalized within two working days of access to the specimen in the laboratory. Code 0550F is used to report for routine specimens for which the recommended cytopathology report was performed. If the nongynecologic specimen is nonroutine, then the measure notes that the report should note this. Code 0551F is used in this circumstance. Because no performance exclusions have been noted for this measure, modifiers 1P, 2P, and 3P may not be used with this code when reporting for this measure.

●**0555F**   Symptom management plan of care documented (HF)[1]

Rationale

Code 0555F has been included for use within the Heart Failure measure set to note compliance with the Symptom Management measure.[1] This is a replacement measure, as all the previous measures included for Heart Failure have been deleted and replaced by new measures. The new measures are intended to more specifically identify the revisions made for the Heart Failure clinical condition. Code 0555F is one of two codes that note compliance for the Symptom Management measure. This measure is used to determine whether patients aged 18 or older with a diagnosis of heart failure and who have had quantitative results of an evaluation of both level of activity and clinical symptoms documented, either (1) have had symptoms that have improved or have remained consistent with the treatment goals since the last assessment; or (2) if the symptoms have demonstrated clinically important deterioration since the last assessment, that the patient has a symptom plan of care that is documented. Code 0555F is used to identify a documented symptom management plan of care. If the patient's symptoms have shown deterioration (as noted above) and a plan of care is documented for management of the symptoms, then code 1451F is reported in addition to code 0555F, as use of

⊘=Modifier 51 Exempt   ⊙=Moderate Sedation   ✚=Add-on Code   �=FDA approval pending

both codes notes: (1) acknowledgement that action is necessary for the condition; and (2) that the practitioner has taken appropriate action by developing a plan of care for the symptoms.

Reporting for the complete measure requires use of other codes that help to separate the patient population and also note the type of test that was used for the symptoms evaluation. Codes 3115F, 3118F, and 3117F identify various acceptable methods that may be used for symptom evaluation for this measure. If any of these methods are used and there are symptoms present, then either code 1450F should be used (to note that the patient's symptoms have improved or have remained consistent with the treatment goals since the last assessment) or codes 1451F and 0555F should be reported (to note that the symptoms had deteriorated and the health professional has taken appropriate action documenting the plan of care for the symptoms). If no evaluation of the level of activity or clinical symptoms was provided, then code 3119F should be reported. The reporting instructions listed within the measure snapshot included in the Alphabetical Clinical Topics Listing for this measure includes instructions that direct users regarding the appropriate codes to report for each circumstance. In addition, because no performance exclusions have been noted for this measure, modifiers 1P, 2P, and 3P may not be used with this code when reporting for this measure.

●**0556F**   Plan of care to achieve lipid control documented (CAD)[1]

●**0557F**   Plan of care to manage anginal symptoms documented (CAD)[1]

Rationale

Codes 0556F and 0557F are both used within separate measures in the Chronic Stable Coronary Artery Disease (CAD) measure set. The CAD measure set is one of a number of measure sets that have been completely revised via deletion of the existing measures and addition of new measures. The new measures, developed by the Physician Consortium for Performance Improvement [PCPI], were included to address the need for updates for these measures. Both codes are used to identify compliance within the respective measures by noting that plans of care have been documented according to the measures requirements.

Code 0556F is used within the Lipid Control[1] measure. This measure identifies whether the patient aged 18 years and older who has a diagnosis of CAD has an low density LDL-C result of less than 100 mg/dL, or, for those patients whose LDL-C is greater than or equal to 100 mg/dL, has a plan of care documented with the inclusion of a prescription of statin (at a minimum). The plan and prescription should have a goal of achieving an LDL-C that is less than 100 mg/dL. A number of codes have been included within the measure snapshot within the Alphabetical Listing to help identify factors that are important for reporting for this measure. This includes: (1) use of code 3048F to identify the most recent LDL-C is less than 100 mg/dL; (2) use of codes 3049F and 3050F to identify most recent LDL-Cs of 100-129 mg/dL (3049F) or an LDL-C that is equal to or greater than 130 mg/dL (3050F); and (3) that statin therapy is either being prescribed by the examining physician or is already being taken by the patient (ie, prescribed by another appropriate health care professional). The measure snapshot notes that exclusions are included for this measure, indicating that medical, patient, and system reasons exist for not prescribing statin to CAD patients who do not meet the appropriate LDL-C criteria for this measure. In addition, reporting instructions included within the Alphabetical Listing provide details regarding appropriate use of these codes and the 1P, 2P, and 3P modifiers (the instructions note that the 1P, 2P, and 3P modifiers may be used for performance exclusions for code 4013F [that is, when statin therapy is not prescribed for the patient]).

Code 0557F is used within the Symptom Management measure. This measure identifies whether the patient aged 18 years and older who has a diagnosis of CAD is receiving appropriate management of their angina symptoms. The measure snapshot includes information that directs users to the measure developer's Web site for a definition of "appropriate management." In addition to this code, there are other codes included for reporting for this measure that are used to separate the patient population. Code 1010F is used to identify assessment of angina according to the level of activity. Codes 1011F and 1012F are used to identify presence (1011F) or absence (1012F) of angina. The measure snapshot notes that exclusions are included for this measure, indicating that medical, patient, and system reasons exist for not managing angina symptoms. In addition, reporting instructions included within the Alphabetical Listing provide details regarding appropriate use of these codes and the 1P, 2P, and 3P modifiers. (The instructions note that the 1P, 2P, and 3P modifiers may be used for performance exclusions for code 0557F.) These instructions also direct users to report this measure with the Symptom and Activity Assessment measure because the two measures are not intended to be reported independently.

The Symptom and Activity Assessment measure is used to determine whether a patient aged 18 years or older with a diagnosis of CAD has results of an evaluation of level of activity and results of evaluation of anginal symptoms documented in the medical record. This measure also uses codes 1010F-1012F. However, because no performance exclusions have been noted for this measure, modifiers 1P, 2P, and 3P may not be used with this code when reporting for this measure.

Patient History

1003F   Level of activity assessed (NMA No Measure Associated)

✍ Rationale

Due to the deletion of a number of existing measures and their replacement by updated measures, a number of codes that were previously listed within the Category II codes set are no longer associated with current measures. Because these codes have been developed for use in future measures, the codes that are no longer associated with a specific measure are now included in the CPT code set as "NMA–No Measure Associated." The code and its descriptor are retained but are now listed with a suffix that notes that these codes are not associated with a measure that is included within the CPT code set (as part of the Alphabetical Clinical

Topics Listing). Because the suffix is not considered part of the code descriptor, the codes are not listed with the "▲" symbol. A notation for the change in the intended use of the code is documented, however, within the CPT code set listings. This allows users the ability to note the change in status for these codes.

●**1010F**   Severity of angina assessed by level of activity (CAD)[1]

●**1011F**   Angina present (CAD)[1]

●**1012F**   Angina absent (CAD)[1]

✍ Rationale

Codes 1010F, 1011F, and 1012F are used in two separate measures that are intended to be reported in conjunction with each other. The Symptom and Activity Assessment includes use of these codes to: (1) determine if a severity of angina is assessed (using level of activity as the criteria for the assessment); and (2) note if angina is either present (1011F) or absent (1012F). These codes are used in a similar manner for the Symptom Management measure; however, the measure goes a step further by including a code that notes the treatment that should be provided in response to the results. To find more information regarding the intended use for these codes, see the rationale for code 0557F.

●**1031F**   Smoking status and exposure to second hand smoke in the home assessed (Asthma)[1]

●**1032F**   Current tobacco smoker OR currently exposed to secondhand smoke (Asthma)[1]

●**1033F**   Current tobacco non-smoker AND not currently exposed to secondhand smoke (Asthma)[1]

✍ Rationale

Codes 1031F, 1032F, and 1033F are used in separate measures included in the Asthma measure set. Code 1031F is used within the Tobacco Use: Screening measure, and codes 1032F and 1033F are used within the Tobacco Use – Intervention measure. These codes are included as part of a new set of measures that have been included for use for the Asthma measure set as the previously existing measure has been replaced. The codes included for these measures serve different purposes within each of the noted measures.

Code 1031F identifies compliance for the Tobacco Use: Screening measure. This measure notes whether the patient aged 5 through 50 years old (or caregiver) with a diagnosis of asthma was queried about tobacco use and exposure to second-hand smoke in his or her home environment. In this particular measure, the use of the code is straightforward: code 1031F is reported for each patient whose smoking status and exposure to second-hand smoke in the home was assessed (as is noted within the code's descriptor). The reporting instructions include directions that make the intent for use of this code clear. Because no performance exclusions have been noted for this measure, modifiers 1P, 2P, and 3P may not be used with this code when reporting for this measure.

Codes 1032F and 1033F are used within the Tobacco Use – Intervention measure. They are used to separate the patient population because the measure is used to determine whether the patient aged 5 through 50 years with a diagnosis of asthma and identified as a tobacco user is receiving tobacco cessation intervention during the measurement period. Code 1033F is used to identify individuals who are current tobacco nonsmokers and are not currently exposed to second-hand smoke (Note: both criteria must be met to use this code). Code 1032F is used to identify either type of patient: those who smoke or those who are exposed to second-hand smoke. If the patient is a smoker or is exposed to smoke, then the measure specifies that the patient should be receiving cessation intervention (using code 4000F to identify counseling intervention and code 4001F for pharmacologic therapy intervention). This measure includes information that further assists users in identifying the targeted population by providing a definition of those considered to be "tobacco users" (ie, patients who currently use tobacco as well as patients who do not currently use tobacco, but are exposed to second-hand smoke in their home environment). Because this measure deals with asthma patients who smoke or who co-habitate with smokers (and are therefore, exposed to second-hand smoking), the measure includes instructions that direct users regarding all options for compliance. As a result, a note has been included within the Alphabetical Clinical Topics Listing snapshot that instructs users that "Practitioners providing tobacco cessation interventions to a pediatric patient's primary caregiver are still numerator compliant whether the primary caregiver is the source of second-hand smoke in the home." In addition, the reporting instructions included within the Alphabetical Listing directs users regarding the appropriate use for these codes, noting use of either code 1032F or 1033F to identify the smoking status and use of either code 4000F or 4001F to identify the type of cessation intervention provided for the patient (or caregiver). In addition, because no performance exclusions have been noted for this measure, modifiers 1P, 2P, and 3P may not be used with this code when reporting for this measure.

The tobacco measure for asthma has been intentionally redeveloped to address this additional issue regarding smoking because this habit does not only affect the smoker but also any household members with conditions that increase their vulnerability to smoking (asthma). As a result, this measure is intended to assist health professionals in addressing causes of asthma symptoms that are related to smoking. By addressing both the asthma patient who smokes and the caregiver of an asthma patient who is exposed to smokers or second-hand smoke, the chances are increased that the smoker may cease his or her behavior (because the caregiver has access to the smoker to note the concerns and detrimental results of their behavior).

1123F Advance Care Planning discussed and documented advance care plan or surrogate decision maker documented in the medical record (DEM)[1] (GER, Pall Cr)[5]

1124F Advance Care Planning discussed and documented in the medical record, patient did not wish or was not able to name a surrogate decision maker or provide an advance care plan (DEM)1 (GER, Pall Cr)[5]

⊘=Modifier 51 Exempt   ⊙=Moderate Sedation   ✚=Add-on Code   ✚=FDA approval pending

✍️ Rationale

Codes 1123F and 1124F are both used to report services for the Dementia measure set. They are existing Category II codes that are now used within the Palliative Care Counseling and Advance Care Planning[5] measure to note whether the patient with a diagnosis of dementia (or their caregiver), regardless of age, either (1) received comprehensive counseling regarding ongoing palliation and symptom management and end-of-life decisions for the condition and has an advance care plan or surrogate decision maker in the medical record or (2) that documentation exists in the medical record that the patient did not wish or was not able to name a surrogate decision maker or provide an advance care plan within two years of initial diagnosis or assumption of care. Codes 1123F and 1124F are used to note compliance for the measure, indicating that: (1) the advance care plan was discussed with the patient or caregiver; and (2) either an advance care plan or surrogate decision maker was documented in the record (specified by code 1123F), or the patient did not wish or was not able to name a surrogate decision maker or provide an advanced care plan (identified by the use of code 1124F). When a plan of care is made, an additional code is intended to be used within the measure. Code 4350F is reported if the patient has received ongoing counseling regarding palliation and symptom management. The measure snapshot also includes a definition of what is considered "Comprehensive counseling regarding end-of-life decisions" noting that it ". . . includes a discussion of the risks and benefits of various medical interventions to address the major clinical issues associated with advanced dementia." Because no performance exclusions have been noted for this measure, modifiers 1P, 2P, and 3P may not be used with this code when reporting for this measure. Additional instructions included in the reporting instructions provided information regarding intended use of code 4350F.

○**1127F** New episode for condition (NMA-No Measure Associated)

○**1128F** Subsequent episode for condition (NMA-No Measure Associated)

✍️ Rationale

Codes 1127F and 1128F have been reinstated as "NMA-No Measure Associated" codes. Originally deleted from the Melanoma Coordination of Care measure (within the Melanoma measure set), these codes have been reinstated for future use with other measures.

●**1175F** Functional status for dementia assessed and results reviewed (DEM)[1]

●**1181F** Neuropsychiatric symptoms assessed and results reviewed (DEM)[1]

●**1182F** Neuropsychiatric symptoms, one or more present (DEM)[1]

●**1183F** Neuropsychiatric symptoms, absent (DEM)[1]

✍ Rationale

Codes 1175F, 1181F, 1182F, and 1183F are all included for use with the Dementia measure set. For more information regarding intent for use of these codes within the Dementia measure set, see the rationale for code 1490F.

● **1450F**   Symptoms improved or remained consistent with treatment goals since last assessment (HF)[1]

● **1451F**   Symptoms demonstrated clinically important deterioration since last assessment (HF)[1]

✍ Rationale

Codes 1450F and 1451F are used to identify compliance for the Symptoms Management measure within the Heart Failure measure set. They are used to identify that symptoms have improved or have remained consistent with treatment goals since the last assessment (1450F) or that the symptoms demonstrate clinically important deterioration since the last assessment was provided (1451F). For more information regarding use of codes 1450F and 1451F within the Symptoms Management measure, see the rationale included for code 0555F.

● **1460F**   Qualifying cardiac event/diagnosis in previous 12 months (CAD)[1]

● **1461F**   No qualifying cardiac event/diagnosis in previous 12 months (CAD)[1]

✍ Rationale

Codes 1460F and 1461F are used within the Cardiac Rehabilitation Patient Referral From an Outpatient Setting measure, which is a measure included within the Chronic Stable Coronary Artery Disease measure set. This measure notes whether a patient aged 18 years and older with a qualifying event or diagnosis of CAD was referred to an outpatient cardiac rehabilitation program (or if they have already participated in an outpatient cardiac rehabilitation program). For this measure, these codes are used to separate the patient population according to whether the patient has had a qualifying cardiac event within the last 12 months. For those patients who have had a qualifying event (identified by the use of code 1460F), either code 4500F or 4510F is used to identify compliance for the measure. Code 4500F indicates that the patient was referred to an outpatient cardiac rehabilitation program, while code 4510F is used to note that a previous cardiac rehabilitation has already been completed for a qualifying event. To assist users in identifying the correct patient population, a note has also been included within the Alphabetical Listing's snapshot directing users to "See [the] ICD-9-CM diagnosis codes and CPT® procedure codes in the measure specifications that define 'qualifying event diagnosis.'" There are also medical, patient, and system exclusions for this measure. As a result, the reporting instructions note provide users with directions to use modifier 1P, 2P, or 3P for qualifying performance exclusions for this measure. In addition, instructions are also provided that guide users to the appropriate method to report these codes when compliance is achieved for this measure, noting the use of code 1460F or 1461F to indicate the presence or absence of a qualifying cardiac event or diagnosis.

⊘=Modifier 51 Exempt   ⊙=Moderate Sedation   ✚=Add-on Code   ⋏=FDA approval pending

●**1490F**   Dementia severity classified, mild (DEM)[1]

●**1491F**   Dementia severity classified, moderate (DEM)[1]

●**1493F**   Dementia severity classified, severe (DEM)[1]

●**1494F**   Cognition assessed and reviewed (DEM)[1]

✎ Rationale

The Dementia measure set is a new clinical topic that has been added to the Category II codes within the CPT code set. This measure set includes a number of different measures that are intended for report for patients with dementia. As is true for other measures included for report, each measure within the dementia measure set is unique and has a specific set of instructions and codes to note compliance.

Codes 1490F, 1491F, and 1493F are all used within the Staging for Dementia[1] measure. The measure notes whether the patient, regardless of age, with a diagnosis of dementia had severity of dementia classified as mild, moderate, or severe at least once within a 12-month period. To ensure that users are familiar with the differences in the levels of dementia, additional information has been included within the Alphabetical Listing measure snapshot directing users to the measure specifications for definitions of "mild," "moderate," and "severe" dementia. In addition, the codes were specifically designed to be particular to each level, allowing use of a separate code according to the level of dementia that is present. Reporting instructions have been provided that direct use of these codes in this manner. In addition, because no performance exclusions have been noted for this measure, modifiers 1P, 2P, and 3P may not be used with this code when reporting for this measure.

Code 1494F is used to note compliance for the Cognitive Assessment[1] measure. This measure notes whether the dementia patient, regardless of age, had an assessment of cognition performed and a review of results at least once within a 12-month period. The measure is intended to allow for medical and patient exclusions. As a result, the reporting instructions note that use of modifiers 1P and 2P are allowed for report for this measure. However, there are no systems exclusions allowed for this measure, and the instructions note that modifier 3P is not allowed for use within this measure.

Code 1175F is used within the Functional Status Assessment[1] measure of the Dementia[1] measure set. This measure notes whether the patient with a diagnosis of dementia, regardless of age, had an assessment of functional status performed and the results reviewed at least once within a 12-month period. This code is specified for use for functional status for dementia only (do **not** use code 1170F for dementia). To assist users regarding compliance for this measure, instruction regarding what is included as part of functional status assessment has been included within the Alphabetical Listing for this measure. The additional instructions provide information regarding: (1) from whom this information may be obtained (ie, direct examination of the patient or a knowledgeable informant); (2) what the assessment should include (ie, an evaluation of the patient's ability to perform instrumental activities of daily living and basic activities of daily living [at minimum]); and (3) additional instruments that may be used to identify functional status (which may include instruments available from medical literature such as the Barthel ADL Index and the Katz Index of Independence in ADL). Because only medical performance exclusions exist for report for this measure, the reporting instructions direct that only modifier 1P may be used for exclusions reporting for this measure.

Code 1181F is used to report compliance for the Neuropsychiatric Symptom Assessment[1] measure. It is the only code included for use for this measure and is used to note whether the dementia patient, regardless of age, had an assessment of neuropsychiatric symptoms performed and results reviewed at least once in a 12-month period. Added instructions have been included within the Alphabetical Listing for this measure noting that "Neuropsychiatric symptoms can be assessed by direct examination of the patient or knowledgeable informant." There is also an instruction, which notes that this measure has to be reported with the Management of Neuropsychiatric Symptoms measure. Because no performance exclusions have been noted for this measure, modifiers 1P, 2P, and 3P may not be used with this code when reporting for this measure.

Codes 1182F and 1183F are both used to differentiate patients who have neuropsychiatric symptoms from those who don't for the Management of Neuropsychiatric Symptoms[1] measure. This measure notes whether the dementia patient, regardless of age, received or was recommended to receive an intervention for neuropsychiatric symptoms within a 12-month period. As was previously noted, this measure is intended to be reported in conjunction with the Neuropsychiatric Symptom Assessment measure. Therefore, both measures should be reported together: (1) to identify assessment of the neuropsychiatric symptoms and review of results; (2) to identify the appropriate patient population (which is done through use of code 1182F to note presence of neuropsychiatric symptoms or by use of code 1183F to identify an absence of symptoms); and (3) to identify the order of neuropsychiatric intervention (4525F) or that this service has already been received by the patient (4526F). The reporting instructions included for this measure direct users regarding the intent of use for both measures, ie, that these measures are required to be used in conjunction with each other. The instructions also indicate the appropriate reporting of codes 4525F and 4526F to note compliance. Because no performance exclusions have been noted for this measure, modifiers 1P, 2P, and 3P may not be used with this code when reporting for this measure.

Physical Examination

2000F   Blood pressure measured (CKD)1(DM)[2,4]

2001F   Weight recorded (PAG)[1]

⊘=Modifier 51 Exempt   ⊙=Moderate Sedation   ✚=Add-on Code   ⊮=FDA approval pending

Rationale

Codes 2000F and 2001F have both been removed from measure sets that were revised to more accurately reflect current medical practice. Because the Chronic Stable Coronary Artery Disease, Heart Failure, and Hypertension measures have all been completely revised by deletion of the old measure information and inclusion of new information, these codes have been removed from use for these measures. Code 2000F is now reported with the Chronic Kidney Disease and Diabetes Mellitus measures, and code 2001F is intended for reporting measures included for the Pediatric Acute Gastroenteritis measure. Additional information is included within the Alphabetical Clinical Topics Listing for these measures on the AMA Web site at www.ama-assn.org/go/cpt.

●**2015F** Asthma impairment assessed (Asthma)[1]

●**2016F** Asthma risk assessed (Asthma)[1]

Rationale

Codes 2015F and 2016F are both used to identify compliance for the Asthma measure set. They are included as part of different measures (code 2016F is used within two measures) within the newly revised asthma measures.

Code 2015F is used within a single measure: Assessment of Asthma Control. This measure notes whether the patient aged 5 through 50 years with a diagnosis of asthma was evaluated at least once for asthma control. Unlike other measures that include codes that note compliance, this measure requires that *both* codes be reported to identify compliance for this measure. This is because the numerator—that is, the patient population for whom the designated action has been performed—notes that the desire is to obtain patients who were evaluated for asthma *control*. To assist users with this intent, instruction has been provided that defines what is meant by asthma control, which notes that it includes: (1) documentation of an evaluation of asthma impairment; *and* (2) documentation of asthma risk. Each of these factors is also defined, noting that asthma impairment must include daytime symptoms *and* nighttime awakenings *and* interference with normal activity *and* short-acting beta$_2$-agonist use for symptom control. It is also noted that documentation of asthma risk must include the number of asthma exacerbations requiring oral systemic corticosteroids in the prior 12 months. Completion of a validated questionnaire is also considered appropriate compliance with assessing asthma impairment. Because of the need that both requirements be met, the reporting instructions for this measure include instructions to indicate that both codes 2015F and 2016F should be reported to note compliance for this measure. Users are also instructed that assessment of both impairment and risk should be done during the same encounter to comply with the measures' requirements. Because no performance exclusions have been noted for this measure, modifiers 1P, 2P, and 3P may not be used with this code when reporting for this measure.

Code 2016F is also reported independently within the Assessment of Asthma Risk measure and is used to note compliance for this measure. The measure notes whether the patient aged 5 through 50 years with a diagnosis of asthma exacerbation was evaluated for the number of asthma exacerbations that required oral systemic corticosteroids (asthma risk). Similar to the Assessment of Asthma Control measure, this measure includes a definition for *asthma risk* as well as reporting instructions to direct users regarding the specific and expected environments and circumstances in which this code is to be reported (ie, all emergency department and inpatient admission encounters for patients with a diagnosis of acute asthma exacerbation). Because no performance exclusions have been noted for this measure, modifiers 1P, 2P, and 3P may not be used with this code when reporting for this measure.

Diagnostic/Screening Processes or Results

●3019F   Left ventricular ejection fraction (LVEF) assessment planned post discharge (HF)[1]

✍ Rationale

Codes 3019F, 3115F, 3118F, 3117F, 3119F, 3055F, and 3056F have all been developed for use for reporting measures included within the new Heart Failure measure set. These codes serve different purposes within different measures and include instructions with each measure that identifies the intended use for each of these codes.

Code 3019F is included for use within the Left Ventricular Ejection Fraction (LVEF) Assessment (Inpatient)[1] measure. This measure notes whether the patient aged 18 years and older with a principal diagnosis of heart failure has a result of LVEF assessment available in hospital medical record or LVEF assessment planned after discharge. If results for an LVEF are obtained, then either code 3021F or 3022F is reported to identify and note if the results have an ejection fraction that is less than 40% (or documented as moderately or severely depressed) or an ejection fraction that is equal to or greater than 40% (or noted as normal or mildly depressed). The reporting instructions included in the Alphabetical Listing for this measure direct users to report this measure for every hospitalization. Additional instructions are also provided, specifying report of code 3021F or 3022F to note the presence of an LVEF result. In addition, the instructions direct users to report code 3019F if an LVEF is planned for after the patient is discharged from the hospital. Because medical exclusions exist for this measure (eg, if the patient expires), modifier 1P may be reported with code 3019F to note the exclusion.

Codes 3115F, 3118F, and 3117F are used to identify acceptable methods that may be used for symptom evaluation for the Symptoms Management measure for the Heart Failure measure set. These codes separate patient population to determine if additional services are needed. Code 3119F is used to identify that no evaluation of the level of activity or clinical symptoms was provided. Codes 3115F, 3118F, and 3117F are intended to be reported with other codes that note whether the symptoms have improved, remained stable, or have deteriorated and require additional action. For more information regarding the intended use of these codes within the Symptoms Management measure, see the rationale included for code 0556F.

⃠=Modifier 51 Exempt   ⊙=Moderate Sedation   ✚=Add-on Code   ⁄=FDA approval pending

Codes 3055F and 3056F are used within the Counseling Regarding Implantable Cardioverter-Defibrillator (ICD) Implantation for Patients with Left Ventricular Systolic Dysfunction on Combination Medical Therapy[1] measure to separate the patient population according to patients who have an LVEF that is less than or equal to 35% and those who have an LVEF that is greater than 35% or do not have an LVEF result available. Two other codes, 4480F and 4481F, are also included for use for this measure to help separate the patient population. These codes are used to identify patients who have been receiving ACE/ARB therapy or a beta-blocker for at least three months (4480F) and those who have been receiving these medications for less than three months (4481F). Because this measure notes whether the patient with a diagnosis of heart failure with a current LVEF of less than or equal to 35% despite ACE/ARB therapy and beta-blocker therapy for three months was counseled regarding implantable cardioverter-defibrillator (ICD) implantation as a treatment option for the prophylaxis of sudden death, each of these codes are used to differentiate the patient population according to whether the patient falls within the ". . . less than or equal to 35% LVEF" population; and if so, whether the patient has been receiving ACE/ARB therapy or a beta-blocker for at least three months. If the patient has not received the indicated medication for at least this amount of time, there is a possibility that the medication may still have an effect on improving the patient's condition without the need for further intervention. If the patient has an LVEF that falls below the 35% threshold and has been receiving these medications for at least three months, then additional intervention is indicated, and the patient should receive counseling regarding the need for use of an ICD to alleviate the symptoms and improve the condition of the patient (**Note:** This counseling is identified by reporting code 4470F). The reporting instructions provided for this measure within the Alphabetical Clinical Topics Listing direct users regarding the appropriate codes to report for each circumstance that exists for the patient with regards to this measure. In addition, medical exclusions exist for this measure. Therefore, only modifier 1P may be reported for performance exclusions that exist for this measure. Modifiers 2P and 3P may not be used.

3048F Most recent LDL-C less than 100 mg/dL (CAD)[1] (DM)[4]

3049F Most recent LDL-C 100-129 mg/dL (CAD)[1] (DM)[4]

3050F Most recent LDL-C greater than or equal to 130 mg/dL (CAD)[1] (DM)[4]

🖎 Rationale

Codes 3048F, 3049F, and 3050F are all existing codes that are being used within the replacement Chronic Stable Coronary Artery Disease[1] measures. These codes are used to differentiate the LDL-C levels for the Lipid Control measure. For more information regarding how these codes are intended to be used for this measure, see the rationale for code 0556F.

●**3055F** Left ventricular ejection fraction (LVEF) less than or equal to 35% (HF)[1]

●**3056F** Left ventricular ejection fraction (LVEF) greater than 35% or no LVEF result available (HF)[1]

✐ Rationale

Codes 3055F and 3056F are used to report measures within the new Heart Failure measure set. These codes identify thresholds for left ventricular ejection fraction. For more information regarding the intended use of these codes, see the rationale for code 3019F.

3074F   Most recent systolic blood pressure less than 130 mm Hg (DM)2,4 (HTN, CKD, CAD)[1]

3075F   Most recent systolic blood pressure 130 - 139 mm Hg (DM)2,4 (HTN, CKD, CAD)[1]

3077F   Most recent systolic blood pressure greater than or equal to 140 mm Hg (HTN, CKD, CAD)1 (DM) [2,4]

3078F   Most recent diastolic blood pressure less than 80 mm Hg (HTN, CKD, CAD)1 (DM) [2,4]

3079F   Most recent diastolic blood pressure 80-89 mm Hg (HTN, CKD, CAD)1 (DM) [2,4]

3080F   Most recent diastolic blood pressure greater than or equal to 90 mm Hg (HTN, CKD, CAD)1 (DM) [2,4]

✐ Rationale

Codes 3074F, 3075F, 3077F, 3078F, 3079F, and 3080F are all existing codes that are being used within the replacement Chronic Stable Coronary Artery Disease (CAD) measures and the Hypertension measure. These codes are used within identical measures within these measures sets, and therefore, serve the exact same purpose for these measures. The measure Blood Pressure Control[1] is used to determine whether a patient aged 18 years and older with a diagnosis of CAD has a blood pressure lower than 140/90 or has a blood pressure greater than or equal to 140/90 and is prescribed two or more antihypertensive agents during the most recent office visit. The codes are intended to be used to differentiate various blood pressures (both systolic and diastolic) for the measure, which utilize a threshold systolic and diastolic pressure (systolic pressure of 140mm Hg or more, identified by code 3077F; with a diastolic pressure of 90mm Hg or more, identified by code 3080F) to note whether treatment needs to be provided for the patient. Code 4145F is used to identify compliance for the measure, indicating that two or more antihypertensive agents have been prescribed or are currently being taken. The measure numerator information identifies that compliance for this measure may be obtained either by: (1) patients who exhibit a blood pressure of less than 140/90 mm Hg; or (2) by patients who have a blood pressure that is 140/90 mm Hg or higher, who are prescribed two or more antihypertensive agents or are currently on the same. The reporting instructions included for this measure includes information to note when each of these codes should be reported. In addition, because medical, patient, and system reasons exist for this measure as used in both measure sets, modifiers 1P, 2P, and 3P are appropriate for use with this measure when reporting for either measure set.

▲**3111F**   CT or MRI of the brain performed in the hospital within 24 hours of arrival OR performed in an outpatient imaging center, to confirm initial diagnosis of stroke, TIA or intracranial hemorrhage (STR)[6]

⊘=Modifier 51 Exempt   ⊙=Moderate Sedation   ✚=Add-on Code   𝒩=FDA approval pending

▲3112F CT or MRI of the brain performed greater than 24 hours after arrival to the hospital OR performed in an outpatient imaging center for purpose other than confirmation of initial diagnosis of stroke, TIA, or intracranial hemorrhage (STR)[5]

 Rationale

Codes 3111F and 3112F have been editorially revised to include language that further specifies the intended use for these codes, adding the term *intracranial* to the descriptor for each code. The measures for which these codes are intended to be used have not changed for 2012. Instead, the included change refers more specifically to the circumstances in which these codes are intended to be used.

●3115F Quantitative results of an evaluation of current level of activity and clinical symptoms (HF)[1]

●3117F Heart Failure disease specific structured assessment tool completed (HF)[1]

●3118F New York Heart Association (NYHA) Class documented (HF)[1]

●3119F No Evaluation of level of activity or clinical symptoms (HF)[1]

Rationale

Codes 3115F, 3117F, 3118F, and 3119F are all included for use in reporting as part of the new Heart Failure measure set. For more information regarding intended use for these codes, see the rationale included for report of code 3019F.

●3125F Esophageal biopsy report with statement about dysplasia (present, absent, or indefinite) (PATH)[9]

●3267F Pathology report includes pT category, pN category, Gleason score, and statement about margin status (PATH)[9]

●3394F Quantitative HER2 immunohistochemistry (IHC) evaluation of breast cancer consistent with the scoring system defined in the ASCO/CAP guidelines (PATH)[9]

●3395F Quantitative non-HER2 immunohistochemistry (IHC) evaluation of breast cancer (eg, testing for estrogen or progesterone receptors [ER/PR]) performed (PATH)[9]

Rationale

Codes 3125F, 3267F, 3394F, and 3395F are all used within the Pathology Measure set. They are included as part of three different measures within the set and note distinct services for each of the measures in which they are reported.

Code 3125F is used within an esophageal biopsy measure titled "Esophageal Biopsies with a Diagnosis of Barrett's Esophagus that also include a Statement on Dysplasia." The measure notes whether an esophageal biopsy report that documents the presence of Barrett's mucosa includes a statement about dysplasia. As a result, code 3125F includes descriptor language that notes this and includes information regarding what should be noted regarding the dysplasia (if it is present, absent, or if the finding is indefinite). The measure specifies that medical exclusions exist (eg, the absence of intestinal metaplasia or the existence of a malignant neoplasm, both of which eliminates the need for documenting a statement regarding dysplasia). As a result, instructions have been included in the Alphabetical

Clinical Topics Listing directing users to report modifier 1P with code 3125F to note the exclusion.

Code 3267F is used within the Pathology measure set to identify items of importance regarding the pathology report as well. Its use for the Radical Prostatectomy Report includes the pT Category, the pN Category, Gleason Score, and a Statement about Margin Status measure, and is used to identify whether a radical prostatectomy pathology report includes the pT category, the pN category, the Gleason score, and a statement about margin status. The measure allows for medical exclusions, and as a result, modifier 1P may be appended to this code to identify medical exclusions that exist for the patient.

Codes 3394F and 3395F are both used within the Quantitative HER2 Evaluation by Immunohistochemistry (IHC) measure, which notes whether a quantitative HER2 Immunohistochemistry (IHC) evaluation was consistent with the scoring system defined in the ASCO/CAP guidelines. The codes are intended to differentiate Quantitative HER2 IHC evaluation (3394F) from Quantitative non-HER2 IHC evaluations of breast cancer. Because there are specific parameters that are defined by the American Society of Clinical Oncology (ASCO) and the College of American Pathologists, use of code 3394F identifies compliance with the guidelines identified by these organizations. Code 3395F identifies non-HER2 IHC breast cancer evaluation provided by other means, such as testing for estrogen or progesterone receptors.

●**3725F**   Screening for depression performed (DEM)[1]

 Rationale

Codes 3725F is used to report compliance for the Screening for Depressive Symptoms measure in the Dementia measure set. This measure notes whether the dementia patient, regardless of age, was screened for depressive symptoms within a 12-month period. It is the only code used to report this measure. As a result, the language in the code descriptor is straightforward, noting that this code is for "screening for depression performed," which is similar to the wording of the measure title. Because no performance exclusions have been noted for this measure, modifiers 1P, 2P, and 3P may not be used with this code when reporting for this measure. This information is noted in the reporting instructions listed with the snapshot of the Alphabetical Listing.

Therapeutic, Preventive, or Other Interventions

4000F   Tobacco use cessation intervention, counseling (COPD, CAP, CAD, Asthma)[1](DM)[4](PV)[2]

4001F   Tobacco use cessation intervention, pharmacologic therapy (COPD, CAD, CAP, PV, Asthma)[1] (DM)4(PV)[2]

 Rationale

Codes 4000F and 4001F have been added to the Asthma measure set. These codes have been included to address issues regarding smoking cessation for asthma patients who smoke and those who are exposed to second-hand smoke. They are used to note compliance for the Tobacco Use – Intervention measure. For more information regarding the intended use of these codes within this measure, see the rationale included for codes 1031F, 1032F, and 1033F.

▶(4002F has been deleted. To report statin therapy, use 4013F)◀

✍ Rationale

Codes 4002F has been replaced by code 4013F. For more information regarding intended use of code 4013F for reporting statin therapy, see the rationale for this code.

▲**4004F**   Patient screened for tobacco use AND received tobacco cessation intervention (counseling, pharmacotherapy, or both), if identified as a tobacco user (PV, CAD)[1]

✍ Rationale

Code 4004F has been editorially revised to include language that reflects the intended use of this code in its previous listing within the Preventive Care measure set and the new **Tobacco Use:** Screening and Cessation Intervention[1] measure included in the Chronic Stable Coronary Artery Disease measure set. The language within the code descriptor was editorially revised to reflect that intervention includes counseling, pharmacotherapy, or both, for patients who have been screened for tobacco use and identified as tobacco users. This measure cites use of another code to note measurement compliance. Because this code is intended to be used for all patients aged 18 years and older who have a diagnosis of coronary heart disease, code 1036F is used to identify those patients who are **not** smokers and to separate them from the patients who should receive treatment (and for whom this measure was developed). As is noted in the numerator, the intent is that both the screening and intervention occur for those patients identified as tobacco users, which (as noted before) may include counseling and/or pharmacotherapy. Because no performance exclusions have been noted for this measure, modifiers 1P, 2P, and 3P may not be used with this code when reporting for this measure.

▶(4006F has been deleted. To report beta blocker therapy, use 4008F.)◀

✍ Rationale

Code 4006F has been removed from use for the Heart Failure and Chronic Stable Coronary Artery Disease measure sets. Because this code is not included as part of any other measure set, and because 4008F has been developed to replace this code to identify the intended use for reporting this measure, code 4006F has been deleted from the CPT code set. This includes deletion from the Category II code section listing, as well as removal from the measures included for the CAD and HF measure sets within the Alphabetical Clinical Topics Listing document.

(4007F has been deleted. To report age related eye disease study (AREDS) formulation prescribed or recommended, use code 4177F)

●**4008F**   Beta blocker therapy prescribed or currently being taken (CAD,HF)[1]

✐ Rationale

Codes 4008F, 4010F, and 4450F are each used within separate measures of the Heart Failure measure set. Each code serves to identify compliance for its respective measure. However, the correct method for reporting each code differs according to the measure in which it is intended to be used.

Code 4450F is intended to note compliance for the Patient Self-Care Education[1], measure of the Heart Failure measure set. It is the only code used to report this measure, which notes whether the patient aged 18 and older with a diagnosis of heart failure was provided self-care education on three or more elements of education. The measure does not allow for performance exclusions. As a result, modifiers 1P, 2P, and 3P may not be used to report performance exclusions for this measure.

Code 4008F is intended to report compliance for the Beta-Blocker Therapy for Left Ventricular Systolic Dysfunction (Outpatient and Inpatient Setting)[1] measure. This measure is intended to be paired for reporting with the Angiotensin-Converting Enzyme (ACE) Inhibitor or Angiotensin Receptor Blocker (ARB) Therapy for Left Ventricular Systolic Dysfunction (Outpatient and Inpatient Setting)[1] measure. The intent is to identify two separate actions that need to be taken for patients who have a left ventricular ejection fraction of less than 40%: (1) to ensure that these patients are on beta-blocker therapy; and (2) to ensure that these patients are also on ACE/ARB therapy (angiotensin converting enzyme/ angiotensin receptor blocker therapy). The intent of the measure is to identify whether the patient aged 18 and older with a diagnosis of heart failure with a current or prior LVEF less than 40% was prescribed beta-blocker therapy. Because this measure is intended to be reported with another measure, as noted above, instructions included in the Alphabetical Listing for this measure direct users in the appropriate reporting method for the use of these codes.

Code 4010F is used to report compliance for the Angiotensin-Converting Enzyme (ACE) Inhibitor or Angiotensin Receptor Blocker (ARB) Therapy for Left Ventricular Systolic Dysfunction (Outpatient and Inpatient Setting)[1] measure. This measure notes whether the patient aged 18 and older with a diagnosis of heart failure with a current or prior LVEF of less than 40% was prescribed an ACE inhibitor or ARB therapy. As was noted for code 4008F, this measure is intended to be reported in conjunction with the Beta-Blocker Therapy for Left Ventricular Systolic Dysfunction (Outpatient and Inpatient Setting)[1] measure. As a result, reporting instructions for this measure are similar to those of the aforementioned measure, ie, the requirement to report the additional measure. As a result, users should consult the measure information listed for both measures to ensure appropriate reporting.

Use of both measures includes the use of modifiers that identify performance exclusions that exist to report these measures. As a result, the reporting

⊘=Modifier 51 Exempt   ⊙=Moderate Sedation   ✚=Add-on Code   ✚=FDA approval pending instructions provide information, which notes that modifiers 1P, 2P, and 3P may be used to identify performance exclusions that exist for the use of these measures.

▶(4009F has been deleted. To report Angiotensin converting enzyme (ACE) inhibitor or angiotensin receptor blocker (ARB) therapy, use 4010F)◀

🖎 Rationale

Code 4009F has been removed from use for the Heart Failure (HF) and Chronic Stable Coronary Artery Disease (CAD) measure sets. As a result, the suffixes that noted use within these measures have been removed. In addition, this code has been removed from the measure included for the CAD and HF measure sets within the Alphabetical Clinical Topics Listing document.

Code 4010F is now included as part of the Chronic Kidney Disease (CKD) and Diabetes Mellitus (DM) measure sets, replacing 4009F.

This code was removed from consideration from the CAD and HF measures sets because code 4010F more appropriately identifies the intended use for these measures. (Ace and ARB therapy should be prescribed or should currently be taken.) See the rationale for code 4010F for more information regarding intended use for this code.

●**4010F** Angiotensin Converting Enzyme (ACE) Inhibitor or Angiotensin Receptor Blocker (ARB) therapy prescribed or currently being taken (CAD, HF)[1]

🖎 Rationale

Code 4010F is used within the Chronic Stable Coronary Artery Disease (CAD) and Heart Failure (HF) measure sets. This code is intended to replace the use of code 4009F within these measure sets as this code is intended be used to identify that angiotensin converting enzyme (ACE) inhibitor or angiotensin receptor blocker (ARB) therapy is being prescribed for the patient or that one of these therapies is currently being taken by the patient. For more information regarding the intended use for code 4010F with the CAD and HF measure sets, see the rationale for code 4008F.

●**4013F** Statin therapy prescribed or currently being taken (CAD)[1]

🖎 Rationale

Code 4013F is a new code that is used within the replacement Chronic Stable Coronary Artery Disease measures. This code is used to note compliance with the Lipid Control measure. For more information regarding how these codes are intended to be used for this measure, see the rationale for code 0556F.

●**4086F** Aspirin or clopidogrel prescribed or currently being taken (CAD)[1]

Rationale

Codes 4086F, 4500F, and 4510F are all used to note compliance for measures included within the Chronic Stable Coronary Artery Disease measure set. Code 4086F is used within the Antiplatelet Therapy measure and codes 4500F and 4510F are used within the Cardiac Rehabilitation Patient Referral From an Outpatient Setting measure. Each of these codes has different circumstances regarding when each of the codes should be used (a factor that is identified by the reporting instructions used for each of the measures).

Code 4086F is the only code that is used for the Antiplatelet Therapy measure. This code notes compliance for this measure, which is used to identify whether the patient aged 18 years and older with a diagnosis of CAD was prescribed aspirin or clopidogrel. The measure allows reporting for performance exclusions, which includes reporting for medical, patient, and system exclusions for this measure. As a result, the reporting instructions included for this measure note that modifiers 1P, 2P, or 3P may be reported for this measure.

Codes 4500F and 4510F are used to identify compliance for the Cardiac Rehabilitation Patient Referral From an Outpatient Setting measure. Code 4500F indicates that the patient was referred to an outpatient cardiac rehabilitation program, while code 4510F is used to note that a previous cardiac rehabilitation has already been completed for a qualifying event. To find more information regarding the intended use for these codes, see the rationale included for codes 1460F and 1461F.

●**4140F**   Inhaled corticosteroids prescribed (Asthma)[1]

●**4144F**   Alternative long-term control medication prescribed (Asthma)[1]

Rationale

Codes 4140F and 4144F are used to report compliance for the Pharmacologic Therapy for Persistent Asthma[1] measure used within the Asthma measure set. The measure notes whether persistent-asthma patient, aged 5 through 50 years old, was prescribed long-term medication. To direct users regarding compliance for this measure, information that notes what is included as part of long-term medication has been added to the listing. This information notes that "Long term medication includes: (1) patients prescribed inhaled corticosteroids (the preferred long-term control medication at any step of asthma pharmacological therapy); or (2) patients prescribed alternative long-term control medications." Users are also directed to the measure specifications to locate the list of preferred and alternative long-term control medications

For this measure, codes 1038F and 1039F are used to identify persistent asthma (1038F) and intermittent asthma (1039F). For patients with persistent asthma that have either an inhaled corticosteroid or alternative long-term control medication prescribed, code 1038F is reported with either code 4140F or 4144F, or both. This information is included in the reporting instructions for the measure, which also provides information regarding the use of modifier 1P or 2P to note performance exclusions that may be reported for this measure.

●**4145F**   Two or more anti-hypertensive agents prescribed or currently being taken (CAD, HTN)[1]

✎ Rationale

Code 4145F is used to note compliance for the Chronic Stable Coronary Artery Disease (CAD) measure set and the Hypertension measure set. This code is used within identical measures within these measures sets and serves the exact same purpose for these measures. The measure Blood Pressure Control[1] is used to determine whether the patient aged 18 years and older with a diagnosis of CAD has a blood pressure lower than 140/90 or has a blood pressure greater than or equal to 140/90, and is prescribed two or more antihypertensive agents during the most recent office visit. For more information regarding the intended use for this code within each measure set, see the rationale included for codes 3074F-3080F.

▶(4275F has been deleted. To report Hepatitis B vaccine injection administered or previously received, use 4149F)◀

✎ Rationale

An editorial revision has been included for code 4149F since the descriptor for this code was made redundant by another code, which was intended to be used for a different measure within a different measure set. As a result, to conform to appropriate CPT Category II convention, code 4275F (formerly listed for use in the HIV measure set) has been deleted and replaced by code 4149F, which now includes a suffix that notes its use for both the HEP C *and* HIV measures sets. To direct users regarding the appropriate codes to use for deleted code 4275F, a parenthetical note has been included to note that Hepatitis B vaccine injection should be reported with code 4149F.

●**4322F**   Caregiver provided with education and referred to additional resources for support (DEM)[1]

●**4350F**   Counseling provided on symptom management, end of life decisions, and palliation (DEM)[1]

✎ Rationale

Code 4350F is used to report services for the Palliative Care Counseling and Advance Care Planning[1] measure within the Dementia measure set. It is one of three codes included to note compliance for this measure. For more information regarding the intended use of this code, see the rationale provided for codes 1123F and 1124F.

Code 4322F is also used with the Dementia measure set. It is used as a singular compliance code for the Caregiver Education and Support[1] measure. This measure notes whether the caregiver for a patient with a diagnosis of dementia, regardless of age, was provided with education on disease management and health behavior changes and referred to additional resources for support within a 12-month period. The measure provides instructions indicating that code 4322F is reported when the caregiver is provided with education *and* referred to additional resources for support (both are required to comply with this measure and to report this code). In addition, the instructions note that medical reasons exist for noncompliance use of this measure (identified by the use of modifier 1P with code 4322F). As a result, modifiers 2P and 3P may not be reported for this measure.

●**4450F**   Self-care education provided to patient (HF)[1]

✐ Rationale

Code 4450F is used to report measure compliance for the Heart Failure measure set. It is used to note compliance for self-care education for the patient. For more information regarding the intended use of code 4450F, see the rationale included for code 4008F.

●**4470F**   Implantable cardioverter-defibrillator (ICD) counseling provided (HF)[1]

●**4480F**   Patient receiving ACE inhibitor/ARB therapy and beta-blocker therapy for 3 months or longer (HF)[1]

●**4481F**   Patient receiving ACE inhibitor/ARB therapy and beta-blocker therapy for less than 3 months or patient not receiving ACE inhibitor/ARB therapy and beta-blocker therapy (HF)[1]

✐ Rationale

Code 4470F is used to note compliance for the Counseling regarding ICD Implantation for Patients with Left Ventricular Systolic Dysfunction on Combination Medical Therapy measure. This measure also uses codes 4480F and 4481F to separate the patient population according to whether the patient has been receiving ACE/ARB therapy or beta-blockers for 3 months. The measure notes whether the patient with a diagnosis of heart failure with a current LVEF ≤ 35% despite ACE/ARB therapy and beta-blocker therapy for 3 months was counseled regarding ICD implantation as a treatment option for the prophylaxis of sudden death. A number of other factors are important to determine if this is an appropriate option for the patient, and separate codes need to first be utilized in order to separate the patients who may need to have this type of counseling from those who do not. For more information regarding this measure and the appropriate use of codes 4470F, 4480F, and 4481F, see the rationale provided for use of codes 3055F and 3056F.

●**4500F**   Referred to an outpatient cardiac rehabilitation program (CAD)[1]

●**4510F**   Previous cardiac rehabilitation for qualifying cardiac event completed (CAD)[1]

✐ Rationale

Codes 4500F and 4510F are used to report measure compliance within the Heart Failure measure set. For more information regarding the intended use for these codes, see the rationale for code 4086F as well as codes 1460F and 1461F.

●**4525F**   Neuropsychiatric intervention ordered (DEM)[1]

●**4526F**   Neuropsychiatric intervention received (DEM)[1]

⊘=Modifier 51 Exempt   ⊙=Moderate Sedation   ✚=Add-on Code   𝒩=FDA approval pending

Rationale

Codes 4525F and 4526F are used to note compliance for the Management of Neuropsychiatric Symptoms measure within the Dementia measure set. They are included to report compliance for a measure that is intended to be reported in conjunction with another dementia measure, Neuropsychiatric Symptom Assessment. For more information regarding the intended use for these codes, see the rationale included for code 1490F.

Follow-up or Other Outcomes

●**5250F**   Asthma discharge plan provided to patient (Asthma)[1]

 Rationale

Code 5250F is used to report compliance for the Asthma Discharge Plan[1] measure within the Asthma measure set. This measure notes whether the patient aged 5 through 50 years old with a diagnosis of asthma exacerbation during an emergency department visit or inpatient admission was discharged with an asthma discharge plan. The measure snapshot notes that the discharge plan must include: (1) instructions regarding inhaled corticosteroid use; (2) information regarding discharge medications and how to use them (eg, instruction on inhaler technique); (3) referral for a follow-up appointment; and (4) instructions for recognizing and managing relapse of exacerbation or recurrence of airflow obstruction. To ensure a thorough understanding of the complete service that should be provided, the listing also includes information regarding the hospital discharge day management services. This information notes that "Hospital discharge day management services codes are to be used to report the total duration of time spent by a physician for final hospital discharge of a patient. The codes include, as appropriate, final examination of the patient, discussion of the hospital stay, even if the time spent by the physician on that date is not continuous, instructions for continuing care to all relevant caregivers, and preparation of discharge records, prescriptions and referral forms." Because no performance exclusions have been noted for this measure, modifiers 1P, 2P, and 3P may not be used with this code when reporting for this measure.

Patient Safety

●**6100F**   Timeout to verify correct patient, correct site, and correct procedure, documented (PATH)[9]

 Rationale

Code 6100F is used to ensure that the correct specimen has been provided for analysis for bone marrow and fine needle aspirations. It is included to be used to identify a patient safety measure developed by the College of American Pathologists (CAP), entitled Bone Marrow and Fine Needle Aspiration (FNA)/ Direct Specimen Acquisition Timeout Procedure[9], and is intended to identify whether the patient undergoing fine needle or bone marrow aspiration or biopsy received a proper timeout procedure to verify correct patient/correct site/correct procedure. Because no performance exclusions have been noted for this measure, modifiers 1P, 2P, and 3P may not be used with this code when reporting for this measure.

● **6101F**   Safety counseling for dementia provided (DEM)[1]

● **6102F**   Safety counseling for dementia ordered (DEM)[1]

● **6110F**   Counseling provided regarding risks of driving and the alternatives to driving (DEM)[1]

Rationale

Codes 6101F, 6102F, and 6110F are used to report compliance for measures included within the Dementia measure set. As a result, separate instructions are provided for each code according to the reported measure.

Codes 6101F and 6102F are used to report the Counseling Regarding Safety Concerns[1] measure. This measure notes whether the dementia patient, regardless of age, (or the patient's caregiver) was counseled or referred for counseling regarding safety concerns within a 12-month period of the last visit. This measure includes information regarding counseling, noting that "Counseling should include a discussion with the patient and their caregiver(s) regarding one or more of the common safety concerns listed in the measure specifications and potential risks to the patient." Because medical and patient reasons exist for not providing the counseling, the reporting instructions note that modifiers 1P and 2P may be used to identify performance exclusions that exist for this measure.

Code 6110F is used to report the Counseling Regarding Risks of Driving[1] measure. This measure is used to identify whether the patient, regardless of age, with a diagnosis of dementia (or their caregiver) was counseled regarding the risks of driving and driving-alternatives within a 12-month period. Medical exclusions exist for this measure. As a result, the reporting instructions direct users to use modifier 1P to identify medical exclusions for this measure. Modifiers 2P and 3P may not be reported for this measure.

    ⊘=Modifier 51 Exempt   ⊙=Moderate Sedation   ✚=Add-on Code   ⅄=FDA approval pending

Category III Codes

Changes that have been made to the Category III section include the addition of 31 codes, revision of 3 codes, and deletion of 9 codes.

The Category III codes' guidelines were revised and expanded to clarify rules for retention and archiving Category III codes.

In accordance with CPT guidelines for archiving Category III codes, 9 codes and related introductory guidelines and parenthetical notes have been deleted for 2012.

Category III Codes

►Services/procedures described in this section make use of alphanumeric characters. These codes have an alpha character as the 5th character in the string, preceded by four digits. The digits are not intended to reflect the placement of the code in the Category I section of CPT nomenclature. Codes in this section may or may not eventually receive a Category I CPT code. In either case, in general, a given Category III code will be archived five years from the date of initial publication or extension unless a modification of the archival date is specifically noted at the time of a revision or change to a code (eg, addition of parenthetical instructions, reinstatement). Services/procedures described by Category III codes, which have been archived after five years, without conversion, must be reported using the Category I unlisted code unless another specific cross reference is established at the time of archiving. New codes in this section are released semi-annually via the AMA/CPT internet site, to expedite dissemination for reporting. The full set of temporary codes for emerging technology, services, and procedures are published annually in the CPT codebook. Go to www.ama-assn.org/go/cpt for the most current listing.◄

🖎 Rationale

The Category III codes guidelines were revised and expanded to clarify rules for retention and archiving Category III codes.

▲**0080T** Endovascular repair using prosthesis of abdominal aortic aneurysm, pseudoaneurysm or dissection, abdominal aorta involving visceral vessels (superior mesenteric, celiac and/or renal artery[s]), radiological supervision and interpretation

🖎 Rationale

Code 0080T has been revised to include descriptor language that more closely matches and notes the procedures that are intended as part of this service. This includes the removal of language that specifies a particular device.

►(0141T-0143T have been deleted)◄

►(To report pancreatic islet cell transplantation, use 48999)◄

►(0155T, 0156T have been deleted)◄

►(For laparoscopic implantation, replacement, revision, or removal of gastric stimulation electrodes, lesser curvature, use 43659)◄

►(0157T, 0158T have been deleted)◄

►(For open implantation, replacement, revision, or removal of gastric stimulation electrodes, lesser curvature, use 43999)◄

►(0160T, 0161T have been deleted. To report, see 90867, 90869)◄

(0162T has been deleted. To report, see 95980-95982)

►(0166T, 0167T have been deleted)◄

►(For transmyocardial transcatheter closure of ventricular septal defect, with implant, including cardiopulmonary bypass if performed, use 33999◄

►(0168T has been deleted)◄

►(For rhinophototherapy, intranasal application of ultraviolet and visible light, use 30999)◄

0169T   Stereotactic placement of infusion catheter(s) in the brain for delivery of therapeutic agent(s), including computerized stereotactic planning and burr hole(s)

🖑 Rationale

In accordance with CPT guidelines for archiving Category III codes, codes 0141T, 0142T, and 0143T and related introductory guidelines and parenthetical notes have been deleted for 2012. These codes were used to report pancreatic islet cell transplantation through a portal vein (0141T percutaneous, 0142T open, and 0143T laparoscopic). A parenthetical note has been added instructing the use of Category I unlisted code 48999 for reporting pancreatic islet cell transplantation.

Codes 0155T, 0156T, 0157T, 0158T have also been deleted in accordance with CPT guidelines for archiving Category III codes. Parenthetical notes have been added instructing the use of Category I unlisted code 43659 for reporting laparoscopic implantation, replacement, revision, or removal of gastric stimulation electrodes, lesser curvature previously described by codes 0155T and 0156T, and 43999 for reporting open implantation, replacement, revision, or removal of gastric stimulation electrodes, lesser curvature, previously described by codes 0157T and 0158T.

Additional codes 0166T and 0167T and related Category I cross-reference notes have been deleted for 2012, in accordance with the Category III archiving guidelines. A parenthetical note has been added instructing the use of Category I unlisted code 33999 for reporting transmyocardial transcatheter closure of ventricular septal defect, with implant, including cardiopulmonary bypass previously described by codes 0166T and 0167T.

Code 0168T and its related Category I cross-reference note have been deleted. A parenthetical note has been added instructing the use of Category I unlisted code 30999 for reporting rhinophototherapy, intranasal application of ultraviolet and visible light previously described by code 0168T.

▲**0240T**   Esophageal motility (manometric study of the esophagus and/or gastroesophageal junction) study with interpretation and report; with high resolution esophageal pressure topography

►(Do not report 0240T in conjunction with 91010 or 91013)◄

+▲**0241T**   with stimulation or perfusion during high resolution esophageal pressure topography study (eg, stimulant, acid or alkali perfusion) (List separately in addition to code for primary procedure)

(Use 0241T in conjunction with 0240T)

►(Do not report 0241T in conjunction with 91010 or 91013)◄

►(Do not report 0241T more than once per session)◄

⊘=Modifier 51 Exempt   ⊙=Moderate Sedation   ✦=Add-on Code   ⊿=FDA approval pending

►(To report esophageal motility studies without high resolution esophageal pressure topography, use 91010 and with stimulant or perfusion, use 91013)◄

✍ Rationale

A change was made to Category III codes 0240T and 0241T (as well as to Category I codes 91010 and 91013 in the Medicine section) to identify the intent of these codes to report 2D or 3D esophageal manometry studies performed with high pressure topography. This included the removal of language that specified either 2D or 3D data for both sets of codes (ie, both in the Category I Medicine and the Category III sections). Clarifications have also been made via use of additions and revisions to parentheticals to: (1) exclude use of codes 0240T and 0241T with code 91010 or 91013; (2) exclude reporting stimulation or perfusion (0241T) more than once per session; and (3) indicate the appropriate method of reporting esophageal motility studies without high resolution esophageal pressure topography (by using code 91010 and additionally reporting code 91013 when stimulant or perfusion are used).

🩺 Clinical Example (0240T)

A 49-year-old female presents with complaints of heartburn and chest pain. Cardiac evaluation and esophagogastroduodenoscopy (EGD) were unremarkable. She has tried a number of pharmacologic agents without relief of symptoms. She is referred for evaluation of esophageal function to assess symptoms in response to stimulation agents.

Description of Procedure (0240T)

Informed consent is obtained. The high resolution esophageal pressure topography (HREPT) recording assembly is set up and calibrated by the physician. Following topical anesthesia to the nares, the HREPT esophageal probe is passed transnasally under direct physician supervision into the esophagus. The proximal pressure sensors are positioned in the hypopharynx and the distal pressure sensors are positioned in the proximal stomach. The patient assumes a supine position. Baseline recordings of sphincter pressure and esophagogastric junction pressure morphology are obtained. A series of water swallow (at least 10) test are obtained by injecting 5 ml water into the subject's mouth. Further series of swallows may be obtained (sitting posture, rapid sequence swallows, larger volumes of water, viscous or solid media) to address specific clinical issues. At the conclusion of the procedure, the probe is removed. The composite results of the 10+ swallows are reviewed and interpreted by the physician according to the Chicago Classification scheme, validated specifically for the interpretation of these studies. The physician reviews and interprets the esophageal pressure and topographical study data and verifies the analysis results. A report is generated.

🩺 Clinical Example (0241T)

A 45-year-old male presents with complaints of heartburn and recurrent dysphagia. Radiological studies, cardiac evaluation, and esophagogastroduodenoscopy (EGD) were unremarkable. He has tried a number of pharmacologic agents without relief of symptoms. The patient is referred for evaluation.

Description of Procedure (0241T)

Informed consent is obtained. The patient is brought to the Gastroenterology Laboratory. After a baseline esophageal motility study with or without pressure, topography is performed, topical anesthesia is administered to the nares, and an additional small infusion catheter is placed into the esophagus to a distance of 30 to 35 cm from the nares. The motility probe is repositioned straddling the distal esophagus, checking pressure measurements. The stimulant is infused through the infusion catheter, and additional pressure measurements are taken. If necessary, a further series of swallows is obtained to address the specific clinical issue. The patient is removed and study completed. The recording is saved for subsequent interpretation. The physician reviews the additional data from the stimulation study and a report is generated.

●0260T   Total body systemic hypothermia, per day, in the neonate 28 days of age or younger

●0261T   Selective head hypothermia, per day, in the neonate 28 days of age or younger

Rationale

Codes 0260T and 0261T have been established to report hypothermia procedures for neonates. These procedures are used as a treatment modality in neonates exposed to serious hypoxia and ischemia at or shortly after delivery. Use of these codes is limited to neonates 28 days of age and younger as these codes are intended for this specific patient population under these specific circumstances. To further exemplify the intended use for these codes, a parenthetical note has been placed within the guideline section of the existing Inpatient Neonatal Intensive Care Services and Pediatric and Neonatal Critical Care Services section directing users to the Category III code section for hypothermia services provided for neonates.

Clinical Example (0260T)

An 8-lb-term infant is born after severe in utero hypoxemia and is admitted to a NICU and receives critical care services. Laboratory, EEG, blood gas, and imaging studies confirm the neonate meets objective criteria for total body cooling. Continuous total body hypothermia is undertaken.

Description of Procedure (0260T)

The procedure is discussed with the parents and consent to move forward with the procedure is obtained. An amplitude integrated EEG is placed by nurse or technician.

The cooling apparatus is placed by the nursing staff. Rectal and esophageal temperature probes are attached and their positions are confirmed by X ray. The cooling is initiated after baseline laboratory studies, including a full coagulation panel, are evaluated. Under neonatologist's supervision, the patient is cooled to a core temperature of 34.5°C and maintained at this temperature. The patient is continued on amplitude integrated EEG looking for evidence of seizures. Sarnat scores are performed by the neonatologist every four hours. Cooling and temperature monitoring are continuous. Adjustments are made by the nurse to the cooling

⊘=Modifier 51 Exempt   ⊙=Moderate Sedation   ✚=Add-on Code   ✗=FDA approval pending

device to keep core temperatures within range. Cooling is continued for a total of 72 hours. After 72 hours under direct supervision by the neonatologist, rewarming is initiated at 0.5° to 1°C per hour to 37°C.

Clinical Example (0261T)

A 2500 g 36-week infant is born after severe in utero hypoxemia. He is admitted to an NICU and critical care is initiated. His gestational age, laboratory work, EEG, and medical imaging confirm he is a candidate for selective head cooling.

Description of Procedure (0261T)

This preterm neonate has been in the NICU receiving critical care with lines placed on a ventilator with frequent monitoring of laboratory data. Laboratory work indicates severe acidemia that is slowing recovering. There are signs of multiorgan injury. The EEG (diagnostic EEG reported separately) shows low voltage activity generalized and CT scan shows some increase in brain water (edema) and blurring on the gray-white interface. It is determined that the child meets criteria for total body cooling. The procedure is discussed with the parents and consent to move forward with the procedure is obtained. An amplitude integrated EEG is placed by the nurse or technician, two leads. The cooling apparatus is placed by the neonatologist after rectal and esophageal temperature probes are attached and their positions are confirmed by X ray. The head cooling is initiated after baseline laboratory studies, including a full coagulation panel, are evaluated. Under neonatologist's supervision, the patient is cooled to a core temperature of 34.5°C and maintained at this temperature. The patient is continued on amplitude integrated EEG looking for evidence of seizures. Sarnat scores are performed by the nurse and neonatologist (has to have either one, not both, for valuation of the code) every four hours. Cooling and temperature monitoring are continuous. Adjustments are made to the cooling device to keep core temperatures within range. Cooling is continued for a total of 72 hours. After 72 hours under direct supervision by the neonatologist, rewarming is initiated at 0.5° to 1°C per hour to 37°C.

●0262T   Implantation of catheter-delivered prosthetic pulmonary valve, endovascular approach

▶(0262T includes all congenital cardiac catheterization[s], intraprocedural contrast injection[s], fluoroscopic radiological supervision and interpretation, and imaging guidance performed to complete the pulmonary valve procedure. Do not report 0262T in conjunction with 76000, 76001, 93530, 93563, 93566-93568)◄

▶(0262T includes percutaneous balloon angioplasty/valvuloplasty of the pulmonary valve/conduit. Do not report 0262T in conjunction with 92990◄

▶(0262T includes stent deployment within the pulmonary conduit. Do not report 37205, 37206, 75960 for stent placement within the pulmonary conduit. Report 92980, 92981, 37205, 37206, 75960 separately when cardiovascular stent placement is performed at a site separate from the prosthetic valve delivery site. Report 92997, 92998 separately when pulmonary artery angioplasty is performed at a site separate from the prosthetic valve delivery site)◄

Rationale

Code 0262T has been established for reporting implantation of a pulmonary valve from an endovascular approach. All catheterizations, injections, and imaging required to implant the prosthetic are included in code 0262T, as indicated in the instructional notes, with the exception of stent placement and pulmonary artery angioplasty that is performed at a site separate from the prosthetic valve delivery site, which may be reported separately.

Clinical Example (0262T)

A 16-year-old patient with a history of total repair of Tetralogy of Fallot has developed shortness of breath and extreme weakness upon exertion believed to be due to a failing pulmonary conduit; cardiac MRI finds severe pulmonary regurgitation and right ventricular dilatation. The patient is found to be a candidate for endovascular pulmonary valve implantation.

Description of Procedure (0262T)

General anesthesia is induced. The patient is intubated and connected to a mechanical ventilator. The patient is further positioned to allow biplanar fluoroscopic capability.

Potential impact to the coronary artery from implantation is accessed. A stiff guidewire is placed across the RV to PA conduit. Under fluoroscopic guidance, an angiographic catheter of choice is placed in position to assess the appropriate site for valve implantation and quantification of pulmonary valve stenosis and/or regurgitation. The angiographic catheter is withdrawn.

A balloon angioplasty catheter is passed over the guidewire and positioned within the RV to PA conduit at the appropriate level, crossing the existing valve within the conduit. Predilation of the conduit and existing valve using the balloon angioplasty/valvuloplasty catheter is performed. Assessment is then undertaken of the size of the newly dilated conduit, waist of the existing valve, and compliance of the conduit to ensure a suitable valve delivery site. Angiography of the area may also be performed at this time to rule out conduit rupture.

When anatomically indicated, the conduit is reinforced by inserting a balloon-expandable stent. Fluoroscopy/angiography may be performed to confirm stent placement.

In preparation for implantation, the percutaneous pulmonary valve is repeatedly rinsed per protocol. The delivery catheter system is vigorously flushed to remove air. The stented valve is crimped onto the delivery catheter system. Correct orientation of the valve on the delivery catheter system is confirmed by the operator and another staff member in the room. Depending on the system, the valve may then be covered with an outer sheath while flushing with saline.

After confirming anticoagulation, the femoral vein or other venous access is sequentially dilated to accept the delivery catheter. Over the guidewire, the delivery system is advanced under fluoroscopy into the right ventricular outflow tract, to the target position within the conduit. Position is confirmed by fluoroscopy and/or by injection of contrast. The stented valve is implanted by successive inflation of balloons on the delivery catheter system. The balloons are deflated and the delivery system is withdrawn.

Repeat angiography and pressure measurements are done to confirm placement. If clinically indicated, an additional high-pressure angioplasty balloon may be used to postdilate the newly implanted stented valve within the conduit.

After confirming satisfactory position and function of the valve, as well as assessing the degree of any paravalvular regurgitation, the guidewire and sheath are removed from the patient. The opening of the access artery is closed via blind closure, manual compression, or a closure device. The venous access may also be closed.

●**0263T** Intramuscular autologous bone marrow cell therapy, with preparation of harvested cells, multiple injections, one leg, including ultrasound guidance, if performed; complete procedure including unilateral or bilateral bone marrow harvest

    ▶(Do not report 0263T in conjunction with 38204-38242, 76942, 93925, 93926)◀

●**0264T**   complete procedure excluding bone marrow harvest

    ▶(Do not report 0264T in conjunction with 38204-38242, 76942, 93925, 93926, 0265T)◀

●**0265T**   unilateral or bilateral bone marrow harvest only for intramuscular autologous bone marrow cell therapy

    ▶(Do not report 0265T in conjunction with 38204-38242, 0264T. For complete procedure, use 0263T)◀

✎ Rationale

Three codes have been established for intramuscular autologous bone marrow cell therapy. Code 0263T is reported for the complete procedure, including a unilateral or bilateral bone marrow harvest. If the procedure is performed by two separate physicians, code 0264T would be reported by the physician performing the intramuscular autologous bone marrow cell therapy, and code 0265T would be reported for the physician performing only the bone marrow harvest. Exclusionary parenthetical notes have also been added for all three new codes, including one precluding the use of code 0264T with code 0265T, as code 0263T should be reported if the complete procedure is performed by the same physician.

🩺 Clinical Example (0263T, 0264T, 0265T)

A 70-year-old male with CAD and a prior failed left leg bypass presents with severe ischemic rest pain and toe gangrene. Angiography reveals infrainguinal arterial occlusive disease. He has no remaining autogenous conduit for bypass.

Description of Procedure (0263T)

Review all relevant office notes, H&P, noninvasive vascular lab studies. Review arteriogram and CT angiogram, and make appropriate preoperative measurements. Order ultrasound equipment and Bone Marrow Harvest Preparation kit from the manufacturer. Review operative plan and informed consent with patient and family. Specifically discuss risk of bleeding, clotting, limb loss, and infection. Discuss patient comorbidities and surgical approach with anesthesiologist. Position patient on bed in pre-op holding area. Perform ultrasound imaging of index limb to confirm operative plan. Determine plan to treat index limb.

Determine primary treatment section by taking into consideration all past imaging studies and real time ultrasound imaging in order to make a clinical judgment of what area(s) have the highest ischemic gradient. For the primary treatment section use tape measure and marking pen to draw line tracing primary arterial branch corresponding to tissue area with highest ischemic gradient. Use clinical judgment to determine spacing of injections along the treatment line. Spacing can be 1 cm, 1.5 cm, or 2 cm. Use tape measure and marker to mark exact site for each injection. Total number of injection sites. If ulcers are present, mark location of all ulcers in patient's operative notes and determine which ulcer(s) would benefit from injection. Mark injection sites around the circumference of the wound. Measure circumference and mark injection sites, spacing the injection sites 1 cm apart.

Change into OR scrubs. Place any needed invasive monitoring lines. Supervise patient positioning, skin preparation, and draping. Scrub and gown. Make a 1 cm incision over right posterior iliac crest. Use aspiration needle to make multiple passes in different areas of the marrow to obtain 120 cc of aspirate. Apply pressure dressing. Hand off the syringe to the scrub tech so that its contents can be put into the blood transfer bag. Make a 1 cm incision over left posterior iliac crest. Use aspiration needle to make multiple passes in different areas of the marrow to obtain 120 cc of aspirate. Apply pressure dressing. Hand off the syringe to the scrub tech so that its contents can be put into the blood transfer bag. Reposition patient from prone to supine position.

Redrape patient and prep index limb. Rescrub and gown. Have the ultrasound machine positioned in the room and drape the ultrasound probe with a sterile cover. Orient ultrasound probe to observe penetration of injection needle through tissue of index limb. Injection procedure at each of marked injection sites (mean of 40 injections). The investigator places his or her finger on the skin surface and pulls the skin and subcutaneous layers out of alignment with the underlying muscle. The skin should be moved about 1 cm. The needle is inserted at a 90-degree angle at the site where the investigator's finger was initially placed, and the progress of the needle through the tissue is monitored by ultrasound imaging. Injections are ideally placed within 1 cm of the targeted vascular bed. Ultrasound guidance is used to localize injections. Although the target areas will typically have occluded arteries, the ultrasound may identify the popliteal or tibial veins, which are always adjacent to the native arteries. To minimize the risk of nerve injury, the injection is placed approximately 5-10 mm away from the neurovascular bundle. When the needle is in its proper position 1 mL of injectate is delivered and the needle is withdrawn. The investigator then removes his or her finger from the skin surface, allowing the layers to return to their normal positions. The needle track is now broken at the junction of each tissue layer, trapping the injectate in the muscle. While inserting the needle, draw back 0.5-1.0 mL on the syringe to prevent intravascular injection.

The injection sites are to be covered with sterile gauze and the leg wrapped loosely with a sterile gauze roll. If wounds are present they will be dressed according to the

⊘=Modifier 51 Exempt   ☉=Moderate Sedation   ✚=Add-on Code   ✗=FDA approval pending attending surgeon's protocol. Apply dressings. Transfer patient to stretcher, accompany patient to recovery area. Write orders. Dictate operative note. Communicate with family, referring and consulting physicians. Participate with the anesthesiologist in the recovery area to ensure smooth emergence from anesthesia. Discuss results of procedure with the patient once he or she is fully awake. When stable, the patient is transferred to the floor.

Description of Procedure (0264T)

Review all relevant office notes, H&P, noninvasive vascular lab studies. Review arteriogram, CT angiogram and make appropriate preoperative measurements. Order ultrasound equipment and Bone Marrow Harvest Preparation kit from the manufacturer. Review operative plan and informed consent with patient and family. Specifically discuss risk of bleeding, clotting, limb loss, and infection. Discuss patient comorbidities and surgical approach with anesthesiologist. Position patient on bed in pre-op holding area. Perform ultrasound imaging of index limb to confirm operative plan. Determine plan to treat index limb.

Determine primary treatment section by taking into consideration all past imaging studies and real time ultrasound imaging in order to make a clinical judgment of what area(s) have the highest ischemic gradient. For the primary treatment section use tape measure and marking pen to draw line tracing primary arterial branch corresponding to tissue area with highest ischemic gradient. Use clinical judgment to determine spacing of injections along the treatment line. Spacing can be 1 cm, 1.5 cm, or 2 cm. Use tape measure and marker to mark exact site for each injection. Total number of injection sites. If ulcers are present, mark location of all ulcers in patient's operative notes and determine which ulcer(s) would benefit from injection. Mark injection sites around the circumference of the wound. Measure circumference and mark injection sites, spacing the injection sites 1 cm apart.

Change into OR scrubs. Place any needed invasive monitoring lines. Supervise patient positioning, skin preparation, and draping. Wait while separate physician performs bone marrow harvest from right iliac crest. Wait while separate physician performs bone marrow harvest from left iliac crest. Reposition patient from prone to supine position.

Redrape patient and prep index limb. Have the ultrasound machine positioned in the room and drape the ultrasound probe with a sterile cover. Orient ultrasound probe to observe penetration of injection needle through tissue of index limb. Injection procedure at each of marked injection sites (mean of 40 injections). The investigator places his or her finger on the skin surface and pulls the skin and subcutaneous layers out of alignment with the underlying muscle. The skin should be moved about 1 cm. The needle is inserted at a 90-degree angle at the site where the investigator's finger was initially placed, and the progress of the needle through the tissue is monitored by ultrasound imaging. Injections are ideally placed within 1 cm of the targeted vascular bed. Ultrasound guidance is used to localize injections. Although the target areas will typically have occluded arteries, the ultrasound may identify the popliteal or tibial veins, which are always adjacent to the native arteries. To minimize the risk of nerve injury, the injection is placed approximately 5-10 mm away from the neurovascular bundle. When the needle is in its proper position 1 mL of injectate is delivered and the needle is withdrawn. The investigator then removes his or her finger from the skin surface, allowing the layers to return to their normal positions. The needle track is now broken at the junction of each tissue layer, trapping the injectate in the muscle. While inserting the needle, draw back 0.5-1.0 mL on the syringe to prevent intravascular injection.

The injection sites are to be covered with sterile gauze and the leg wrapped loosely with a sterile gauze roll. If wounds are present they will be dressed according to the attending surgeon's protocol. Apply dressings. Transfer patient to stretcher, accompany patient to recovery area. Write orders. Dictate operative note. Communicate with family, referring and consulting physicians. Participate with the anesthesiologist in the recovery area to ensure smooth emergence from anesthesia. Discuss results of procedure with the patient once he or she is fully awake. When stable, the patient is transferred to the floor.

Description of Procedure (0265T)
Review all relevant office notes, H&P, noninvasive vascular lab studies. Review operative plan and informed consent with patient and family. Specifically discuss risk of bleeding, clotting, limb loss, and infection. Discuss patient comorbidities and surgical approach with anesthesiologist. Position patient on bed in pre-op holding area. Change into OR scrubs. Supervise patient positioning, skin preparation, and draping. Make a 1 cm incision over right posterior iliac crest. Use aspiration needle to make multiple passes in different areas of the marrow to obtain 120 cc of aspirate. Apply pressure dressing. Hand off the syringe to physician performing the injection therapy. Make a 1 cm incision over left posterior iliac crest. Use aspiration needle to make multiple passes in different areas of the marrow to obtain 120 cc of aspirate. Apply pressure dressing. Hand off the syringe to physician performing the injection therapy.

Write orders. Dictate operative note. Communicate with family, referring and consulting physicians. Participate with the anesthesiologist in the recovery area to ensure smooth emergence from anesthesia. Discuss results of procedure with the patient once he or she is fully awake. When stable, the patient is transferred to the floor.

●**0266T** Implantation or replacement of carotid sinus baroreflex activation device; total system (includes generator placement, unilateral or bilateral lead placement, intra-operative interrogation, programming, and repositioning, when performed)

●**0267T** lead only, unilateral (includes intra-operative interrogation, programming, and repositioning, when performed)

▶(For bilateral lead implantation or replacement, use 0267T with modifier 50)◀

●**0268T** pulse generator only (includes intra-operative interrogation, programming, and repositioning, when performed)

▶(Do not report 0267T, 0268T in conjunction with 0266T, 0269T-0273T)◀

⊘=Modifier 51 Exempt   ⊙=Moderate Sedation   ✦=Add-on Code   𝗡=FDA approval pending

●**0269T**   Revision or removal of carotid sinus baroreflex activation device; total system (includes generator placement, unilateral or bilateral lead placement, intra-operative interrogation, programming, and repositioning, when performed)

▶(Do not report 0269T in conjunction with 0266T-0268T, 0270T-0273T)◀

●**0270T**   lead only, unilateral (includes intra-operative interrogation, programming, and repositioning, when performed)

▶(Do not report 0270T in conjunction with 0266T-0269T, 0271T-0273T)◀

▶(For bilateral lead removal, use 0270T with modifier 50)◀

▶(For removal of total carotid sinus baroreflex activation device, use 0269T)◀

●**0271T**   pulse generator only (includes intra-operative interrogation, programming, and repositioning, when performed)

▶(Do not report 0271T in conjunction with 0266T-0270T, 0272T, 0273T)◀

▶(For removal and replacement, see 0266T, 0267T, 0268T)◀

●**0272T**   Interrogation device evaluation (in person), carotid sinus baroreflex activation system, including telemetric iterative communication with the implantable device to monitor device diagnostics and programmed therapy values, with interpretation and report (eg, battery status, lead impedance, pulse amplitude, pulse width, therapy frequency, pathway mode, burst mode, therapy start/stop times each day);

▶(Do not report 0272T in conjunction with 0266T-0271T, 0273T)◀

●**0273T**   with programming

▶(Do not report 0273T in conjunction with 0266T-0272T)◀

✍ Rationale

Eight Category III codes have been established to describe carotid sinus baroreflex activation device services. These services represent the use of a new technology. The carotid sinus baroreflex activation device is used to treat cardiac conditions such as hypertension and heart failure. Implantation of this device involves placing the electrodes directly around the carotid arteries. The eight new codes describe implantation, replacement, revision, removal, and interrogation of the device. The codes are structured based on whether the services are provided for the total system, lead only, or pulse generator only. Several parenthetical notes have been added to provide clarification of appropriate reporting of these codes.

Codes 0266T-0268T describe implantation or replacement of the carotid sinus baroreflex activation device. Code 0266T describes implantation of the total system. Code 0267T is reported for implantation or placement of the lead only. Modifier 50 should be appended to code 0267T when bilateral lead implantation or replacement is performed. Code 0268T describes implantation or replacement of the pulse generator only. Codes 0269T-0271T describe revision or removal of the carotid sinus baroreflex activation device. Code 0270T is reported for revision or removal of the lead only. Modifier 50 should be appended to code 0270T when bilateral lead removal is performed. Code 0271T describes revision or removal of the pulse generator only.

It is important to note that when removal and replacement are performed, the appropriate code from the 0266T-0268T series should be reported. When the device is removed but not replaced, the appropriate code from the 0269T-0271T series should be reported.

Codes 0272T and 0273T describe an in-person interrogation device evaluation. Code 0273T includes programming. It is important to note that codes 0272T and 0273T should not be reported in conjunction with codes 0266T-0271T, as codes 0266T-0271T include interrogation and programming. Codes 0272T and 0273T should not be reported together.

Clinical Example (0266T)

A 53-year-old adult presents with a long history of resistant hypertension. The patient is currently on medical therapy including maximal doses of a diuretic and two other classes of antihypertensive agents. Despite medications, the patient's blood pressure is still 178/103 and the patient is at a high risk for stroke, myocardial infarction, renal damage, and other sequellae of uncontrolled hypertension. The physician managing the patient's hypertension prescribes treatment with baroreflex activation therapy.

Description of Procedure (0266T)

Please note that every surgeon has his or her preferred method to perform an open surgical operation. In addition, each patient's anatomy and pathology require individualization. Thus, the following is a generic description. Individual procedures will vary.

On both sides of neck: incise skin from ear lobe to clavicle. On both sides: dissect through soft tissues until common carotid artery is located. On both sides: circumferentially dissect artery and pass two soft rubber loops around. On both sides: dissect to expose carotid bifurcation, including distal common carotid, proximal external and internal carotid arteries. Pass loops around each artery for control. Incise the chest wall and create subcutaneous pocket in the pectoral region for placement of the implantable pulse generator. Create tunnel from each neck incision to the pulse generator pocket.

Tunnel each lead subcutaneously to the pulse generator pocket. Attach leads to the pulse generator. The optimal location for attaching each lead to the carotid sinus is determined by placing the lead on the carotid sinus, electrically activating it, and monitoring the blood pressure response of the patient. Several different lead positions are evaluated by rotating the lead slightly and moving it upward and downward on the carotid sinus. The location associated with the optimal blood pressure response is selected for permanent attachment of the lead. The lead is secured in place by suturing to the carotid artery wall, wrapping the lead around the sinus, and suturing the lead back onto itself. This procedure is repeated for the contralateral carotid artery. The pulse generator is inserted into the pocket.

⊘ =Modifier 51 Exempt   ⊙=Moderate Sedation   ✚ =Add-on Code   𝑵 =FDA approval pending

Irrigate incisions copiously with sterile saline. Use electrocautery or suture ligation to achieve final hemostasis. Close incisions in multiple layers with special attention. Close skin.

Clinical Example (0267T)

A 58-year-old adult is being treated for hypertension with a carotid sinus baroreflex activation device. The patient received the total device system five years previously and has responded favorably to the therapy. One or both of the leads have lost function. Possible reasons for this include trauma or damage during surgery in proximity to the device for an unrelated medical problem. Based on the patient's positive response to therapy, the health care provider made the decision to replace the lead(s).

Description of Procedure (0267T)

Please note that every surgeon has his or her preferred method to perform an open surgical operation. In addition, each patient's anatomy and pathology require individualization. Thus, the following is a generic description. Individual procedures will vary. The side of the neck with a malfunctioning lead is incised from ear lobe to clavicle. The soft tissue and scar are dissected until the common carotid artery is located, avoiding the adherent neurovascular structures in the redo field. Circumferentially dissect artery and pass two soft rubber loops around. Dissect to expose carotid bifurcation, including distal common carotid, proximal external and internal carotid arteries. Pass loops around each artery for control. Incise the chest wall and open the subcutaneous pocket in the pectoral region for isolation of the implantable pulse generator. Free malfunctioning lead from tunnel from neck incision to the pulse generator pocket.

Tunnel new lead subcutaneously to the pulse generator pocket. Attach lead to the pulse generator. The optimal location for attaching each lead to the carotid sinus is determined by placing the lead on the carotid sinus, electrically activating it, and monitoring the blood pressure response of the patient. Several different lead positions are evaluated by rotating the lead slightly and moving it upward and downward on the carotid sinus. The location associated with the optimal blood pressure response is selected for permanent attachment of the lead. The lead is secured in place by suturing to the carotid artery wall, wrapping the lead around the sinus, and suturing the lead back onto itself. This procedure is repeated for the contralateral carotid artery.

Irrigate incisions copiously with sterile saline. Use electrocautery or suture ligation to achieve final hemostasis. Close incisions in multiple layers with special attention. Close skin.

Clinical Example (0268T)

A 58-year-old adult is being treated for hypertension with a carotid sinus baroreflex activation device. The patient was previously implanted with a total carotid sinus baroreflex activation system and has responded favorably to the therapy. The pulse generator has reached the end of its battery life and needs to be replaced in order for the patient to continue to receive therapy.

Description of Procedure (0268T)

Please note that every surgeon has his or her preferred method to perform an open surgical operation. In addition, each patient's anatomy and pathology require individualization. Thus, the following is a generic description. Individual procedures will vary. Incise the chest wall and subcutaneous pocket in the pectoral region for isolation of the implantable pulse generator. Remove malfunctioning device from pocket and disconnect leads.

Insert new device. Attach leads to the pulse generator. The pulse generator is inserted into the pocket.

Irrigate incisions copiously with sterile saline. Use electrocautery or suture ligation to achieve final hemostasis. Close incisions in multiple layers with special attention. Close skin.

Clinical Example (0269T)

A 58-year-old adult is being treated for hypertension with a carotid sinus baroreflex activation device. The patient was previously implanted with a total carotid sinus baroreflex activation system. The patient has developed an infection that has localized to the area of the implant. Based on medical necessity in treating the infection, the patient's physician has determined that the device system must be completely removed.

Description of Procedure (0269T)

Please note that every surgeon has his or her preferred method to perform an open surgical operation. In addition, each patient's anatomy and pathology require individualization. Thus, the following is a generic description. Individual procedures will vary. Both sides of the neck are incised from ear lobe to clavicle. The soft tissue and scar are dissected until the common carotid artery is located avoiding the adherent neurovascular structures in the redo field. Circumferentially dissect artery. Dissect to expose carotid bifurcation, including lead attachment site. Repeat for contralateral neck/carotid artery. Incise the chest wall and open the subcutaneous pocket in the pectoral region for isolation of the implantable pulse generator. Free the lead from tunnel from neck incision to the pulse generator pocket. Repeat for contralateral neck/carotid artery. Remove implantable generator.

Irrigate incisions copiously with sterile saline. Use electrocautery or suture ligation to achieve final hemostasis. Close incisions in multiple layers with special attention. Close skin.

Clinical Example (0270T)

A 58-year-old heart failure patient was previously implanted with an entire carotid sinus baroreflex activation system and has responded favorably to the therapy. The patient's lead positioning has begun to cause discomfort, possibly due to movement, scar formation, or patient weight gain/loss, and needs to be corrected.

Description of Procedure (0270T)

Please note that every surgeon has his or her preferred method to perform an open surgical operation. In addition, each patient's anatomy and pathology

⊘=Modifier 51 Exempt   ⊙=Moderate Sedation   ✚=Add-on Code   ⊬=FDA approval pending

require individualization. Thus, the following is a generic description. Individual procedures will vary. The side of the neck with a malfunctioning lead is incised from ear lobe to clavicle. The soft tissue and scar are dissected until the common carotid artery is located avoiding the adherent neurovascular structures in the redo field. Dissect to expose carotid bifurcation, including distal common carotid, proximal external and internal carotid arteries. Incise the chest wall and open the subcutaneous pocket in the pectoral region for isolation of the implantable pulse generator. Free malfunctioning lead from tunnel from neck incision to the pulse generator pocket.

Irrigate incisions copiously with sterile saline. Use electrocautery or suture ligation to achieve final hemostasis. Close incisions in multiple layers with special attention. Close skin.

 ### Clinical Example (0271T)

A 58-year-old adult patient was previously implanted with a total carotid sinus baroreflex activation system and has responded favorably to the therapy. The pulse generator has begun to cause the patient discomfort, possibly due to migration, scar formation, or patient weight gain/loss, and needs to be corrected.

Description of Procedure (0271T)

Please note that every surgeon has his or her preferred method to perform an open surgical operation. In addition, each patient's anatomy and pathology require individualization. Thus, the following is a generic description. Individual procedures will vary. Incise the chest wall and subcutaneous pocket in the pectoral region for isolation of the implantable pulse generator. Remove malfunctioning device from pocket and disconnect leads.

Irrigate incisions copiously with sterile saline. Use electrocautery or suture ligation to achieve final hemostasis. Close incisions in multiple layers with special attention. Close skin.

Clinical Example (0272T)

A 53-year-old hypertensive patient was implanted with a total carotid sinus baroreflex activation system five months ago and is receiving baroreflex activation therapy. A programming device evaluation had been performed two months earlier. The patient returns to her physician for routine evaluation but not for therapy adjustment.

Description of Procedure (0272T)

The programmer head is placed on the patient's skin over the implantable pulse generator to establish a telemetry communication. Information is retrieved from the pulse generator regarding the longevity of the pulse generator battery, the integrity of the implanted leads, and the full set of therapy programmed parameters. The documented information is interpreted by the physician and, based on the results, no programming is required.

Clinical Example (0273T)

A 53-year-old hypertensive patient was implanted with a total carotid sinus baro-reflex activation system three months ago and is receiving baroreflex activation therapy. The patient returns to his or her physician for routine evaluation and therapy optimization.

Description of Procedure (0273T)

A patient has been implanted with a carotid sinus baroreflex activation therapy system. Either bedside for patients with a new implant or in the physician's office for existing patients, the programmer head is placed on the patient's skin over the implantable pulse generator to establish a telemetry communication. Software commands are issued through the programmer computer to the implantable pulse generator with a selected therapy. The patient's blood pressure and heart rate response are continuously monitored. The physician documents the results of the evaluation and interprets the results to determine the optimal setting parameters for the patient. Once determined, the device is programmed and the programmer head is removed from the pulse generator to discontinue communication.

●**0274T** Percutaneous laminotomy/laminectomy (interlaminar approach) for decompression of neural elements, (with or without ligamentous resection, discectomy, facetectomy and/or foraminotomy), any method, under indirect image guidance (eg, fluoroscopic, CT), with or without the use of an endoscope, single or multiple levels, unilateral or bilateral; cervical or thoracic

●**0275T**   lumbar

▶(For laminotomy/hemilaminectomy performed using an open and endoscopically-assisted approach, see 63020-63035)◀

▶(For percutaneous decompression of the nucleus pulposus of intervertebral disc utilizing needle based technique, use 62287)◀

Rationale

Category III codes 0274T and 0275T have been added to identify percutaneous laminotomy/laminectomy procedures. These codes include specific language that notes ". . . any method under indirect imaging guidance . . ." (which includes fluo-roscopic and computerized tomography [CT] imaging and may include the use of an endoscope to complete the procedure). Parenthetical notes have been placed following these codes in the Category III section that direct users to the appro-priate codes to use to identify open and endoscopically assisted decompression procedures (63020-63035) and the correct code to use to identify percutaneous decompression of the nucleus pulposus using needle-based techniques (62287). For more information regarding the appropriate method of reporting hemilaminec-tomy/laminotomy procedures, see the Rationale included for code 62287.

Clinical Example (0274T)

A 45-year-old male presents with a six-week history of right arm pain consistent with a right C-6 radiculitis. Imaging of the cervical spine reveals cervical right-side disc protrusion and spondylosis at C-5-6 consistent with the patient's

---

○=Modifier 51 Exempt   ⊙=Moderate Sedation   ✚=Add-on Code   𝒩=FDA approval pending

C-6 symptoms. The patient has not improved despite nonoperative measures. Because of the patient's persistent symptoms, he elects to undergo a surgical intervention.

Description of Procedure (0274T)

The patient was brought to the operating room after obtaining informed consent. IV access was placed to provide moderate conscious sedation. Appropriate prophylactic antibiotics were administered. Vital signs and continuous pulse oximetry were used throughout the procedure. The patient was sterilely prepped and draped in the prone position on a radiolucent table. "Time out" was performed. Under fluoroscopic guidance to verify the spinal target level, the skin and subcutaneous tissues were anesthetized with 1% lidocaine. A 16-gauge port was inserted via stab incision, and docked on the inferior vertebral segment lamina, using fluoroscopic guidance. The decompression of thecal sac was performed by removal of bone and ligamentum flavum via various instruments through the small port. Decompression was confirmed with epidurogram. The process was completed bilaterally. The instruments and port were removed, and the incision was closed. The bandage was applied, and the patient was taken to the recovery area for approximately 30 minutes of monitoring prior to being discharged with instructions.

Clinical Example (0275T)

A 75-year-old male developed progressive leg pain with walking, over several months, consistent with neurogenic claudication. Lumbar MRI demonstrates focal L4-5 stenosis due to ligamentous thickening (central lumbar stenosis). His leg symptoms are thought to be concordant with the imaging findings of lumbar stenosis. Conservative measures did not alleviate symptoms satisfactorily. The patient is a good candidate for a percutaneous decompressive laminectomy.

Description of Procedure (0275T)

The patient was brought to the operating room after obtaining informed consent. IV access was placed to provide moderate conscious sedation. Appropriate prophylactic antibiotics were administered. Vital signs and continuous pulse oximetry were used throughout the procedure. The patient was sterilely prepped and draped in the prone position on a radiolucent table. "Time out" was performed. Under fluoroscopic guidance to verify the spinal target level, the skin and subcutaneous tissues were anesthetized with 1% lidocaine. A 16-gauge port was inserted via stab incision and docked on the inferior vertebral segment lamina, using fluoroscopic guidance. The decompression of thecal sac was performed by removal of bone and ligamentum flavum via various instruments through the small port. Decompression was confirmed with epidurogram. The process was completed bilaterally. The instruments and port were removed, and the incision was closed. The bandage was applied, and the patient was taken to the recovery area for approximately 30 minutes of monitoring prior to being discharged with instructions.

⊙●0276T   Bronchoscopy, rigid or flexible, including fluoroscopic guidance, when performed; with bronchial thermoplasty, 1 lobe

Rationale

Codes 0276T and 0277T are both used to identify bronchial thermoplasty. This is a therapeutic procedure that reduces the airway smooth muscles by applying radiofrequency energy throughout all of the central airways that are reachable by a standard bronchoscopy. Both services include conscious sedation and fluoroscopic guidance when performed. The services are differentiated according to the number of lobes for which the procedure is provided.

Clinical Example (0276T)

A 40-year-old female presents with a history of poorly controlled severe asthma. Bronchial thermoplasty is performed on either lower lobe.

Description of Procedure (0276T)

In this procedure, the physician uses the energy created from high-frequency radio waves to reduce airway smooth muscle tissue in the bronchial walls of the lung. The physician skilled in bronchoscopy, working with a skilled bronchoscopic assistant, directs the bronchoscope and operates the catheter. Effective treatment with the radiofrequency catheter requires appropriate patient sedation throughout the procedure. A standard patient return electrode is affixed to the patient to provide a complete circuit. After the attending physician or anesthesiologist administers appropriate sedation, a standard flexible bronchoscope is inserted through the nose or mouth for access to the lung. A detailed inspection of the targeted lobe(s) of the lung is performed to plan the application of bronchial thermoplasty, thereby ensuring that the entire length of each and every accessible bronchial tube in the targeted lobe(s) is treated. A small radiofrequency catheter with an expandable electrode array is advanced through the accessory channel of a standard bronchoscope and positioned under direct bronchoscopic visualization into the first treatment area of the targeted lobe(s). The electrode array is then expanded and held in contact with the bronchial wall for up to 10 seconds while the radio-frequency controller delivers energy to the location. The bronchoscope and catheter are repositioned systematically approximately 55 times such that the electrode array is brought into contact with the entire length of each and every accessible bronchial tube in the targeted lobe(s), thereby providing consistent and thorough thermal treatment throughout the targeted lung region.

 ### Clinical Example (0277T)

A 40-year-old female presents with a history of poorly controlled severe asthma. Bronchial thermoplasty is performed on either lower lobe.

Description of Procedure (0277T)

The procedure is similar to above, but is longer in scope, as it involves navigating the tortuous anatomy of the upper airways and covers more geography than either lower lobe. The bronchoscope and catheter are repositioned systematically approximately 75 times such that the electrode array is brought into contact with the entire length of each and every accessible bronchial tube in the targeted lobe(s), thereby providing consistent and thorough thermal treatment throughout the targeted lung region.

● **0278T** Transcutaneous electrical modulation pain reprocessing (eg, scrambler therapy), each treatment session (includes placement of electrodes)

✍ Rationale

Code 0278T is used to report transcutaneous electrical modulation pain reprocessing. Transcutaneous electrical modulation pain reprocessing (also known as TEMPR and includes "scrambler therapy") is a procedure that is administered in the office under direct supervision for the treatment of europathic pain, which includes pain associated with chemo-induced peripheral neuraopathy. For this service, pain is treated by the practitioner through the use of a device that uses 16 different wave forms with small 5.5 mA currents that are tailored to the individual patient's circumstances across up to five stimulation areas. Instead of simply using a "jolt" of electricity to stimulate the nerve receptors that sense pain (thereby "masking" the pain), this pain modulation procedure is designed to stimulate a paresthesia response that helps the patient synthesize new neural signals.

The service is provided in the office setting, is identified by treatment sessions, and includes the placement of the electrodes for the service.

To assist in reporting for this service, a parenthetical note has been included in the Medicine section to direct users to the correct code to use to identify this type of service.

🩺 Clinical Example (0278T)

A 62-year-old female suffers from chronic pain (average daily pain rating of 8 using the pain NRS) and symptoms of peripheral neuropathy of 8 months' duration attributed to chemotherapy-induced peripheral neuropathy. The severe peripheral neuropathy in her hands and legs is attributed to previous treatment for breast cancer. The patient received Adriamycin and cyclophosphamide x4 followed by weekly Taxol x12.

She is currently on Tamoxifen. The patient is ambulatory though restricted in physically strenuous activity and has a life expectancy greater than 5 years. To relieve her pain, the patient has tried numerous pain relievers, including Cymbalta and Neurotonin; medication adjustments and different medication regimens have failed to relieve the pain.

Description of Procedure (0278T)

The patient undergoes transcutaneous electrical modulation pain reprocessing treatment.

● **0279T** Cell enumeration using immunologic selection and identification in fluid specimen (eg, circulating tumor cells in blood);

● **0280T** interpretation and report

►(Use 0280T in conjunction with 0279T)◄

►(For flow cytometric immunophenotyping, see 88184-88189. For flow cytometric quantitation, see 86355-86357, 86359-86361, 86367)◄

Rationale

Two Category III codes have been established to report cell enumeration using immunologic selection and identification. This test is also referred to as circulation tumor cells (CTC) enumeration. The purpose of this test is to determine disease prognosis in cancer patients and for use in determining the course of treatment. Two parenthetical notes have been added following code 0280T. The first note indicates that code 0280T should be reported in conjunction with 0279T. Code 0280T describes interpretation and report of the enumeration procedure. When performed in conjunction with the actual procedure, both 0279T and 0280T should be reported.

Clinical Example (0279T)

A female with metastatic breast cancer presents to her physician for follow-up. An anticoagulated blood sample is submitted to the laboratory for cell enumeration using immunologic selection and identification in fluid specimen (eg, circulating tumor cells in blood).

Description of Procedure (0279T)

Following centrifugation of 10 mL of patient blood received in an EDTA tube with special preservative, the buffy coat and plasma are separated from red blood cells and placed in buffer. A semi-automated system is used to separate, stain, and fluorescently label cells from the buffy coat and packed red cells. The resulting mixture of fluorescently labeled cells is disbursed onto a flat plane for image analysis. A series of fluorescent images are recorded at high magnification by a photographic scanning device in each of four channels for cytokeratin, DAPI, white cell marker, and controls. The resulting images are compiled by a computer and presented as an image gallery. Cells conforming to the characteristic immunofluorescent pattern are scored. A final circulating epithelial cell count is enumerated and the results are entered into the laboratory information system (LIS).

Clinical Example (0280T)

A female with metastatic breast cancer presents to her physician for follow-up. Results of the cell enumeration using immunologic selection and identification in fluid specimen (eg, circulating tumor cells in blood) require interpretation by physician.

Description of Procedure (0280T)

The physician scans the entire image file and classifies circulating cells as epithelial tumor cells, white blood cells, or other, based on strict cytomorphologic criteria and experience in fluorescent microscopy. The physician prepares and signs an interpretive written report.

⊘=Modifier 51 Exempt   ⊙=Moderate Sedation   ✚=Add-on Code   𝒩=FDA approval pending

●**0281T**   Percutaneous transcatheter closure of the left atrial appendage with implant, including fluoroscopy, transseptal puncture, catheter placement(s), left atrial angiography, left atrial appendage angiography, radiological supervision and interpretation

►(Do not report 0281T in conjunction with 93462 [left heart catheterization by transseptal puncture])◄

►(Report cardiac catheterization procedures [93451-93461, 93530-93533] separately for indications distinct from the left atrial appendage closure procedure)◄

►(For left ventriculography performed by transseptal approach for indications distinct from the left atrial appendage closure procedure, use 93565◄

►(Do not report 0281T in conjunction with 93452, 93453, 93458-93461, 93531-93533 unless catheterization of the left ventricle is performed by a non-transseptal approach for indications distinct from the left atrial appendage closure procedure)◄

►(Do not report 0281T in conjunction with 93451, 93453, 93456, 93460, 93461, 93530-93533 unless complete right heart catheterization is performed for indications distinct from the left atrial appendage closure procedure)◄

✐ Rationale

Category III code 0281T has been established to report a new technology involving percutaneous transcatheter closure of the left atrial appendage with an implant. The purpose of the implant is to deter the formation of emboli in the left atrial appendage. The implant is inserted percutaneously over a catheter and implanted in the left atrial appendage. As stated in the code descriptor, code 0281T includes fluoroscopy, transseptal puncture, catheter placements, left atrial angiography, left atrial appendage angiography, and radiological supervision and interpretation.

The first parenthetical note following code 0281T directs users not to report left heart catheterization by transseptal puncture (code 93462) with code 0281T, as transseptal puncture is included. The remaining parenthetical notes provide instructions for reporting cardiac catheterization for indications that are distinct from the left atrial appendage closure procedure but that are performed at the same session.

⚕ Clinical Example (0281T)

A 76-year-old female with diabetes, hypertension, and congestive heart failure suffering from nonvalvular paroxysmal, persistent, or permanent atrial fibrillation (AF) requires long-term anticoagulant therapy to reduce her risk of stroke. She has no other medical conditions that require long-term anticoagulation therapy. She is eligible for anticoagulation, but due to her general frailty and risk for falls, her physicians are concerned about the potential for long term bleeding complications. Left atrial appendage closure with an implantable device is recommended.

Description of Procedure (0281T)

A "time out" occurs during which confirmation of critical information is ensured, such as the patient's identity, planned procedure, access route, allergies, completion of the consent process, availability of proper equipment, and any unusual circumstances which might influence the procedure. The physician observes while transesophageal echo (TEE) is performed by an echocardiographer to confirm that the patient's anatomy is suitable for an LAA implant. The echocardiographer performs TEE imaging throughout the procedure to provide guidance for transseptal puncture, LAA imaging, and device placement.

Percutaneous venous access is obtained, typically through the femoral vein. A thin-walled needle is inserted percutaneously into the vein, through which a flexible guidewire is inserted into the vein. The needle is removed over the wire, a sheath/dilator system is inserted over the guidewire, the dilator is removed, and the sidearm of the sheath is flushed to remove any clot or air. Percutaneous arterial access is obtained, typically through the femoral artery. A thin-walled needle is inserted percutaneously into the artery, through which a flexible guidewire is inserted into the artery. The needle is removed over the wire, a sheath/dilator system is inserted over the guidewire, the dilator is removed, and the sidearm of the sheath is flushed to remove any clot or air. An appropriate catheter is inserted over a wire through the venous sheath into the venous system and advanced under fluoroscopic guidance up to the superior vena cava. The wire is removed. A rigid transseptal puncture needle is carefully advanced through the catheter stopping just short of the end of the catheter. The needle-catheter unit is flushed and attached to a second pressure manifold and then withdrawn to the level of the fossa ovalis in the interatrial septum under fluoroscopic guidance. The imaging system is rotated in both the anterior and lateral positions to confirm proper positioning with respect to the arterial wire or catheter, which has been positioned just above the aortic valve. Exquisite precision of the needle-catheter unit is imperative as improper positioning can lead to puncture of the aorta or perforation through the atrial wall into the pericardium. Continuous arterial pressure monitoring is maintained. Typically, the needle-catheter unit may not be positioned properly on the first attempt and one or more repositionings of the unit may be required. This typically requires removal of the needle, reinsertion of the guidewire, readvancement of the wire and catheter to the superior vena cava, removal of the wire, reinsertion of the needle and then repeating the process of positioning the needle-catheter unit in the proper spot on the interatrial septum. Once successful positioning is achieved, the needle-catheter unit is then advanced several millimeters across the interatrial septum to the left atrium while observing the pressure waveform. The transseptal puncture is achieved. Left atrial position is confirmed by pressure waveform analysis, oxygen saturation measurement, and contrast injection through the system. If the needle-catheter unit has not traversed the septum properly, complications are first excluded and then the device is repositioned and a repeat attempt is performed until successful. Once the needle is confirmed to be safely in the left atrium, the transseptal dilator is advanced over the needle into the left atrium, the needle withdrawn to the right atrial side, and then the transseptal sheath is telescoped over the dilator into the left atrium. The transseptal needle is removed from the sheath/dilator apparatus, which is now in the left atrium. The dilator is then removed while infusing saline through it to minimize risk of air introduction. The access sheath and dilator are prepped and inserted over the guidewire into the left atrium. The dilator and wire are removed and the pigtail catheter is inserted into the access sheath and into the left

⃠=Modifier 51 Exempt   ☉=Moderate Sedation   ✚=Add-on Code   𝑵=FDA approval pending

atrium/left atrial appendage under fluoroscopy. Left atrial appendage angiography is performed.

The access sheath is advanced over the pigtail catheter into the left atrial appendage under fluoroscopic guidance and the pigtail is removed. Fluoroscopy and contrast angiography are used to assess the anatomy of the LAA and to define if it is multilobed. The echocardiographer uses TEE to measure the LAA ostium width and length in at least three to four views (0°, 45°, 90°, 135°). Appropriate size implant based on the maximum LAA ostium width is recorded. The catheter used to deliver the LAA closure implant is prepped and inserted into the access sheath and advanced under fluoroscopic guidance into the left atrial appendage.

The device is delivered into the left atrial appendage and assessed under fluoroscopy to confirm release criteria are met. While observing under fluoroscopy, implant stability is confirmed by gently pulling back on the deployment knob and visualizing the proximal movement of the implant and the LAA. Appropriate implant size selection is also confirmed by measuring the deployed diameter of the implant in situ using TEE. The device is released. Implant stability is assessed under fluoroscopy. Images are reviewed to ensure no additional views are required before leaving the procedure suite. The echocardiographer separately performs TEE imaging to independently confirm release criteria are met, to assess implant stability, and to ensure appropriate implant size selection. Patient is awakened from anesthesia by anesthesiology on the table and transferred to stretcher and sent to recovery.

⊙●**0282T** Percutaneous or open implantation of neurostimulator electrode array(s), subcutaneous (peripheral subcutaneous field stimulation), including imaging guidance, when performed, cervical, thoracic or lumbar; for trial, including removal at the conclusion of trial period

⊙●**0283T**   permanent, with implantation of a pulse generator

⊙●**0284T** Revision or removal of pulse generator or electrodes, including imaging guidance, when performed, including addition of new electrodes, when performed

●**0285T** Electronic analysis of implanted peripheral subcutaneous field stimulation pulse generator, with reprogramming when performed

▶(Do not report 0282T-0285T in conjunction with 64550-64595, 77002, 77003, 95970-95973)◀

✍🏿 Rationale

Four Category III codes have been established for reporting peripheral field stimulation. Peripheral field stimulation is a new technology for the treatment of chronic cervical, thoracic, or lumbar pain. Electrode leads are placed in subcutaneous tissue around the painful area, and electrical current is applied to create stimulation in the area, or "field," of pain. This technique is different from peripheral nerve stimulation, in which specific peripheral nerves are targeted. In peripheral field stimulation, a field of pain is targeted rather than specific nerves. The electrodes are placed in the skin either through an open or percutaneous approach. Imaging guidance is included, when performed.

Code 0282T describes implantation of trial electrode arrays and includes removal of the electrodes at the end of the trial period. Code 0283T is reported for permanent implantation of electrode arrays with implantation of a pulse generator. Revision or removal of the pulse generator or electrodes is reported with code 0284T and includes addition of new electrodes, when performed. Code 0285T describes electronic analysis of the pulse generator and includes reprogramming, when performed. An exclusionary parenthetical note precludes the reporting of codes 0282T-0285T with the peripheral nerve neurostimulator codes 64550-64595, fluoroscopic guidance codes 77002 and 77003, or electronic analysis of neurostimulator pulse generator codes 95970-97973.

Clinical Example (0282T)

A 66-year-old male who previously underwent a lumbar discectomy presents with chronic low back pain without radiculopathy. He has no lower extremity symptoms. He denies any bowel or bladder symptoms. Physical examination reveals no neurological abnormalities but lumbar spine range of motion is restricted by pain. He complains of low back pain upon palpation at approximately L3, L4, and L5 bilateral paraspinal muscles. Plain film radiographs of the lumbar spine demonstrated degenerative disc disease and spondylosis at multiple levels. Lumbar spine MRI demonstrates multilevel disc bulges and mild multilevel facet hypertrophy. Despite treatment with physical therapy, nonsteroidal anti-inflammatory medications, opiate therapy, facet joint steroid injections, and epidural steroid injections, no improvement in pain or function was obtained. Due to the patient's failure with conservative treatments and his persistent complaints of diffuse low back pain, a trial of peripheral field stimulation is indicated to attempt to relieve patient's pain and improve function.

Description of Procedure (0282T)

Prior to sedation, the area of pain is carefully outlined and patient receives preoperative intravenous antibiotics. Under sterile conditions, with minimal sedation and appropriate monitoring, a needle is placed subcutaneously, using a small amount of lidocaine at the insertion point. Subcutaneous electrode leads are placed centrally in the area of greatest pain. On-the-table stimulation ensures the correct depth of the leads and adequate stimulation over the area of pain. The leads are then sutured to the skin and dressing is applied. Average trial duration is five to seven days.

Clinical Example (0283T)

A 66-year-old male who previously underwent lumbar discectomy presents with chronic low back pain without radiculopathy. He has no lower extremity symptoms. He denies any bowel or bladder symptoms. Physical examination reveals no neurological abnormalities but lumbar spine range of motion is restricted by pain. He complains of low back pain upon palpation at approximately L3, L4, and L5 bilateral paraspinal muscles. Plain film radiographs of the lumbar spine demonstrated degenerative disc disease and spondylosis at multiple levels. Lumbar spine MRI demonstrates multilevel disc bulges and mild multilevel facet hypertrophy. Despite treatment with physical therapy, nonsteroidal anti-inflammatory medications, opiate therapy, facet joint steroid injections, and epidural steroid injections,

⊘=Modifier 51 Exempt   ⊙=Moderate Sedation   ✦=Add-on Code   𝒩=FDA approval pending

no improvement in pain or function was obtained. Due to the patient's failure with conservative treatments and his persistent complaints of diffuse low back pain, he had undergone a trial of peripheral field stimulation and received significant relief during the trial. Permanent placement of a peripheral field stimulator is indicated.

Description of Procedure (0283T)

Prior to sedation, the area of pain is carefully outlined and patient receives preoperative intravenous antibiotics. Under sterile conditions, with minimal sedation and appropriate monitoring, a needle is placed subcutaneously, using a small amount of lidocaine at the insertion point. Subcutaneous electrode leads are placed centrally in the area of greatest pain and in the same region as the trial electrode leads had been placed. On-the-table stimulation ensures the correct depth of the leads and adequate stimulation over the area of pain. The leads are then sutured to the fascia. The pulse generator or receiver is then implanted by a separate incision by establishing a subcutaneous pocket. The electrode array is tested to verify proper connection and the device is programmed to begin stimulation. The wound is closed and dressing is applied.

 Clinical Example (0284T)

A 66-year-old male presents with an implanted peripheral field stimulator for pain control, which initially provided good coverage and control of pain in the affected area. Over time, the stimulator no longer provided coverage to the affected area and removal of the electrode array and generator is indicated.

Description of Procedure (0284T)

Prior to sedation, the area of pain is carefully outlined and patient receives preoperative intravenous antibiotics. Under sterile conditions, with minimal sedation and appropriate monitoring, the old skin incision of the generator is reopened and the wound checked for hemostasis. The old generator is dissected out of its subcutaneous pocket and delivered onto a sterile towel. The lead terminals are carefully disconnected from the expired generator. The subcutaneous pocket is then irrigated and closed. Dressing is applied. The anchoring site of the previous stimulator lead is localized and the overlying soft tissue structures are anesthetized. An incision is made to expose the leads. The lead is cut at the site and removed via gentle traction. The incision is closed and dressing is applied.

 Clinical Example (0285T)

A 66-year-old male has undergone implantation of a peripheral field stimulator for pain control of his low back pain. Analysis and programming of the pulse generator to correctly address the region of his pain is indicated.

Description of Procedure (0285T)

Electronic analysis and programming of an implanted permanent single array electrode system and subcutaneous generator/transmitter is performed. The physician tests a limited combination of the implant parameters while assessing the degree of symptom and side effect improvement or worsening after each programming change.

●0286T   Near-infrared spectroscopy studies of lower extremity wounds (eg, for oxyhemoglobin measurement)

 Rationale

In response to new technology and changes in clinical practice, CPT 2012 has added a new Category III code (0286T) to report near-infrared spectroscopy studies of lower extremity wounds. Other changes in CPT 2012 related to the establishment of code 0286T is the addition of a new subsection in the Medicine/Noninvasive Vascular Diagnostic Studies subsection entitled Other Noninvasive Vascular Diagnostic Studies. A Category I code for reporting unlisted noninvasive vascular diagnostic studies (93998) has been added under this heading. Finally, related cross-reference notes preceding laboratory code 88720 and following Medicine codes 93922 and 93923 have been added instructing users to report code 0286T for transcutaneous oxyhemoglobin measurement in a lower extremity wound by near-infrared spectroscopy.

 Clinical Example (0286T)

A 65-year-old female presents with a heel ulcer with an area of approximately 10 cm^2, which hasn't progressed to healing in the past two weeks. Patient has a history of heart disease and diabetes mellitus (Type II) with related complications including diabetic neuropathy. Patient is being seen by the clinician on a weekly or biweekly basis for evaluation, which includes measurements of wound size and photographic documentation, debridement, and treatment that can include moist wound healing protocols, offloading, active wound healing agents, and/or active therapies such as hyperbaric oxygen and/or negative pressure therapy. Near-infrared spectroscopy will be used to assess tissue beneath the surface in order to guide the treatment.

Description of Procedure (0286T)

A noninvasive near-infrared spectroscopy is performed. The near-infrared spectroscopy device is turned on, warmed up, and calibrated prior to patient measurement. The patient is placed on the examination table, positioning the injured leg or foot at the distal end of the table, and removing any existing wound dressings. Clinician cleans the wound and assesses it visually, including surrounding tissue. Size measurements and pictures are taken. Patient data is then entered into the device computer. A sterile single-use cover is placed on the device (to prevent cross-contamination) and the patient's wound is interrogated using the device in up to 10 different locations. Data outputs are in the form of concentrations of oxygenated hemoglobin and total hemoglobin in the blood vessels in the wound. The clinician evaluates these outputs to assess wound healing progression, comparing results on a weekly or biweekly basis, to determine the need for changes in clinical approach.

●0287T   Near-infrared guidance for vascular access requiring real-time digital visualization of subcutaneous vasculature for evaluation of potential access sites and vessel patency

Rationale

Code 0287T is used to report near-infrared guidance for vascular access of subcutaneous vasculature. This code is used to identify use of near-infrared real-time digital projection of subcutaneous structures to decrease difficulty in locating hard-to-locate vessels. This procedure is intended for use by clinicians who have difficulty accessing an appropriate vessel for IV access and venipuncture. This procedure includes guidance only. As a result, vascular services provided during the encounter should be separately reported.

Clinical Example (0287T)

A 6-year-old female presents to the ER with a severe allergic reaction. Patient is dehydrated, hypotensive, and in respiratory distress. A peripheral IV is necessary for urgent/emergent treatment and resuscitation. Patient has small veins, excess subcutaneous tissue that obscures veins, and/or due to distress, has increased vasoconstriction.

Description of Procedure (0287T)

Patient's arm is held steady. Clinical protocol is used while applying a tourniquet. A clinician attempts to visually and with palpation determine an appropriate vein for venous access via traditional method, but is unsuccessful in locating an appropriate vein. Near-infrared device is used to provide near-infrared light that penetrates the skin and subcutaneous fat, which is detected with video camera. A projected image of veins under the skin is then reflected directly onto the surface of the skin in real time. Medical personnel assess image on skin to determine greater number of venous options, valve location, and vessel flushing after venous access is obtained for IV placement or blood draw.

Note: Needle placement for blood draw is reported separately.

●0288T   Anoscopy, with delivery of thermal energy to the muscle of the anal canal (eg, for fecal incontinence)

▶(Do not report 0288T in conjunction with 46600-46615)◀

Rationale

A Category III code, 0288T, has been established for radiofrequency energy treatment of the anal canal for fecal incontinence with an instructional note directing users not to report code 0288T in addition to codes 46600-46615. A cross-reference parenthetical note was also added following code 46615 directing users to the new code for delivery of thermal energy to the muscle of the anal canal.

Clinical Example (0288T)

A 54-year-old female, with no past medical history, has had increasingly greater difficulty with fecal incontinence to flatus, liquid, and solid stool. She is gravida 5, para 5, and all deliveries were normal spontaneous vaginal deliveries without significant perineal injury or protracted labor. She has decreased rectal tone, 2-cm perineal descent with Valsalva, and poor motion of the pelvic floor with straining. Anal manometry and pudendal nerve terminal motor latency testing were consistent with significant neuropathic related reduction in anal sphincter tone and contraction. She undergoes radiofrequency energy treatment of the anal canal.

Description of Procedure (0288T)
The patient is placed in lithotomy position. The perineum is anesthetized with lidocaine injected circumferentially. The anal canal is gently dilated and the treatment anoscope is inserted with the intent of beginning therapy 0.5 cm distal to the dentate line in the posterior midline. The needles are deployed into the sphincter muscle, and the appropriate tissue temperature and electrical imped- ance are confirmed to be within normal range. The energy is then administered according to the instrument based algorithm, taking care to monitor the tem- perature and electrical impedance. The needles are withdrawn, the anoscope is advanced 0.5 cm in the posterior midline, and the treatment cycle is repeated for four more cycles. The entire process is then replicated at the same five locations in the remaining three quadrants of the anal canal. The anal canal is inspected for hemostasis or evidence of thermal injury. The perineum is cleansed.

+●0289T   Corneal incisions in the donor cornea created using a laser, in preparation for penetrating or lamellar keratoplasty (List separately in addition to code for primary procedure)

▶(Use 0289T in conjunction with 65710, 65730, 65750, 65755)◀

+●0290T   Corneal incisions in the recipient cornea created using a laser, in preparation for penetrating or lamellar keratoplasty (List separately in addition to code for primary procedure)

▶(Use 0290T in conjunction with 65710, 65730, 65750, 65755)◀

 Rationale
Two Category III codes, 0289T and 0290T, for reporting both donor and recipient corneal incisions using a laser in preparation for penetrating or lamellar kera- toplasty, have been established. Codes 0289T and 0290T describe a new way of making corneal incisions in preparation for a corneal transplant that utilizes a femtosecond laser. These incisional procedures are usually done in the laser suite, and the keratoplasty itself is performed in the hospital or an ambulatory surgery center (ASC). Thus the add-on code designation and reference to use codes 65710, 65730, 65750, and 65755 in conjunction with codes 0289T and 0290T have been added.

 Clinical Example (0289T and 0290T)
A 40-year-old female presents with advanced keratoconus OD > OS and poor uncorrected visual acuity in OD that cannot be improved with glasses. Her right eye also cannot be adequately fit with a contact lens. She is a candidate for pen- etrating keratoplasty OD with femtosecond laser corneal incisions.

Description of Procedure (0289T)
The femtosecond laser is preprogrammed in the laser suite in order to create stan- dardized, zigzag configuration incisions of the same shape and diameter in both the donor and host corneas. Using sterile technique, the donor cornea is then mounted on an artificial anterior chamber and brought to the femtosecond laser

⊘=Modifier 51 Exempt   ⊙=Moderate Sedation   ✛=Add-on Code   ◪=FDA approval pending

in the laser suite, and a full thickness zigzag configuration incision is created with the laser. The donor tissue is placed in a sterile container to await transplantation.

Description of Procedure (0290T)

The femtosecond laser is programmed for the patient's cornea to retain a 70-μm issue bridge of uncut posterior stroma to maintain the integrity of the globe and allow safe transport of the patient from the laser suite to the operating room. The patient's cornea is then treated with the femtosecond laser with sterile technique under topical anesthesia and with prophylactic antibiotics. Once the host cornea had been incised, further antibiotic drops are administered, the patient's eye is patched, a firm shield is taped in place, and the patient is transported to the operating room to proceed with the penetrating keratoplasty. The surgeon then proceeds with the keratoplasty (separately reported) as follows. Retrobulbar anesthesia is then administered to the surgical eye in the operating room, then, with sterile technique, the host corneal button is separated by blunt dissection with a microsurgical hook to reveal the incisions made by the laser. Penetrating keratoplasty is then completed with alignment of the donor and host corneal zigzag incisions in a tongue-in-groove fashion.

Appendix A

For CPT 2012, Appendix A has been updated in response to the Patient Protection and Affordable Care Act (PPACA) by adding a new modifier 33 to identify a preventive service. This appendix was also updated with a revision to modifier 92.

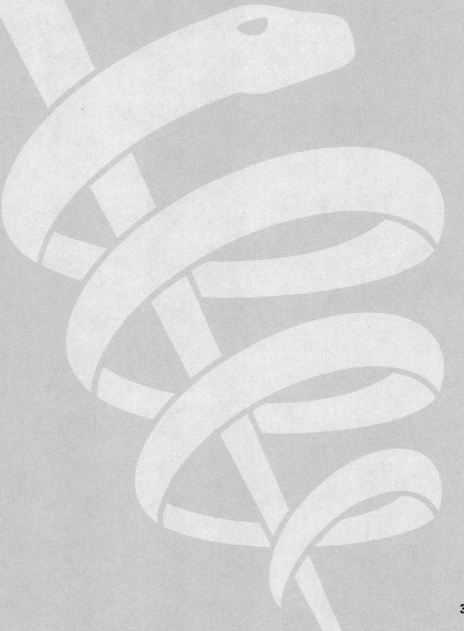

Appendix A

Modifiers

33 ▶Preventive Services: When the primary purpose of the service is the delivery of an evidence based service in accordance with a US Preventive Services Task Force A or B rating in effect and other preventive services identified in preventive services mandates (legislative or regulatory), the service may be identified by adding 33 to the procedure. For separately reported services specifically identified as preventive, the modifier should not be used.◀

✐ Rationale

In response to the Patient Protection and Affordable Care Act (PPACA) which requires all health care plans to begin covering immunizations and preventive services without any cost sharing, modifier 33 has been added to identify a service as a preventive service. The modifier allows providers to identify to payers that the service was preventive under applicable laws and patient cost sharing does not apply. For more information, please see the December 2010 issue of the *CPT Assistant* newsletter.

92 ▶**Alternative Laboratory Platform Testing:** When laboratory testing is being performed using a kit or transportable instrument that wholly or in part consists of a single use, disposable analytical chamber, the service may be identified by adding modifier 92 to the usual laboratory procedure code (HIV testing 86701-86703, and 87389). The test does not require permanent dedicated space, hence by its design may be hand carried or transported to the vicinity of the patient for immediate testing at that site, although location of the testing is not in itself determinative of the use of this modifier.◀

✐ Rationale

In support of the addition of code 87389 for reporting HIV-1 antigen(s), with HIV-1 and HIV-2 antibodies, single result and the revision of code 86703, modifier 92, Alternative Laboratory Platform Testing, has been updated to include 87389.

Tabular Review of the Changes

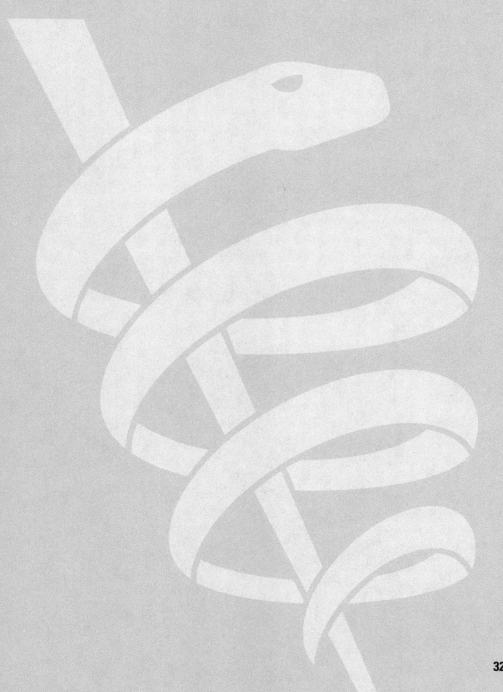

Evaluation and Management

Hospital Observation Services

Initial Observation Care

New or Established Patient					
99218			X		
99219			X		
99220			X		

Prolonged Services

Prolonged Service With Direct Patient Contact

99354			X		
99355			X		
99356			X		
99357			X		

Prolonged Service Without Direct Patient Contact

99358			X		
99359			X		

Surgery

Integumentary System

Introduction

11975		X			
11977		X			

Repair (Closure)

Skin Replacement Surgery

Surgical Preparation

Autografts/Tissue Cultured Autograft

15121					X
15150			X		

Section/Code	Added	Deleted	Revised	Grammatical Revision	Cross-reference
15151			X		
15152			X		
15155			X		
15156			X		
15157			X		
15261					X

Skin Replacement Surgery and Skin Substitutes

Grafts

Acellular Dermal Replacement

15170		X			
15171		X			
15175		X			
15176		X			

Skin Substitute Grafts

15271	X				
15272	X				X
15273	X				
15274	X				X
15275	X				
15276	X				X
15277	X				
15278	X				

Skin Replacement Surgery and Skin Substitutes

Grafts

Allograft/Tissue Cultured Allogeneic Skin Substitute

15300		X			
15301		X			
15320		X			
15321		X			

⊘=Modifier 51 Exempt   ⊙=Moderate Sedation   ✚=Add-on Code   ✱=FDA approval pending

Section/Code	Added	Deleted	Revised	Grammatical Revision	Cross-reference
15330		X			
15331		X			
15335		X			
15336		X			
15340		X			
15341		X			
15360		X			
15361		X			
15365		X			
15366		X			

Xenograft

15400		X			
15401		X			
15420		X			
15421		X			
15430		X			
15431		X			

Other Flaps and Grafts

15777	X				X

Other Procedures

15830	X				X

Musculoskeletal System

General

Introduction or Removal

20527					X

Spine (Vertebral Column)

Incision

22010					X

Section/Code	Added	Deleted	Revised	Grammatical Revision	Cross-reference
Vertebral Body, Embolization or Injection					
22520			X		
22521			X		
22522			X		
22525					X
Arthrodesis					
Posterior, Posterolateral or Lateral Transverse Process Technique					
22610			X		
22612			X		X
22614					X
22632					X
22633	X				
22634	X				X

Hand and Fingers

Section/Code	Added	Deleted	Revised	Grammatical Revision	Cross-reference
Repair, Revision, and/or Reconstruction					
26341	X				

Pelvis and Hip Joint

Section/Code	Added	Deleted	Revised	Grammatical Revision	Cross-reference
Introduction or Removal					
27096			X		X

Application of Casts and Strapping

Section/Code	Added	Deleted	Revised	Grammatical Revision	Cross-reference
Lower Extremity					
Strapping—Any Age					
29540					X
29580					X
29581			X		
29582	X				X
29583	X				X
29584	X				X

⊘=Modifier 51 Exempt ⊙=Moderate Sedation ✚=Add-on Code ⊅=FDA approval pending

Section/Code	Added	Deleted	Revised	Grammatical Revision	Cross-reference
Endoscopy/Arthroscopy					
29826			X		
29880			X		
29881			X		

Respiratory System

Lungs and Pleura

Incision

Section/Code	Added	Deleted	Revised	Grammatical Revision	Cross-reference
32095					X
32096	X				
32097	X				X
32098	X				
32100			X		
32110			X		
32120			X		
32124			X		
32140			X		
32141			X		
32150			X		
32151			X		
32160			X		

Excision/Resection

Section/Code	Added	Deleted	Revised	Grammatical Revision	Cross-reference
32402		X			
32405			X		

Removal

Section/Code	Added	Deleted	Revised	Grammatical Revision	Cross-reference
32440			X		
32442			X		
32445			X		X
32480			X		
32482			X		

Section/Code	Added	Deleted	Revised	Grammatical Revision	Cross-reference
32484			X		
32486			X		
32488			X		
32491			X		
32500		X			
32505	X				
32506	X				X
32507	X				X

Thoracoscopy (Video-assisted thoracic surgery [VATS])

Section/Code	Added	Deleted	Revised	Grammatical Revision	Cross-reference
32601			X		
32607					X
32608	X				
32609	X				
32655			X		X
32663			X		X
32665					X
32666					X
32667					X
32668					X
32669	X				
32670	X				
32671	X				
32672	X				
32673					X
32674					X

Endoscopy

Section/Code	Added	Deleted	Revised	Grammatical Revision	Cross-reference
32602		X			
32603		X			
32605		X			

⊘=Modifier 51 Exempt ⊙=Moderate Sedation ✚=Add-on Code ✗=FDA approval pending

Section/Code	Added	Deleted	Revised	Grammatical Revision	Cross-reference
32606					
32657		X			
32660		X			

Cardiovascular System

Heart and Pericardium

Pericardium

33050			X		X

Pacemaker or Pacing Cardioverter-Defibrillator

33206			X		X
33207			X		
33208			X		
33212			X		
33213			X		
33218			X		
33220			X		
33221	X				
33224			X		
33225			X		X
33226			X		
33227	X				
33228	X				
33229	X				
33230	X				
33231	X				X
33233			X		
33240			X		
33241			X		
33249			X		
33250					X

Section/Code	Added	Deleted	Revised	Grammatical Revision	Cross-reference
33262	X				
33263	X				
33264	X				X

Cardiac Assist

Section/Code	Added	Deleted	Revised	Grammatical Revision	Cross-reference
33960			X		
33961			X		

Arteries and Veins

Endovascular Repair of Abdominal Aortic Aneurysm

Section/Code	Added	Deleted	Revised	Grammatical Revision	Cross-reference
34808					
34813					X
34826					

Bypass Graft

Vein

Section/Code	Added	Deleted	Revised	Grammatical Revision	Cross-reference
35500					X
35548		X			
35549		X			
35551		X			

Other Than Vein

Section/Code	Added	Deleted	Revised	Grammatical Revision	Cross-reference
35651		X			

Adjuvant Techniques

Section/Code	Added	Deleted	Revised	Grammatical Revision	Cross-reference
35686					X

Excision, Exploration, Repair, Revision

Section/Code	Added	Deleted	Revised	Grammatical Revision	Cross-reference
35700					X

Vascular Injection Procedures

Intra-Arterial—Intra-Aortic

Interventions for Arteriovenous (AV) Shunts Created for Dialysis (AV Grafts and AV Fistulae)

Section/Code	Added	Deleted	Revised	Grammatical Revision	Cross-reference
36200			X		
36245			X		
36246			X		

⃠=Modifier 51 Exempt   ⊙=Moderate Sedation   ✚=Add-on Code   𝑵=FDA approval pending

Section/Code	Added	Deleted	Revised	Grammatical Revision	Cross-reference
36247			X		
36248			X		
36251	X				
36252	X				
36253	X				
36254	X				
Venous					
36476					X
36479					X

Transcatheter Procedures

Other Procedures					
37191	X				X
37192	X				X
37193	X				

Ligation					
37619	X				
37620		X			

Hemic and Lymphatic Systems

General

Bone Marrow or Stem Cell Services/Procedures					
38205				X	
38208			X		
38209			X		
38230			X		X
38232	X				
38240				X	

Lymph Nodes and Lymphatic Channels

Radical Lymphadenectomy (Radical Resection of Lymph Nodes)					
38746			X		

Section/Code	Added	Deleted	Revised	Grammatical Revision	Cross-reference
Introduction					
38792			X		

Mediastinum and Diaphragm

Mediastinum

Section/Code	Added	Deleted	Revised	Grammatical Revision	Cross-reference
Excision/Resection					
39200			X		
39220			X		
Endoscopy					
39400			X		

Digestive System

Stomach

Section/Code	Added	Deleted	Revised	Grammatical Revision	Cross-reference
Laparoscopy					
43648					X
Other Procedures					
43882					X

Liver

Section/Code	Added	Deleted	Revised	Grammatical Revision	Cross-reference
Incision					
47000			X		

Abdomen, Peritoneum, and Omentum

Section/Code	Added	Deleted	Revised	Grammatical Revision	Cross-reference
Incision					
49080		X			
49081		X			
49082	X				
49083	X				
49084	X				

Female Genital System

Section/Code	Added	Deleted	Revised	Grammatical Revision	Cross-reference
56405					X

Corpus Uteri

⃠=Modifier 51 Exempt ⊙=Moderate Sedation ✚=Add-on Code ⑂=FDA approval pending

Section/Code	Added	Deleted	Revised	Grammatical Revision	Cross-reference
Introduction					
58300					X

Nervous System

Skull, Meninges, and Brain

Section/Code	Added	Deleted	Revised	Grammatical Revision	Cross-reference
Neurostimulators (Intracranial)					
61886					X

Spine and Spinal Cord

Section/Code	Added	Deleted	Revised	Grammatical Revision	Cross-reference
Injection, Drainage, or Aspiration					
62287			X		
62310			X		
62311			X		
62318			X		
62319			X		
Reservoir/Pump Implantation					
62367			X		
62369	X				
62370	X				

Posterior Extradural Laminotomy or Laminectomy for Exploration/Decompression of Neural Elements or Excision of Herniated Intervertebral Discs

Section/Code	Added	Deleted	Revised	Grammatical Revision	Cross-reference
63020			X		
63030			X		
63035			X		

Extracranial Nerves, Peripheral Nerves, and Autonomic Nervous System

Section/Code	Added	Deleted	Revised	Grammatical Revision	Cross-reference
Introduction/Injection of Anesthetic Agent (Nerve Block), Diagnostic or Therapeutic					
Paravertebral Spinal Nerves and Branches					
64490					X
Neurostimulators (Peripheral Nerve)					
64553			X		
64555			X		

Section/Code	Added	Deleted	Revised	Grammatical Revision	Cross-reference
64560		X			
64561			X		
64565			X		
64575			X		
64577		X			
64580			X		
64581			X		
64585			X		

Destruction by Neurolytic Agent (eg, Chemical, Thermal, Electrical or Radiofrequency)

Somatic Nerves

Section/Code	Added	Deleted	Revised	Grammatical Revision	Cross-reference
64622		X			
64623		X			
64626		X			
64627		X			
64633	X				X
64634	X				X
64635	X				X
64636	X				

Eye and Ocular Adnexa

Anterior Segment

Cornea

Other Procedures

Section/Code	Added	Deleted	Revised	Grammatical Revision	Cross-reference
65775					X

Auditory System

Inner Ear

Incision and/or Destruction

Section/Code	Added	Deleted	Revised	Grammatical Revision	Cross-reference
69802		X			

⊘=Modifier 51 Exempt   ⊙=Moderate Sedation   ✚=Add-on Code   𝒩=FDA approval pending

Section/Code	Added	Deleted	Revised	Grammatical Revision	Cross-reference

Radiology

Diagnostic Radiology (Diagnostic Imaging)

Head and Neck

Section/Code	Added	Deleted	Revised	Grammatical Revision	Cross-reference
70355			X		

Chest

Section/Code	Added	Deleted	Revised	Grammatical Revision	Cross-reference
71090		X			

Spine and Pelvis

Section/Code	Added	Deleted	Revised	Grammatical Revision	Cross-reference
72114			X		
72120			X		
72191					X

Lower Extremities

Section/Code	Added	Deleted	Revised	Grammatical Revision	Cross-reference
73542		X			

Abdomen

Section/Code	Added	Deleted	Revised	Grammatical Revision	Cross-reference
74174	X				X
74175					X

Vascular Procedures

Aorta and Arteries

Section/Code	Added	Deleted	Revised	Grammatical Revision	Cross-reference
75722		X			
75724		X			

Transcatheter Procedures

Section/Code	Added	Deleted	Revised	Grammatical Revision	Cross-reference
75940		X			
75952					X
75962			X		
75964			X		

Other Procedures

Section/Code	Added	Deleted	Revised	Grammatical Revision	Cross-reference
76376					X
76377					X

Section/Code	Added	Deleted	Revised	Grammatical Revision	Cross-reference
Diagnostic Ultrasound					
76506					X
Ultrasonic Guidance Procedures					
76937					X
76942					X
Radiologic Guidance					
Fluoroscopic Guidance					
77003			X		X
Bone/Joint Studies					
77079		X			
77083		X			
Radiation Oncology					
Radiation Treatment Delivery					
77424	X				
77425	X				
Radiation Treatment Management					
77469	X				
77470			X		
Nuclear Medicine					
Diagnostic					
Gastrointestinal System					
78220		X			
78223		X			
78226	X				
78227	X				
Cardiovascular System					
78466					X
78481					X

⊘=Modifier 51 Exempt   ⊙=Moderate Sedation   ✚=Add-on Code   ✗=FDA approval pending

Section/Code	Added	Deleted	Revised	Grammatical Revision	Cross-reference
Respiratory System					
78579	X				
78580			X		X
78582	X				
78584		X			
78585		X			
78586		X			
78587		X			
78588		X			
78591		X			
78593		X			
78594		X			
78596		X			
78597	X				
78598	X				X

Pathology and Laboratory

Molecular Pathology

Tier 1 Molecular Pathology Procedures

Section/Code	Added	Deleted	Revised	Grammatical Revision	Cross-reference
81200	X				
81205	X				
81206	X				
81207	X				
81208	X				
81209	X				
81210	X				
81211	X				
81212	X				
81213	X				
81214	X				X

Section/Code	Added	Deleted	Revised	Grammatical Revision	Cross-reference
81215	X				
81216	X				
81217	X				
81220	X				
81221	X				
81222	X				
81223	X				
81224	X				
81225	X				
81226	X				
81227	X				
81228	X				
81229	X				X
81240	X				
81241	X				
81242	X				
81243	X				
81244	X				
81245	X				
81250	X				
81251	X				
81255	X				
81256	X				
81257	X				
81260	X				
81261	X				
81262	X				
81263	X				
81264	X				X
81265	X				

⊘=Modifier 51 Exempt   ⊙=Moderate Sedation   ✚=Add-on Code   ⁄\=FDA approval pending

Section/Code	Added	Deleted	Revised	Grammatical Revision	Cross-reference
81266	X				
81267	X				
81268	X				X
81270	X				
81275	X				
81280	X				
81281	X				
81282	X				
81290	X				
81291	X				
81292	X				
81293	X				
81294	X				
81295	X				
81296	X				
81297	X				
81298	X				
81299	X				
81300	X				
81301	X				
81302	X				
81303	X				
81304	X				
81310	X				
81315	X				
81316	X				X
81317	X				
81318	X				
81319	X				
81330	X				

Section/Code	Added	Deleted	Revised	Grammatical Revision	Cross-reference
81331	X				
81332	X				
81340	X				
81341	X				
81342	X				
81350	X				
81355	X				
81370	X				
81371	X				
81372	X				X
81373	X				X
81374	X				X
81375	X				X
81376	X				X
81377	X				
81378	X				
81379	X				
81380	X				
81381	X				X
81382	X				X
81383	X				X

Tier 2 Molecular Pathology Procedures

Section/Code	Added	Deleted	Revised	Grammatical Revision	Cross-reference
81400	X				
81401	X				
81402	X				
81403	X				
81404	X				
81405	X				
81406	X				

⊘=Modifier 51 Exempt   ⊙=Moderate Sedation   ✚=Add-on Code   ⃕=FDA approval pending

Section/Code	Added	Deleted	Revised	Grammatical Revision	Cross-reference
81407	X				
81408	X				

Immunology

Section/Code	Added	Deleted	Revised	Grammatical Revision	Cross-reference
86386	X				
86703			X		X

Tissue Typing

Section/Code	Added	Deleted	Revised	Grammatical Revision	Cross-reference
86822					X

Microbiology

Section/Code	Added	Deleted	Revised	Grammatical Revision	Cross-reference
87389	X				
87502				X	

Cytopathology

Section/Code	Added	Deleted	Revised	Grammatical Revision	Cross-reference
88107		X			

Surgical Pathology

Section/Code	Added	Deleted	Revised	Grammatical Revision	Cross-reference
88312			X		X
88313			X		X
88314			X		X
88318		X			
88319			X		X

Medicine

Immunization Administration for Vaccines/Toxoids

Section/Code	Added	Deleted	Revised	Grammatical Revision	Cross-reference
90460			X		
90461			X		
90470		X			

Vaccines, Toxoids

Section/Code	Added	Deleted	Revised	Grammatical Revision	Cross-reference
90581			X		
90644			X		

Section/Code	Added	Deleted	Revised	Grammatical Revision	Cross-reference
90654	X				
90663		X			

Psychiatry

Psychiatric Therapeutic Procedures

Other Psychiatric Services or Procedures

90867			X		
90868			X		
90869	X				X

Gastroenterology

91010			X		
91013			X		

Ophthalmology

Special Ophthalmological Services

92070		X			
92071	X				X
92072	X				
92120		X			X
92130		X			

Contact Lens Services

92310					X

Special Otorhinolaryngologic Services

Audiologic Function Tests

92558	X				
92587			X		
92588			X		

Evaluative and Therapeutic Services

92605			X		
92618	X				

⊘=Modifier 51 Exempt   ⊙=Moderate Sedation   ✚=Add-on Code   🖉=FDA approval pending

Section/Code	Added	Deleted	Revised	Grammatical Revision	Cross-reference
92621			X		

Cardiovascular

Cardiography

Cardiovascular Monitoring Services

93271				X	

Echocardiography

93351					X

Cardiac Catheterization

93451				X	
93455				X	
93456				X	

Injection Procedures

93561			X		
93562			X		X

Noninvasive Physiologic Studies and Procedures

93720		X			
93721		X			
93722		X			

Noninvasive Vascular Diagnostic Studies

Cerebrovascular Arterial Studies

93875		X			

Other Noninvasive Vascular Diagnostic Studies

93998	X				

Pulmonary

Other Procedures

94240		X			
94260					
94350		X			

Section/Code	Added	Deleted	Revised	Grammatical Revision	Cross-reference
94360		X			
94370		X			
94720		X			
94725		X			

Pulmonary Diagnostic Testing and Therapies

Section/Code	Added	Deleted	Revised	Grammatical Revision	Cross-reference
94726					X
94727	X				
94728	X				
94729	X				
94780	X				
94781	X				

Neurology and Neuromuscular Procedures

Electromyography

Section/Code	Added	Deleted	Revised	Grammatical Revision	Cross-reference
95885	X				
95886					X
95887	X				

Nerve Conduction Tests

Section/Code	Added	Deleted	Revised	Grammatical Revision	Cross-reference
95905					X

Evoked Potentials and Reflex Tests

Section/Code	Added	Deleted	Revised	Grammatical Revision	Cross-reference
95938	X				
95939					X

Neurostimulators, Analysis-Programming

Section/Code	Added	Deleted	Revised	Grammatical Revision	Cross-reference
95970			X		
95971			X		
95972			X		
95973			X		
95974			X		
95975			X		

⊘=Modifier 51 Exempt   ⊙=Moderate Sedation   ✚=Add-on Code   ⊘=FDA approval pending

Section/Code	Added	Deleted	Revised	Grammatical Revision	Cross-reference
Other Procedures					
95990					
95991			X		X
Central Nervous System Assessments/Tests (eg, Neuro-Cognitive, Mental Status, Speech Testing)					
96110			X		
96111			X		
Hydration, Therapeutic, Prophylactic, Diagnostic Injections and Infusions, and Chemotherapy and Other Highly Complex Drug or Highly Complex Biologic Agent Administration					
Therapeutic, Prophylactic, and Diagnostic Injections and Infusions (Excludes Chemotherapy and Other Highly Complex Drug or Highly Complex Biologic Agent Administration)					
96367			X		X
96368					X
Special Services, Procedures and Reports					
Miscellaneous Services					
99090					X

Category II Codes

Composite Codes

0001F				X	

Patient Management

0550F	X				
0551F	X				
0555F	X				
0556F	X				
0557F	X				

Patient History

1003F				X	

Section/Code	Added	Deleted	Revised	Grammatical Revision	Cross-reference
1010F	X				
1011F	X				
1012F	X				
1031F	X				
1032F	X				
1033F	X				
1123F				X	
1124F				X	
1175F	X				
1181F	X				
1182F	X				
1183F	X				
1450F	X				
1451F	X				
1460F	X				
1461F	X				
1490F	X				
1491F	X				
1493F	X				
1494F	X				

Physical Examination

Section/Code	Added	Deleted	Revised	Grammatical Revision	Cross-reference
2000F				X	
2001F				X	
2015F	X				
2016F	X				

Diagnostic/Screening Processes or Results

Section/Code	Added	Deleted	Revised	Grammatical Revision	Cross-reference
3019F	X				
3048F				X	
3049F				X	

⊘=Modifier 51 Exempt   ⊙=Moderate Sedation   ✚=Add-on Code   ⊅=FDA approval pending

Section/Code	Added	Deleted	Revised	Grammatical Revision	Cross-reference
3050F				X	
3055F	X				
3056F	X				
3074F				X	
3075F				X	
3077F				X	
3078F				X	
3079F				X	
3080F				X	
3111F			X		
3112F			X		
3115F	X				
3117F	X				
3118F	X				
3119F	X				
3125F	X				
3267F	X				
3394F	X				
3395F	X				
3725F	X				

Therapeutic, Preventive, or Other Interventions

Section/Code	Added	Deleted	Revised	Grammatical Revision	Cross-reference
4000F				X	
4001F				X	
4002F		X			
4004F			X		
4006F		X			
4008F	X				
4009F		X			
4010F	X				

Section/Code	Added	Deleted	Revised	Grammatical Revision	Cross-reference
4013F	X				
4086F	X				
4140F	X				
4144F	X				
4145F	X				
4275F		X			
4322F	X				
4350F	X				
4450F	X				
4470F	X				
4480F	X				
4481F	X				
4500F	X				
4510F	X				
4525F	X				
4526F	X				

Follow-up or Other Outcomes

Section/Code	Added	Deleted	Revised	Grammatical Revision	Cross-reference
5250F	X				

Patient Safety

Section/Code	Added	Deleted	Revised	Grammatical Revision	Cross-reference
6100F	X				
6101F	X				
6102F	X				
6110F	X				

Category III Codes

Section/Code	Added	Deleted	Revised	Grammatical Revision	Cross-reference
0080T			X		
0141T		X			
0142T		X			
0143T		X			

⊘=Modifier 51 Exempt ⊙=Moderate Sedation ✚=Add-on Code ⊼=FDA approval pending

Section/Code	Added	Deleted	Revised	Grammatical Revision	Cross-reference
0155T		X			
0156T		X			
0157T		X			
0158T		X			
0166T		X			
0167T		X			
0168T		X			

Remote Real-Time Interactive Videoconferenced Critical Care Services

Atherectomy (Open or Percutaneous) for Supra-Inguinal Arteries

0240T			X		
0241T			X		
0260T	X				
0261T	X				
0262T	X				X
0263T	X				
0264T	X				
0265T	X				
0266T	X				
0267T	X				X
0268T	X				X
0269T	X				X
0270T	X				X
0271T	X				X
0272T	X				X
0273T	X				X
0274T	X				
0275T	X				X
0276T	X				
0277T	X				

Section/Code	Added	Deleted	Revised	Grammatical Revision	Cross-reference
0278T	X				
0279T	X				
0280T	X				
0281T	X				X
0282T	X				
0283T	X				
0284T	X				
0285T	X				
0286T	X				
0287T	X				
0288T	X				
0289T	X				X
0290T	X				X

⃠=Modifier 51 Exempt   ⊙=Moderate Sedation   ✚=Add-on Code   ✍=FDA approval pending

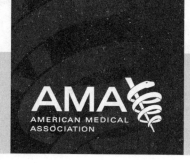
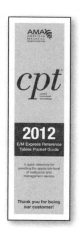
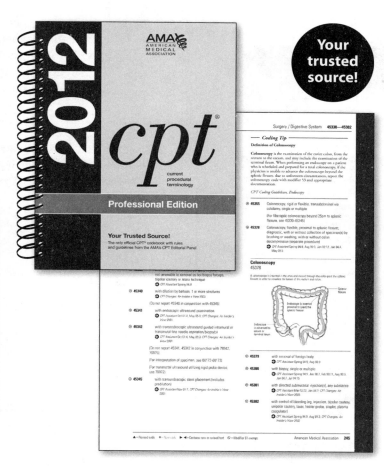

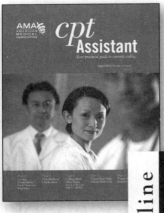
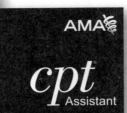
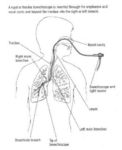
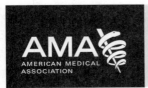

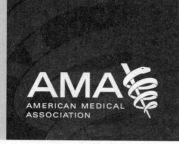

Get answers to your most challenging CPT® coding questions

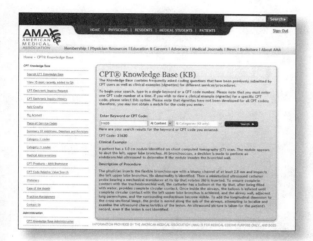

Your online solution to quickly research "Knowledge Base," the AMA's CPT® database of more than 5,000 commonly asked coding questions and answers. In addition to finding answers to your questions, **CPT® Network** subscribers can submit electronic inquiries directly to a CPT expert for a timely and accurate solution to their coding question.

Features include:

- "Pay as you go"—convenient single electronic inquiry option as well as new inquiry packages for customer flexibility

- Quick access to AMA webinars—obtain relevant information on the latest coding news

- Enhanced search functionality—quickly search by CPT code or keyword

- Newly added clinical vignettes—increase your coding expertise

- Monthly case scenarios—test your coding knowledge

- Category II and III code updates—stay current on the latest changes

For complete details, or to choose the subscription package that best fits your needs visit *cptnetwork.com* today.

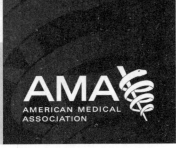
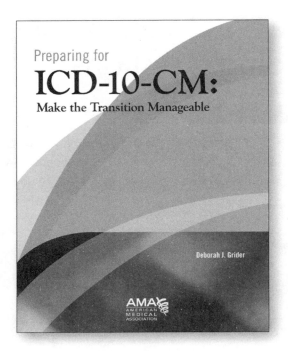

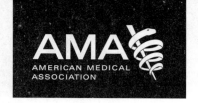

CODING *with* MODIFIERS:

A Guide to Correct CPT® and HCPCS Level II Modifier Usage, fourth edition

Modifier changes:
- **One new**
- **One deleted**
- **Four revised**

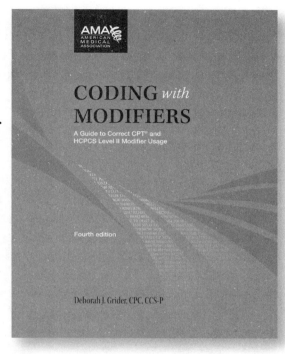

The ultimate modifiers resource—revised. Essential components to the coding process, modifiers help create clear and concise communications between the provider and payer. *Coding with Modifiers* provides guidance on how and when to use modifiers in order to avoid costly payment delays and denials.

Using the 2012 code set, the fourth edition contains new, deleted and revised modifiers, along with updates to Centers for Medicare & Medicaid Services, third-party payer, and AMA-modifier guidelines to assist with coding accuracy.

- **Coding tips**—explain how to use specific modifiers to help clear up confusion surrounding modifier usage

- **Modifiers approved for hospitals and ASCs**—provide information for professional service and hospital reporting requirements

- **Teaching tools**—allow you to create and administer tests using questions and answers developed by the AMA

- **Clinical examples**—guide readers in determining the correct modifier to use with helpful scenarios

- **Test-Your-Knowledge questions**—test your comprehension of the material with more than 190 questions

Visit amabookstore.com for more information or call (800) 621-8335 to order!

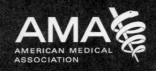
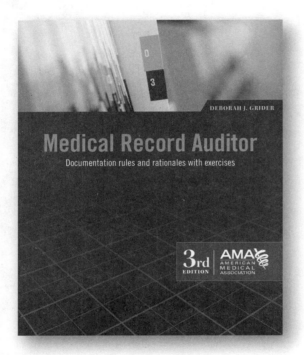